BASES
OF
FITNESS

Edward L. Fox

Late of The Ohio State University

Timothy E. Kirby

The Ohio State University

Ann Roberts Fox

The Ohio State University

MACMILLAN PUBLISHING COMPANY

New York

Copyright © 1987, Macmillan Publishing Company, a division of Macmillan, Inc.

Printed in the United States of America

Macmillan Publishing Company
866 Third Avenue, New York, New York 10022

Collier Macmillan Canada, Inc.

Library of Congress Cataloging-in-Publication Data

Fox, Edward L.
    Bases of fitness.

    Includes bibliographies and indexes.
    1. Exercise—Physiological aspects.   2. Physical
fitness.   I. Kirby, Timothy E.   II. Fox, Ann Roberts.
III. Title.
QP301.F67   1986   613.7′1   85–23154
ISBN   0-02-339190-1

Printing: 2 3 4 5 6 7   Year: 7 8 9 0 1 2 3

ISBN   0-02-339190-1

*Dedicated
to the Memory
of
Edward L. Fox, Ph.D.*

Preface

THIS text has been developed to provide an interpretation of fitness for persons beginning an exercise program and for those who have been involved in exercise but are not sure of why they are exercising or if their methods are correct. It was particularly designed for students who do not have a background in the science of exercise but who have an interest in developing an appropriate and well-rounded fitness program.

We have tried to meet these goals by presenting the book's information in a very readable form—remembering the words of Dr. Arthur H. Steinhaus, "Never before has man been in greater need of what education for health and fitness has to offer. . . . First we must ourselves gain a clearer understanding and then we must tell others in a language they will understand. This is Interpretation." It is hoped that the reader will find in these pages information that will provide an adequate interpretation of fitness; this in turn will hopefully foster an appreciation of the value of fitness and promote a style of living that will result in fitness.

Acknowledgments

We wish to thank our editor, James D. Anker, for his support and encouragement during the writing of *Bases of Fitness*. To Pat Kirby go many thanks for her typographical skills in all stages of the preparation of the manuscript. She and our children have been extremely cooperative in helping us to meet deadlines. We greatly appreciate the photography of Catherine Hunter and the time and efforts of Megan Markwood and Eric Miller, who modeled for all the flexibility and weight training photographs. We also wish to thank Julie Pulcipher, Steve Nary, Steve McKenzie, Leslie Pruitt, Kathy Greaves, and Kim Herling; their talents were willingly shared for other photos in the book.

Most of all, we acknowledge Edward Fox, who had just begun this manuscript when his untimely death occurred. We honor and miss him as a husband, colleague, teacher, researcher, and friend.

Timothy E. Kirby
Ann Roberts Fox

Contents

Chapter 1 ◇ **Introduction** 1

Chapter 2 ◇ **Scientific Bases of Fitness** 15

Chapter 3 ◇ **Cardiorespiratory (Endurance) Fitness** 47

Chapter 10 ◇ **Lifetime Sports and Fitness**   199

Appendix A ◇ **Commonly Asked Questions and Answers About Fitness**   209

Appendix B ◇ **Caloric and Other Values for Selected Common Foods, Including "Fast" Foods**   215

Appendix C ◇ **Caloric Costs of Selected Activities**   249

Appendix D ◇ **Fitness Evaluation Forms**   257

Glossary   273

Index   283

Chapter 1
Introduction

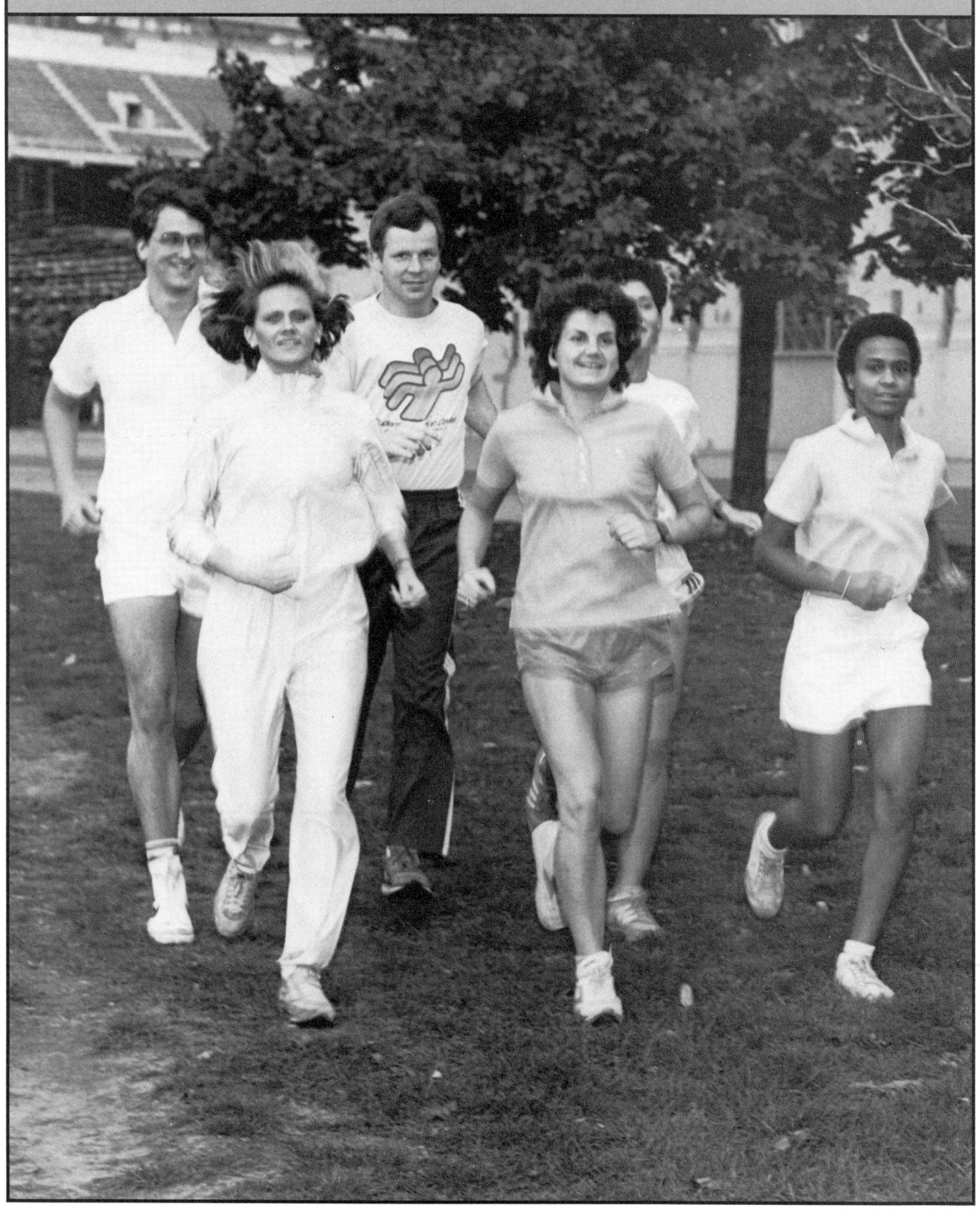

Chapter Outline

Learning Objectives

◇ To understand that a sedentary life-style can lead to poor health and to a low level of fitness.

◇ To understand that fitness is a physiological or functional capacity that improves the quality of life.

◇ To understand that cardiorespiratory endurance, muscular strength and endurance, joint flexibility, nutritional fitness, mental and emotional fitness, and motor fitness are the components of total fitness.

◇ To understand that quality of life refers to an overall positive feeling and enthusiasm for life.

Key Words and Phrases

cardiorespiratory fitness

cardiovascular fitness

fitness

functional capacity

joint flexibility

mental and emotional fitness

motor fitness

muscular fitness

muscular endurance

muscular strength

nutritional fitness

overfat

overweight

physical fitness

quality of life

sedentary life-style

Sedentary Living

TECHNOLOGY has come a long way in this century—from the horse-drawn buggy to the automobile, from the prop-driven airplane to jet propulsion to the exploration of space. It is generally believed that many of these technological advances have made our lives more comfortable or easier. However, with all the advancement in technology and the so-called ease of living has come a drastic change from an active to an inactive life-style. How many of us have seriously thought about this? Examples of inactive or **sedentary life-styles** are all around us (Figure 1–1). We drive to the supermarket in the shopping center rather than walking to the neighborhood grocery store. The cars we drive to the shopping center are even equipped with power steering and power brakes. We sit or lie down and watch television rather than jogging or cycling with the family. We drive to work and park as close as possible to the office door, thus minimizing the walk from the car to the office. We ride elevators in department stores and office buildings. We ride lawnmowers rather than pushing them, and we even ride golf carts around the course rather than walking. And what about sports fans? They sit in front of television sets watching others being active while their most vigorous activity is "bending the elbow" as they drink another beer. With modern technology, sports fans don't even have to get up from their chairs or couches to change the television channel. If that isn't enough, cable television now provides a channel that telecasts sports on a twenty-four-hour basis.

Let's go back for a moment to the idea that technological advances have made our lives more comfortable and easier. This is a common misconception. Have our lives actually been made easier and more comfortable as a result of our inactivity? Easier, yes, in the sense of human energy expenditure; but more comfortable—not really. The fact of the matter is that a sedentary life-style has led to a decline in our overall health and fitness level. Because of this the risk of certain diseases is greater. Perhaps the best example of this is the risk of cardiovascular disease, which is the number one cause of death in America today. For example, as shown by Borhani (1977) in Figure 1–2, of all deaths in the United States, more than half are caused by cardiovascular diseases (heart attack, stroke, and high blood pressure, in that order). One of the several known risk factors of cardiovascular disease is lack of regular exercise.

Another common health problem associated with inactivity in the United States today is obesity. Obesity is not only being **overweight,** but **overfat** as well. As with cardiovascular disease, more than 50 percent of all adults are afflicted with obesity. Furthermore, the incidence of cardiovascular disease is statistically and physiologically related to obesity. For example, if you are obese, your chance of dying of cardiovascular disease is 2½ times

3

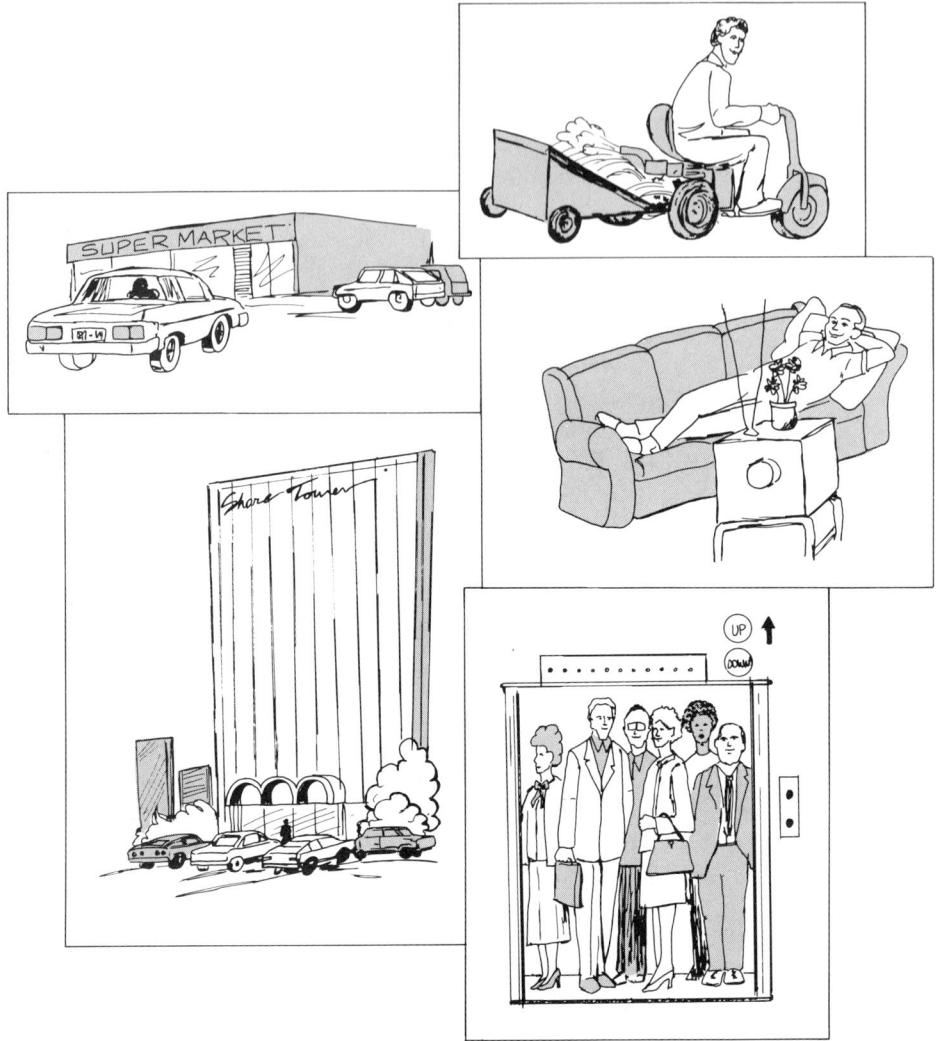

Figure 1–1. The "easy life."

greater than that of a contemporary who has an average or below average amount of body fat (Figure 1–3). Therefore, since the major cause of obesity is physical inactivity, regular physical exercise can significantly reduce the problems of obesity and promote **cardiovascular fitness.** Are our lives easier and more comfortable as a result of inactivity? Think about it.

Figure 1–2. The percentage of deaths caused by cardio-vascular diseases as compared with the percentage of deaths from all other causes.

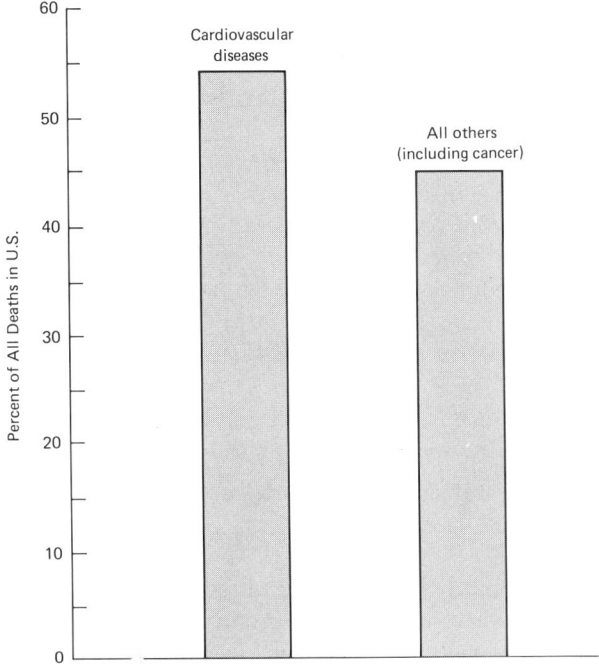

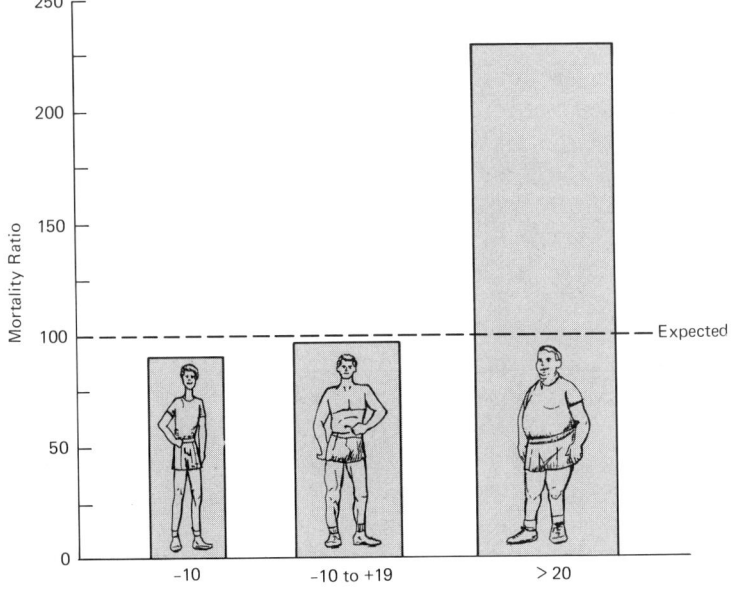

Figure 1–3. The influence of being overweight on the risk of death from heart attack. The expected average ratio is 100. (Based on data from Kannel, W. B.: Medical evaluation for physical exercise programs. In R. L. Morris (ed.), Exercise and the Heart, 1972. Reprinted courtesy of Charles C. Thomas Publisher, Springfield, Ill.)

Fitness—What Is It?

Fitness has several different definitions. We will not, however, need to spend a lot of time discussing them. Any word or concept that has different meanings to different people needs only to be defined in a functional sense, in this case, functional with respect to the purpose of this book. The sole purpose of this book is to help you improve the quality of your life. A good working definition of *fitness* therefore is *a physiological or functional capacity that allows for an improved quality of life.*

Components of Fitness

Two key phrases in our definition of fitness are **functional capacity** and **quality of life.**

Functional Capacity.   Functional capacity most often refers to physiological capacity or fitness. For example, the ability of the cardiorespiratory or heart-lung system to deliver oxygen to working muscles during prolonged periods of exercise is a physiological capacity. The higher this capacity, the greater the endurance fitness level. Other examples are **muscular strength, muscular endurance,** and **joint flexibility.** In these cases, the physiological capacities are how much force a muscle or muscle group can exert (strength), how long it can continue to exert force without fatiguing (endurance), and how much range of motion is possible in the joint over which the muscle works (flexibility). The greater these capacities, the greater is the level of muscular fitness. **Cardiorespiratory fitness** and **muscular fitness** are sometimes referred to collectively as **physical fitness.**

Other components of fitness are not necessarily related to specific physiological functions as are cardiorespiratory fitness or muscular fitness. Instead, the fitness is more general, involving many physiological functions. **Nutritional fitness** is a good example. All bodily functions rely upon nutrition. Thus, sound nutrition promotes optimal body growth and development and prevents a host of diseases. It also contributes to proper body composition and control of body weight. In other words, good nutritional habits along with good exercise habits help ward off excessive accumulations of body fat.

Mental and emotional fitness and **motor fitness** are also good examples of general rather than specific fitness components. Mental and emotional stress or tension are frequent by-products of today's society. Such tensions and stresses are quite often associated with anxiety, depression, muscular weakness, and even loss of appetite. One of the ways to relieve built-up tension is through physical activity. In fact some physicians and psychologists have found that exercise is a better prescription than any chemical medication for many of their emotionally stressed patients. The good feeling or "high" experienced by many joggers and other regular exercisers may very well be a result of temporary relief from mental and emotional stress.

Motor fitness refers to one or more qualities or abilities associated with physical skills such as endurance, strength, agility, flexibility, balance, and coordination. This component of fitness is associated with high-level athletic performance.

Quality of Life. The second key phrase in our definition of fitness is quality of life. Quality of life generally refers to an overall positive feeling and enthusiasm for life. An ability to easily perform daily tasks with enthusiasm and to go beyond the requirements of one's routine exemplify what is meant by quality of life. How many of you who are working your way through college come home at night and collapse from exhaustion? How often have you heard one of your parents say "Let's not go out tonight, I'm too tired." Such feelings of exhaustion resulting from routine day-to-day activities prevent us from increasing the quality of our lives. An increased fitness level that changes our physical and mental pace will help us to endure the physical demands of our responsibilities as well as alleviate the exhaustion associated with the boredom of routine tasks. As a result, we can look forward to participation in activities we enjoy. More about the quality of life will be discussed in Chapter 10.

Overview of the Text

With this general idea of what really constitutes fitness, let's take a closer look at some of its components. This book focuses on the following components of fitness: (1) cardiorespiratory fitness; (2) muscular strength; (3) muscular endurance; (4) flexibility; (5) nutrition; and (6) body composition.

Chapter 2: Scientific Bases of Fitness

Before meaning and understanding can be given to the components of fitness, a review of their basic structures and functions is necessary. The primary systems reviewed are the cardiorespiratory system, the muscular system, and the metabolic or energy-producing system. The review of the cardiorespiratory system involves the functioning of the heart, the blood vessels, and the lungs in supplying oxygen to and removing carbon dioxide from the muscles. The major function of the muscles is to impart bodily movement and maintain stability. These functions depend upon the availability of energy within the cells. Therefore, a review of how the body metabolically produces energy is also necessary in order to establish a good scientific basis for fitness.

The scientific basis for nutritional fitness is also related to energy production. Certain foods provide the chemical energy needed to ensure that a supply of useful energy is always readily available to the cells. Another link that energy and nutrition have to fitness is control of body weight. The basic scientific rule regulating your body weight is the relationship between the amount of energy taken in as food calories and the amount of energy or calories expended through activity. When the two are equal body weight does not change; when the number of calories taken in exceeds those expended body weight increases; when the number of calories expended exceeds those taken in body weight decreases.

Chapter 3: Cardiorespiratory Fitness

The prefix *cardio* refers to the heart and blood vessels (cardiovascular would be more precise), whereas the term *respiratory* or *respiration* refers to the lungs and the exchange of oxygen and carbon dioxide between the lungs and the blood and the blood and the muscles. Thus, cardiorespiratory fitness has a direct relationship with cardiovascular diseases such as coronary heart disease. For example, a high degree of cardiorespiratory fitness usually correlates with a low incidence of coronary heart disease.

Other names for cardiorespiratory fitness include *cardiovascular fitness*, *endurance fitness*, and *aerobic fitness*. In this text, we will use the term cardiorespiratory fitness more often than the others. As previously mentioned, cardiorespiratory fitness refers to the ability of the heart-lung system to deliver oxygen to and remove carbon dioxide from the working skeletal muscles during prolonged exercise activities. The greater this ability, the higher the cardiorespiratory fitness level.

Chapter 4: Exercise Prescription for Cardiorespiratory Fitness

The physiological benefits of chronic exercise programs are specific. That is to say, the particular benefits desired must be precisely matched with a particular kind of exercise, which is performed on a regular basis, at a particular intensity, and for a particular duration. Therefore, exercise programs for the purpose of increasing cardiorespiratory fitness must be prescribed. This is similar to a physician prescribing a medicine to reduce or minimize symptoms caused by disease. In this case, the "disease" is a low cardiorespiratory fitness level and some of the symptoms are breathlessness upon exertion, chronic or persistent fatigue, and overweight. The correct prescription, of course, is regular participation in an exercise program involving activities that are carried out over prolonged periods of time and that sufficiently tax or stress the heart-lung system.

An important ingredient in the exercise prescription is your exercise *target heart rate.* The target heart rate is defined as the heart rate during exercise that will assure you that you are exercising at the proper intensity to stimulate improvement in your heart-lung or cardiorespiratory fitness level. This rate is individually determined, being calculated on the basis of your age, sex, resting heart rate, and maximal attainable heart rate during exercise. Besides the intensity of exercise, other important components of the exercise prescription include a medical examination, proper frequency per week of the exercise sessions, and proper warm-up and cool-down activities.

Chapter 5: Muscular Strength and Endurance Fitness—Weight-Training Programs

A common misconception about fitness programs is that any form of exercise, whether it be jogging or lifting weights, will improve your total level of fitness. This is not true. As just emphasized, fitness is specific in that improvement in a particular form of fitness requires a particular kind of exercise program. Thus, weight-training or weight-resistance programs are necessary for improvement in muscular strength and muscular endurance. Here too such factors as intensity (amount of resistance or weight lifted), repetitions (number of times a given load or weight is lifted), and frequency and duration of the lifting sessions are important in determining how much improvement will take place in the muscular system.

With weight-resistance training, the intensity of the program is determined by the amount of resistance or weight lifted. These two factors when combined are referred to as the *repetition maximum.* The repetition maximum is the maximal load that a muscle or muscle group can lift over a given number of repetitions before fatiguing. Generally speaking, increases in muscular strength result from programs in which a relatively heavy load is coupled with few repetitions, whereas increases in muscular endurance result from programs in which a relatively light load is coupled with many repetitions.

Chapter 6: Muscular and Joint Flexibility

Flexibility is the range of motion of a joint. Often this particular type of fitness is ignored. It is, however, an important fitness component that is relatively easily attained and maintained. For example, flexibility has been found to be important in performing certain sports or motor skills. In addition, flexibility exercises have been successfully prescribed for relief of dysmenorrhea (painful menstruation), general neuromuscular tension, and low back pains. If athletes maintain a satisfactory degree of flexibility, they will be less susceptible to certain muscular injuries. The best exercises for the development of flexibility are stretching exercises.

Chapter 7: Nutrition and Fitness

Today more than ever before scientists recognize that nutrition is functionally linked to health and fitness. Not only does a nutritionally sound daily diet help you ward off many diseases, but it also aids in the ever-increasing battle against obesity. Of the many popular diets on the market today, do you know which ones, if any, are nutritionally sound? Do you know how many calories you need as a daily minimum? What is the total amount of fats, proteins, or carbohydrates that you need? How many calories are contained in an 8-ounce steak? How much fat? What kinds of foods, when consumed on a regular basis, contribute to high blood levels of cholesterol? Do all forms of cholesterol contribute to the threat of heart attack? Are vegetarian diets nutritionally sound? It is now possible to answer most of these questions. Just a few years ago they were not answerable, at least not on the basis of sound scientific information.

Other important questions about nutrition focus on sports performances. For example, of what should the pregame diet or meal consist? What is glycogen or carbohydrate loading and can it improve endurance performance? What is the basic difference between an athlete's diet and a non-athlete's diet?

Proper nutrition is also concerned with water intake (hydration) and vitamins and minerals. Americans are hooked on vitamin and mineral supplements. Are they necessary?

Chapter 8: Exercise, Body Composition, and Body Weight Control

It has been said that if you intend to maintain an average body weight and at the same time lead a sedentary life, you will have to literally starve yourself for the majority of your life. How true this is. Contrary to popular belief, the single greatest cause of obesity is probably physical inactivity, not overeating. This is supported by evidence from population studies that show that the leanest members of the population have the highest caloric intake. This is exemplified by athletes who consume anywhere from 5,000 to 10,000 kilocalories of food a day during the sports season but do not gain a single pound. As a matter of fact, some of these athletes may even lose a few pounds over the season. Exercise is an effective tool for the control and maintenance of body weight.

Obesity is usually defined as a body weight 20 percent or more above ideal weight. Based on this definition and recognizing the difficulty in establishing ideal weight, there are probably between fifty and eighty million obese persons in the United States today. Obesity can also be defined on the basis of body composition. Body composition refers to how much of your body is fat tissue and how much is nonfat tissue. Approximately one half of the nonfat tissue is muscle and therefore is often referred to as *lean body weight* or *lean body mass.* The average college-aged man has between 12 and 15 percent body fat. In other words, if he has a total body weight of 160 pounds, 19 to 24 pounds* would be fat and the rest (136 to 141 pounds) would be lean body weight. The average college-aged woman has between 22 and 25 percent fat.

If you are obese, you have an excess of fat weight, not lean body weight; hence the term *overfat* rather than *overweight;* overfat is more accurate in describing obesity. For example, a 250-pound football player who has 8 percent body fat (20 pounds of fat tissue and 230 pounds of lean body weight) would probably be considered overweight by most clinicians. However, with only 8 percent fat, he definitely would not be overfat or obese.

Other considerations discussed in Chapter 8 are anorexia nervosa and bulimia. These diet-related illnesses primarily affect young women in late adolescence and their early twenties. Both conditions require medical supervision and treatment.

How do you correctly go about losing body fat or gaining lean body weight? As mentioned earlier, the basic principle involved in losing or gaining body weight is the balance between energy taken in as food and energy expended through physical activity.

Chapter 9: Evaluation of Fitness

One of the purposes of any evaluation program is to measure improvement. Evaluation of a fitness program therefore involves measuring the change in fitness resulting from the program. Not all benefits derived from fitness programs are immediately apparent, nor are they necessarily recognizable by the participant. Thus, an evaluation program is needed in order to provide tangible evidence that fitness benefits are indeed being gained. Such tangible evidence is usually helpful in providing further motivation for you to continue your exercise program. If no fitness gains are made, then the evaluation process serves another very important purpose—the evaluation of the effectiveness of the fitness program itself.

Another purpose of an evaluation program is to give quantitative values to the fitness benefits gained. Comparisons then can be made with other persons of the same age and sex. In other words, you can find out where you stand on a wider scale with regard to your level of fitness. For example, several sets of standards or norms are available, many of which are based on national data. Forms are provided in Appendix D to aid you in your fitness evaluation process.

---

* $160 \times 0.12 = 19$ pounds and $160 \times 0.15 = 24$ pounds

Chapter 10: Lifetime Sports and Fitness

Certain sports, when engaged in on a regular basis, can help to improve your level of fitness or at least maintain your present fitness status. Perhaps the best way to keep fit the year around is to combine a good three-day-a-week fitness program with a sport played two or three times a week. The fitness program, in all likelihood, will get you into shape so that your skill in the sport improves and you can enjoy the sport more.

Not all sports help you to maintain your fitness. For example, the less active sports such as bowling, archery, and golf (particularly when an electric golf cart is used) will probably not provide activity intensive enough to maintain or improve either muscular or cardiorespiratory fitness. As a matter of fact, an activity such as bowling may even be a waste of time with regard to fitness, because people very often consume beer, potato chips, and other high-calorie foods while participating.

Appendices

Four appendices are presented. The first contains commonly asked questions and answers about fitness; the second gives the caloric values and other values of some common foods; the third lists the caloric costs or energy expenditures of various activities and exercises; and as mentioned previously, the fourth provides fitness evaluation forms to help you in your evaluation process.

SUMMARY

◇ Advances in technology have led to a sedentary life-style and in turn to low levels of fitness and relatively high risks of developing certain cardiovascular disease and obesity.

◇ Fitness can be defined as a physiological or functional capacity that allows for an improved quality of life.

◇ Functional capacity refers to physiological capacity or fitness such as cardiorespiratory (heart-lung) fitness and muscular fitness.

◇ The components of fitness are cardiorespiratory endurance, muscular strength, muscular endurance, joint flexibility, body composition, nutritional fitness, mental and emotional fitness, and motor fitness.

◇ Quality of life refers mainly to an overall positive feeling and enthusiasm for life.

STUDY QUESTIONS

1. How have advances in technology been detrimental to society?
2. Define fitness.

3. What is meant by functional capacity?

4. List and briefly define each of the components of fitness.

5. Discuss what is meant by "quality of life."

REFERENCES AND SELECTED READINGS

Allsen, P.; Harrison, J.; and Vance, B.: *Fitness for Life.* Dubuque, Iowa: Wm. C. Brown, 1980.

Borhani, N. D.: Epidemiology of coronary heart disease. In E. A. Amsterdam, J. H. Wilmore, and A. N. de Maria (eds.): *Exercise in Cardiovascular Health and Disease.* New York: Yorke Medical Books, 1977, pp. 1–12.

Corbin, C.; and Lindsey, R.: *Fitness for Life.* Glenview, Ill.: Scott, Foresman and Co., 1979.

Falls, H. B.; Baylor, A. M.; and Dishman, R. K.: *Essentials of Fitness.* Philadelphia: Saunders College Publishing, 1980.

Fisher, A. G.; and Conlee, R.: *The Complete Book of Physical Fitness.* Salt Lake City, Utah: Brigham Young University Press, 1979.

Fox. E. L.: *Lifetime Fitness.* Philadelphia: Saunders College Publishing, 1983.

Getchell, B.: *Physical Fitness: A Way of Life,* 2nd ed. New York: John Wiley & Sons, 1979.

Hockey, R. V.: *Physical Fitness,* 3rd ed. St. Louis: C. V. Mosby, 1978.

Katch, F. I.; and McArdale, W. D.: *Nutrition, Weight Control and Exercise,* Boston: Houghton Mifflin, 1977.

Melograno, V.; and Klinzing, J.: *An Orientation to Total Fitness.* Dubuque, Iowa: Kendall/Hunt Publishing Co., 1974.

Miller, D. K.; and Allen, T. E.: *Fitness: A Lifetime Commitment.* Minneapolis: Burgess Publishing Co., 1979.

Pollock, M. L.; Wilmore, J. H.; and Fox, S. M.: *Health and Fitness Through Physical Activity.* New York: John Wiley & Sons, 1978.

Stokes, R.; Moore, A. C.; Moore, C.; and Williams, C.: *Fitness: The New Wave.* Winston-Salem: Hunter Publishing Company, 1981.

Chapter 2
Scientific
Bases of Fitness

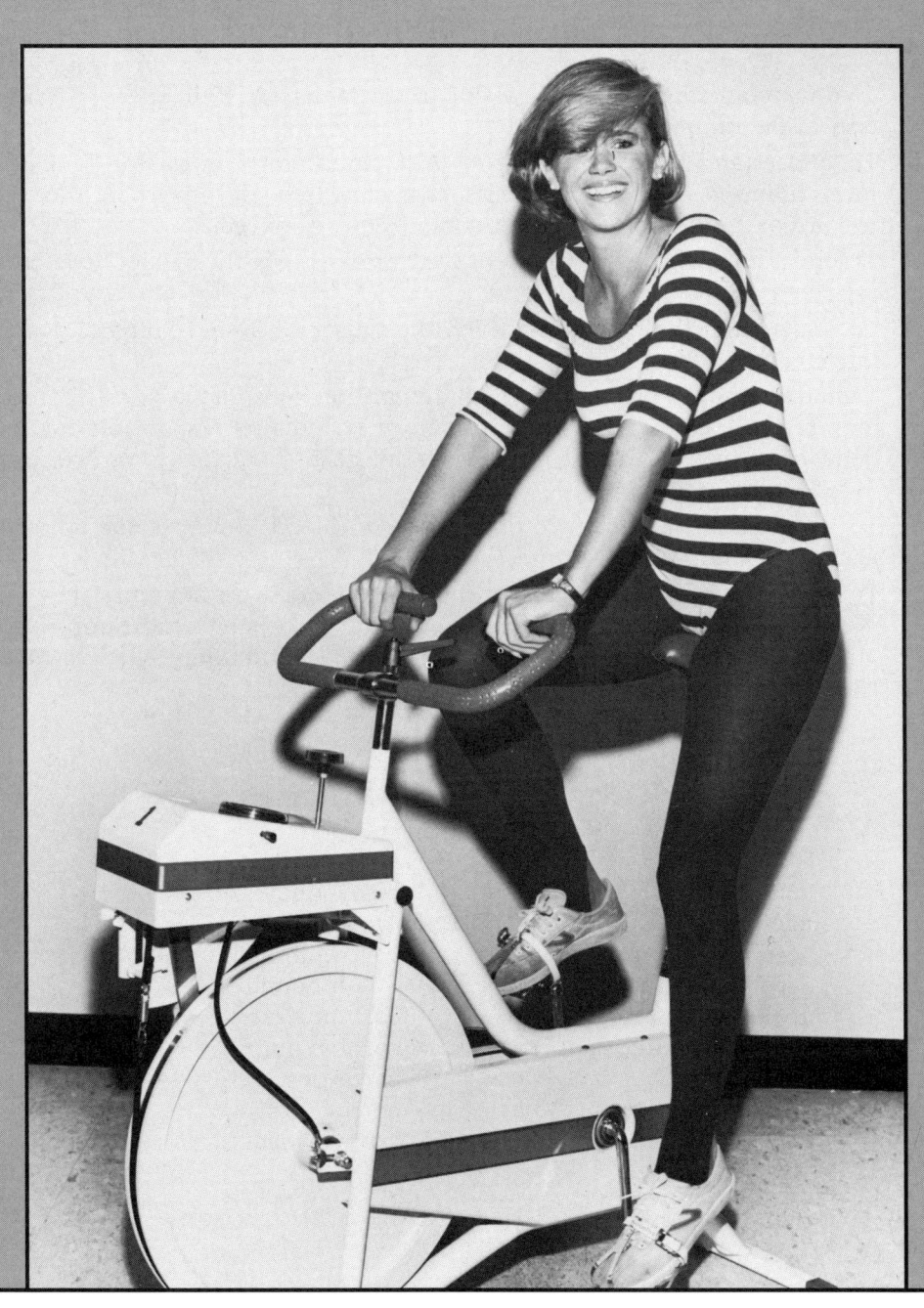

Chapter Outline

Learning Objectives

◇ To understand the role of adenosine triphosphate (ATP) in energy production in the human body.

◇ To understand the relationship of ATP, muscular contraction, and the three different metabolic systems, two of which are anaerobic (do not require oxygen) and the third aerobic (requires oxygen).

◇ To understand the relationship of nutritional fitness to metabolic energy production.

◇ To understand the means by which the muscular system imparts bodily movement.

◇ To understand the process by which the cardiorespiratory system (a combination of the respiratory and circulatory systems) is responsible for the delivery of oxygen to and the removal of carbon dioxide from working muscle cells.

◇ To understand the influence of exercise on blood flow (cardiac output), heart rate, and stroke volume.

◇ To learn that maximal oxygen consumption refers to the amount of oxygen the body can use during maximal exercise. It is the single most important physiological measure of the ability of the heart and lungs to deliver oxygen to the working muscles.

Key Words and Phrases

A band

actin

adenosine triphosphate (ATP)

aerobic

aerobic capacity

alveoli

alveolocapillary membrane

anaerobic

aorta

ATP-PC system

atrium

bicarbonate ion

blood pressure

carbaminohemoglobin
   compound

carbohydrates

cardiac output

cardiorespiratory system

coronary artery

cross-bridges

diffusion
eccentric contraction
endomysium
energy
energy continuum
epimysium
fasciculus
fast-twitch (FT) fibers
fats
flexibility
gas exchange
gas transport
heart rate
hemoglobin
hypertension
hypertrophy
H zone
I band
isokinetically
isometric contraction
isotonic contraction
kilocalorie
lactic acid (LA) system
maximal aerobic power
maximal oxygen consumption
metabolism

motor unit
muscle bundle
myocardial infarction
myofibril
myosin
negative contraction
partial pressure
perimysium
phosphocreatine (PC)
plasma
pulmonary arteries
pulmonary ventilation
pulse
sarcolemma
sarcomere
sliding filament theory
slow-twitch (ST) fibers
stroke volume
systole
systolic pressure
tissue–capillary membrane
vena cava
ventilation
ventricle
Z line

Introduction

A S mentioned in Chapter 1, a thorough understanding of what fitness is all about cannot be fully appreciated without a comprehension of its scientific bases. The purpose of this chapter therefore is to discuss the physiological aspects of fitness.

Our discussion will focus on three major physiological systems: (1) the metabolic or energy-producing system; (2) the muscular system; and (3) the cardiorespiratory or heart-lung system.

The Metabolic or Energy-Producing System—The Production of ATP

The word **metabolism** refers to all the chemical reactions in the body that occur in the production of **energy** for work. Contrary to popular belief, the food we eat is not directly used for energy by the cells. Instead, the energy released from the metabolic breakdown of food is used to manufacture another chemical compound, **adenosine triphosphate,** or, more simply, **ATP.** ATP is a complex compound that belongs to a class of compounds known as nucleotides. It is found in all cells of the body but chiefly in

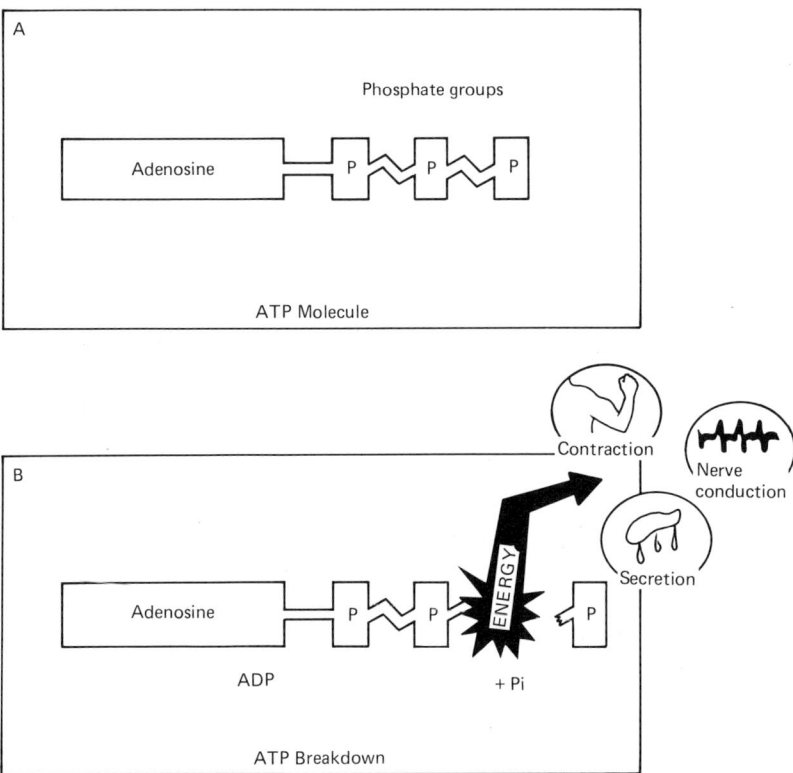

Figure 2–1. (A) ATP consists of a large molecule called adenosine and three simpler components called phosphate groups. (B) The energy released from the breakdown of ATP is used to perform biological work. (From Sports Physiology, *second ed. by E. L. Fox. Copyright © 1984 by CBS Publishing. Copyright 1979 by W. B. Saunders Co. Reprinted by permission of CBS College Publishing.)*

muscle tissue. When ATP breaks down into adenosine diphosphate (ADP) and inorganic phosphate (Pi), energy is released (Figure 2–1). It is this energy that is directly used by the cells to perform their work. ATP is the immediate energy reserve for all tissues. Whenever there is a need for energy for any biological function, such as muscular contraction, conduction of a nerve impulse, glandular secretion, and cellular growth, ATP is the only compound in the body that can provide this immediate energy.

Our major concern now is how ATP is supplied to the muscle cells. There are three ways in which this occurs. Two of the systems are **anaerobic** because the oxygen we breathe is not required for the chemical reactions that manufacture ATP. Anaerobic literally means *without oxygen* (*an* = without, *aerobic* = oxygen or air). The third system, which is perhaps most familiar to us, is **aerobic** because oxygen is a necessary ingredient for manufacturing ATP. As just mentioned, aerobic means with or in the presence of oxygen or air.

The three metabolic systems for ATP production are (1) the adenosine triphosphate-phosphocreatine (ATP-PC) system (anaerobic); (2) the lactic acid (LA) system (which is also anaerobic); and (3) the oxygen or aerobic system.

The ATP-PC System

PC is a chemical abbreviation for the compound **phosphocreatine.** It, like ATP, is also stored in muscle cells. After we use the ATP stored in a muscle (which happens after only a few seconds of intense activity) the muscle must break down phosphocreatine (PC). When PC breaks down, it releases enough energy so that adenosine triphosphate (ATP) can be manufactured (Figure 2–2). This process is almost instantaneous and thereby serves as the most readily available source of ATP energy to the muscle cells. Activities such as the 100-meter dash, the shot-put, the discus throw, the javelin throw, pitching, diving, and climbing stairs performed at maximum intensities over periods of a few seconds derive ATP energy predominately through the ATP-PC system.

The **ATP-PC system** is a valuable energy system for the entire animal kingdom. The tiger springing to its food, the flushed bird flying from its hiding place, the ground hog scurrying to its den, and the Olympic athlete sprinting to a gold medal are all good illustrations. Like most good things, however, there are limitations. The ATP-PC mechanism suffers in that only relatively small quantities of both ATP and PC can be stored in muscles. Thus, while readily available, the supply does not last long—probably 10 seconds or less. However, certain training programs have been shown to increase muscular stores of both ATP and PC. Such programs will be discussed in Chapter 5.

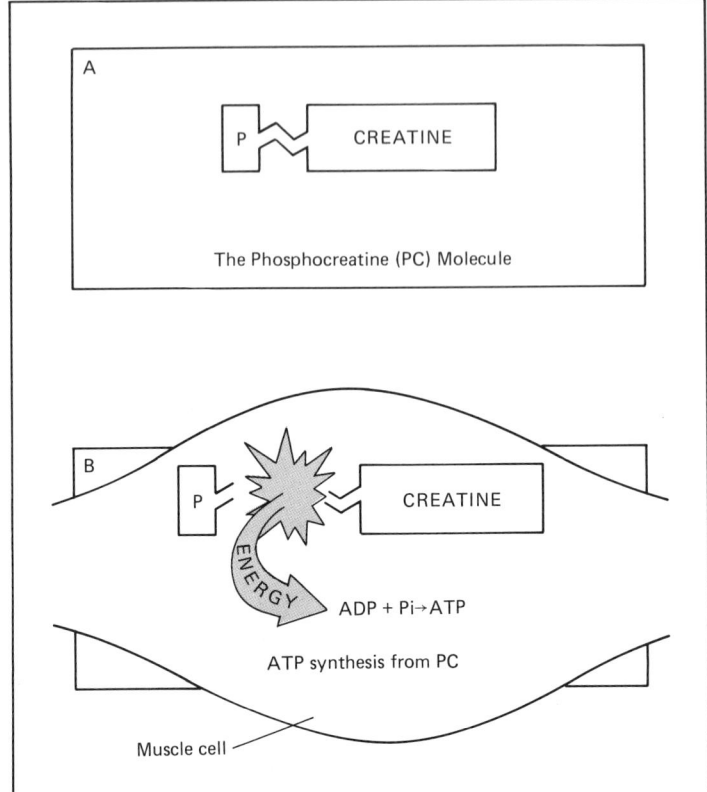

Figure 2–2. The ATP-PC system, also called the phosphagen system. (A) Phosphocreatine, which is stored in muscle cells, contains a high-energy bond. (B) When ATP is broken down during muscular contraction, it is rapidly reformed by the energy liberated during the breakdown of PC. (From Sports Physiology, *second ed. by E. L. Fox. Copyright © 1984 by CBS Publishing. Copyright 1979 by W. B. Saunders Co. Reprinted by permission of CBS College Publishing.)*

The Lactic Acid System

In the 400-meter and 800-meter sprints, as well as during the latter part of a 1,500-meter run, the **lactic acid** or **LA system** is the predominant source for ATP replenishment. The LA system derives its name from the excessive amounts of lactic acid that accumulate in the blood and muscles during activity. Properly associated with painful muscular fatigue, lactic acid accumulates because there is an inadequate amount of oxygen available in the muscle cells. The stored ATP and PC have been depleted and the only way for additional ATP to be produced is through the release of energy from the breakdown of food. In this case, **carbohydrates** (other names for carbo-

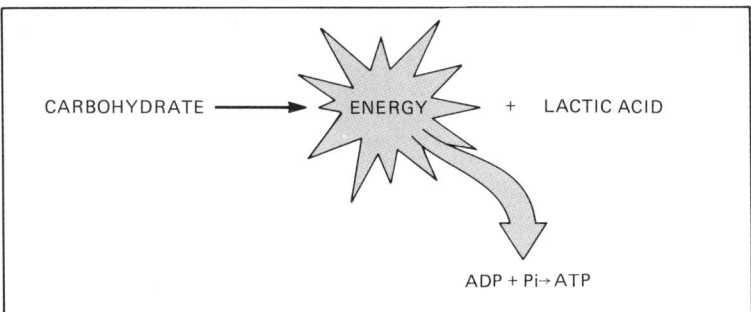

Figure 2–3. The chemical breakdown of carbohydrate yields energy and the byproduct lactic acid. *The energy produced is used for the synthesis of ATP.*

hydrates are sugar, glucose, glycogen, and starch) are the only food source for the LA system. Chapter 7 includes additional information about carbohydrates in our diets. Carbohydrates are also stored in muscles in the form of glycogen. When the oxygen supply is inadequate, carbohydrates are chemically broken down to lactic acid, thus releasing enough energy for some ATP to be manufactured (Figure 2–3). The lactic acid that accumulates as a result causes temporary muscular fatigue. It is real fatigue—ask any athlete, particularly a participant in the 400-meter dash.

High-intensity efforts of short duration primarily draw energy from the LA system. Properly designed training programs for these activities will not only increase the amount of carbohydrate stored in the muscles, but, more importantly, will also develop greater efficiency on the part of muscle cells to anaerobically break down the carbohydrate, thus allowing for greater production of ATP energy. Training programs are discussed in Chapters 4 and 5.

The Oxygen or Aerobic System

Does it seem strange to you that oxygen was not required in the first two energy systems? No animals, especially humans, however, can survive for long without it. After a few minutes without oxygen there will be no ATP production, no energy, and no life. In the presence of oxygen, the foods we eat, especially carbohydrates and **fats**, provide energy for the constant production of ATP for use by the muscle cells (Figure 2–4). The aerobic system, which is a prime factor in ATP production, is essential for our continuous existence. It not only produces ATP most efficiently and most abundantly but it is also the primary energy source during what we shall call endurance events, e.g., 2-mile, cross-country, and marathon (26 miles) performances. The aerobic system is also the prime energy source for low-level activities such as sitting, note-taking, and walking to class.

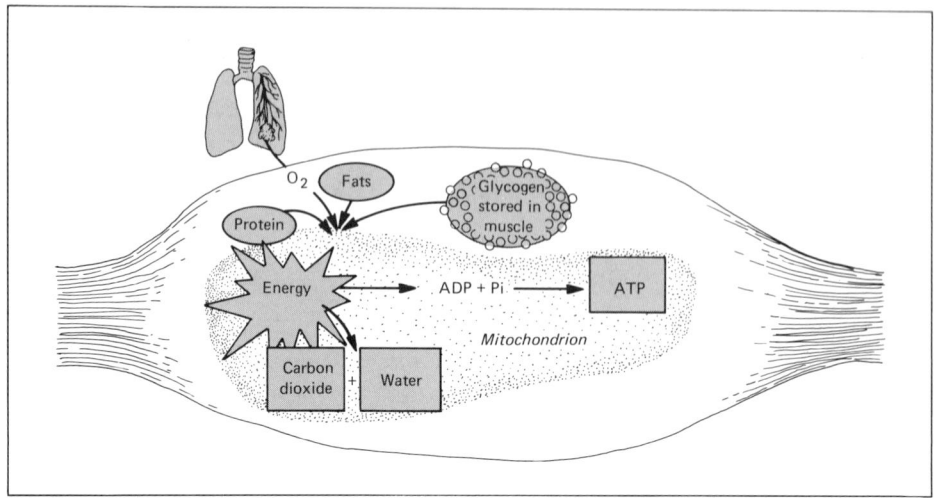

Figure 2–4. The oxygen, or aerobic, system. The aerobic breakdown of carbohydrates, fats, and even proteins provides energy for ATP resynthesis. (From Sports Physiology, *second ed. by E. L. Fox. Copyright © 1984 by CBS Publishing. Copyright 1979 by W. B. Saunders Co. Reprinted by permission of CBS College Publishing.)*

A training program designed specifically for endurance events will enhance the storage of foodstuffs and increase the ability of muscle cells to consume oxygen and thus to aerobically manufacture ATP.

A summary of the characteristics of the three energy systems is given in Table 2–1.

Table 2–1. General Characteristics of the Three Energy (ATP) Producing Systems.

Characteristic	System		
	ATP-PC	*LA*	*O₂*
Speed of reaction	Very rapid	Rapid	Slow
Fuel	Phosphocreatine (PC)	Carbohydrate (glucose and glycogen)	Carbohydrate, fat, and protein
Amount of ATP produced	Very Limited	Limited	Unlimited
Fatiguing by-products	None	Lactic Acid	None
Oxygen required	No	No	Yes
Type of activity supported	Sprint or high-power, short-duration activities	Activities of 1- to 3-minutes duration	Endurance or long-duration activities

The Energy Continuum Idea

Let's review for a moment. ATP is the immediate form of cellular energy. It is supplied in three ways: (1) by the oxygen system; (2) by the LA system; and (3) by the ATP-PC system. The capability of each system to supply the major portion of the ATP required is related to the specific activity or event performed. For example, in short-term, high-intensity activities such as the 100-meter dash the total amount of ATP required is supplied almost entirely by the rapid ATP-PC system. On the other hand, long-term, low-intensity activities such as a marathon race (in which participants do not aim for speed) are supported almost exclusively by the oxygen system. In the middle is the LA system, with the major portion of its ATP production used to support activities such as the 400-meter and 800-meter dashes.

We have tried to develop here the idea of an **energy continuum,** by demonstrating the relationship between the way in which ATP is made available and the type of activity performed. Such a continuum is depicted in Figure 2–5. Observe that all three energy systems contribute ATP during the performance of nearly every activity. Also notice that one system usually contributes more (as indicated by the heavier shaded areas) during one type of activity than do the other systems. This is significant: if the predominant energy system for any given activity is improved, performance in that activity will also be improved.

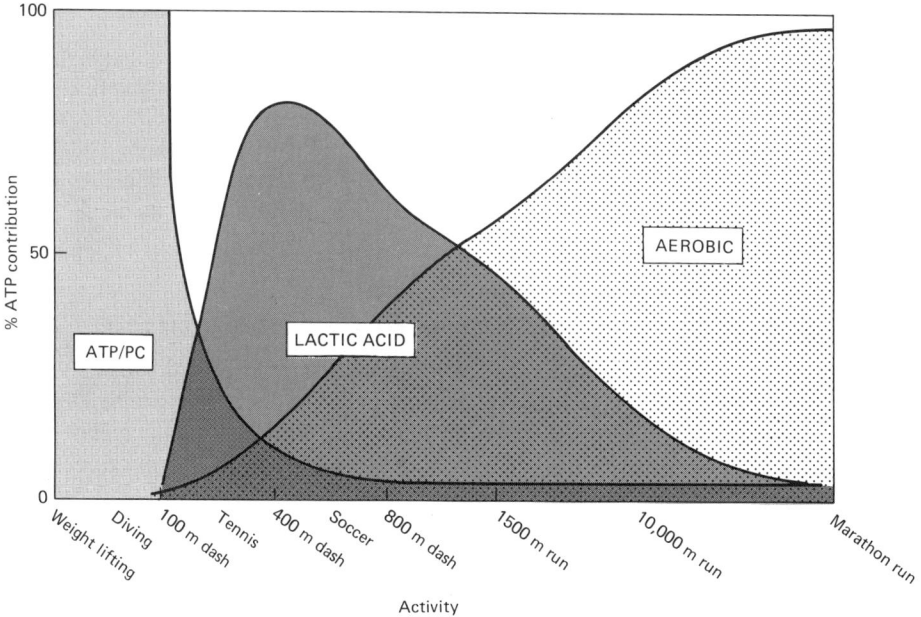

Figure 2–5. The continuum of energy system contributions to activities.

Relationship Between Energy Production and Nutritional Fitness

As mentioned in the first chapter, the scientific basis for nutritional fitness is also related to metabolic energy production. As we have just learned, the foods we eat provide us with the chemical energy needed for the production of ATP. Remember, ATP is the only directly usable form of energy in the human body.

Another link that metabolic energy production has to nutritional fitness is the control of body weight. When a given amount of oxygen is used in the aerobic system to help break down a given amount of carbohydrate or fat, a specific amount of energy is released. For example, when 192 g of oxygen (just under 7 ounces) break down 180 g of glycogen (just over 6 ounces), 686 kcal of heat energy are released. In other words, 686 kcal of energy have been expended. A **kilocalorie** (kcal), by the way, is the amount of heat required to raise the temperature of 1 kg of water (2.2 pounds) one degree centigrade (1.8 degrees Fahrenheit). The basic scientific rule regulating body weight is energy balance. If more energy is expended than is taken in, body weight decreases; if more energy is taken in as food than expended through activity, body weight increases.

The Muscular System

The major job of the muscular system is to impart bodily movement. To understand how this is done, we need to discuss the basic structure and function of the skeletal muscles. Also, since flexibility involves the bony joints and to a certain extent, the muscular tissue that spans the joints, we will want to discuss some basic information about flexibility as well.

Structure and Function of Skeletal Muscle

Skeletal muscle is surrounded by a connective tissue called the **epimysium** (Figure 2–6). The largest subunit of a muscle is the **muscle bundle** or **fasciculus** (plural: fasciculi). A muscle bundle is composed of anywhere from one to several hundred muscle fibers and is surrounded by a connective tissue called the **perimysium.** The individual muscle fibers or cells contained within the bundles are also surrounded by a connective tissue, the **endomysium.** The muscle cell membrane is called the **sarcolemma.**

The component of a muscle cell that distinguishes it from all other cells is the **myofibril.** A myofibril contains two protein filaments, a thicker one called **myosin** and a thinner one called **actin.** These proteins are geometri-

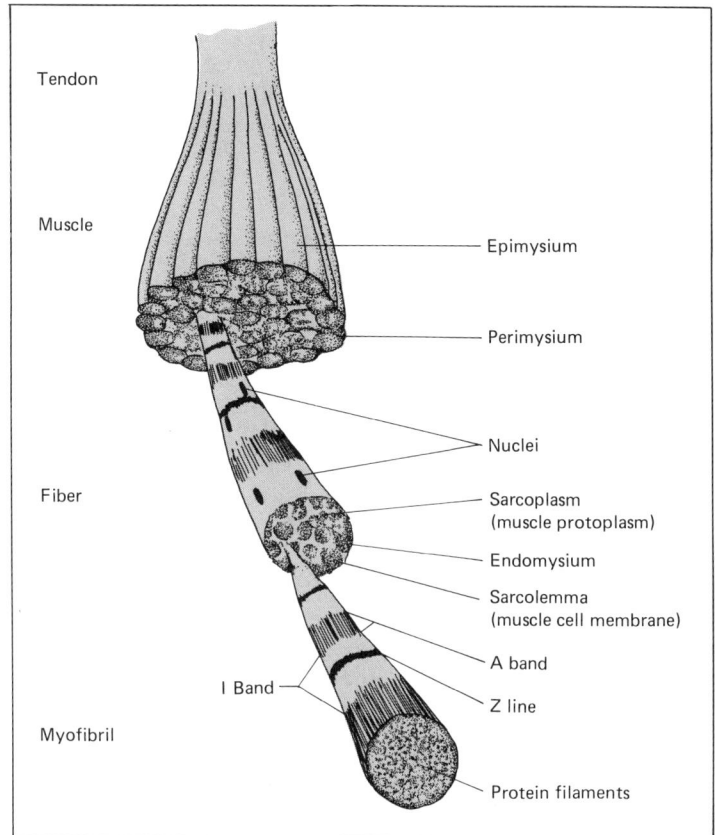

Figure 2–6. The structural and functional subunits of skeletal muscle. (From Sports Physiology, *second ed. by E. L. Fox. Copyright © 1984 by CBS Publishing. Copyright 1979 by W. B. Saunders Co. Reprinted by permission of CBS College Publishing.)*

cally aligned throughout the muscle as shown in Figure 2–7. Such an arrangement gives skeletal muscle its striped or striated appearance.

The smallest functional unit of the myofibril is the **sarcomere,** which is the distance between two **Z lines.** The sarcomere will contract when stimulated. The **I band** of a sarcomere is composed only of actin filaments that extend from the Z lines toward the center of the sarcomere. The **A band** consists of both actin and myosin filaments. The tiny projections extending from the myosin filaments toward the actin filaments are called **crossbridges.** These cross-bridges are instrumental in effecting the shortening of the muscle during contraction. The area in the center of the A band where the cross-bridges are absent is called the **H zone.**

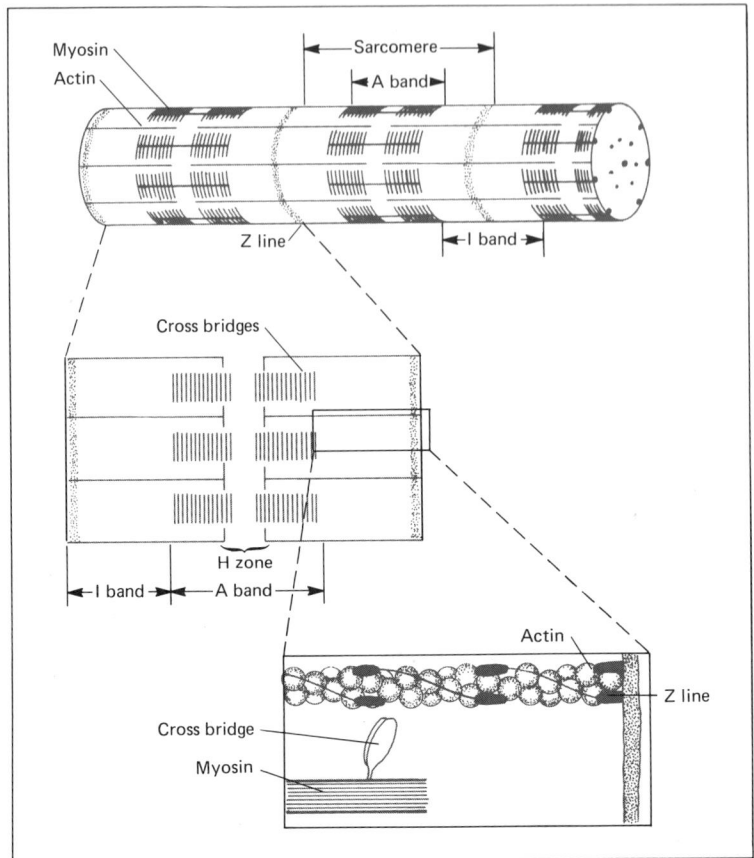

Figure 2–7. The detailed structure of the myofibril. (From Sports Physiology, *second ed. by E. L. Fox. Copyright © 1984 by CBS Publishing. Copyright 1979 by W. B. Saunders Co. Reprinted by permission of CBS College Publishing.)*

Types of Muscular Contraction and the Sliding Filament Theory

There are several types of muscular contractions. The most familiar is perhaps **isotonic contraction** where the muscle shortens as it develops tension. An example of this type of contraction is that seen in most lifting activities. If the lifting movement is performed at a constant speed, then the muscles are said to be contracting **isokinetically.**

Another type of contraction, which is also probably familiar to you, is the **isometric contraction.** Although the muscle develops tension, it does not shorten during an isometric contraction. Your muscles contract isometrically, for example, when you hold a weight stationary at arm's length in front of you.

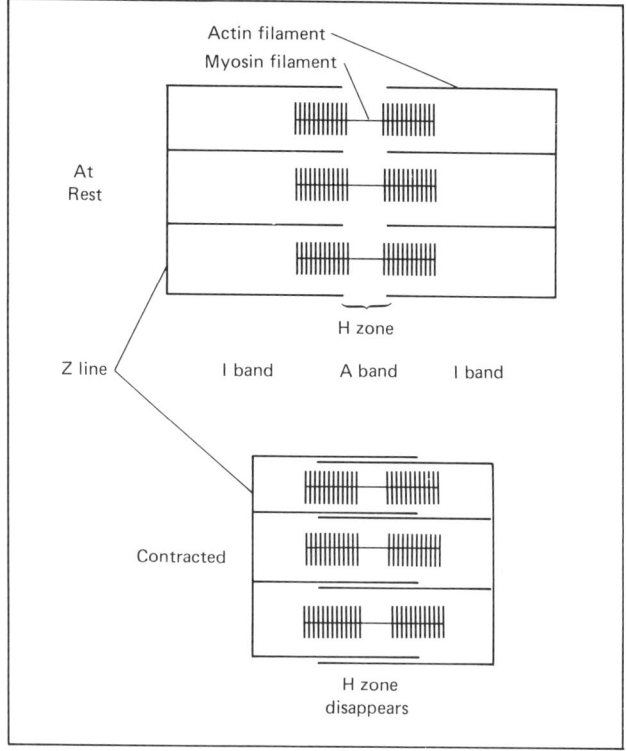

Figure 2–8. The sliding filament theory of muscular contraction. When a muscle contracts isotonically, the actin filaments slide over the myosin filaments. (From Sports Physiology, *second ed. by E. L. Fox. Copyright © 1984 by CBS Publishing. Copyright 1979 by W. B. Saunders Co. Reprinted by permission of CBS College Publishing.)*

An **eccentric** or **negative contraction** is one in which the muscle develops tension, but rather than shortening it lengthens during contraction to resist some force that causes motion. Lowering a weight that was lifted or walking down stairs are common situations in which muscles undergo negative or eccentric contractions. More will be said about the various types of muscular contractions in Chapter 5.

When a muscle shortens, the actin filaments slide over the myosin filaments toward the center of the sarcomere. This is known as the **sliding filament theory** of muscular contraction and is shown schematically in Figure 2–8. The mechanism involved in the sliding process is not exactly known; however, it is fairly well agreed that when a muscle is stimulated, the myosin cross-bridges form a type of bond with selected sites on the actin filaments. Under resting conditions, the cross-bridges are extended toward the actin filaments but are not attached to them. Once attached, the cross-bridges swivel in such a way that the actin filaments are pulled over the myosin filaments and toward the center of the sarcomere. During this process, ATP is broken down and energy is released, the muscle shortens, and tension is developed. When stimulation stops, the muscle relaxes and returns to the resting state.

The Motor Unit

A motor nerve is a nerve that innervates or stimulates a skeletal muscle to contract. Most single motor nerves entering a muscle have many branches and thus innervate many muscle fibers. A motor nerve and all the muscle fibers it innervates are called a **motor unit** (Figure 2–9). The motor unit is the basic functional unit of skeletal muscle. When a motor unit is stimulated, all of the muscle fibers within that unit contract. If there are many muscle fibers in the unit and many units are stimulated, the contraction of the muscle will be maximal. However, if there are only a few muscle fibers within a single stimulated unit, the contraction will be minimal. The response of the muscle can thus be graded depending upon the size and number of motor units stimulated. Such an arrangement allows for fine, delicate movements such as movements of the eye as well as for gross, coarse movements such as in the large muscles of the leg.

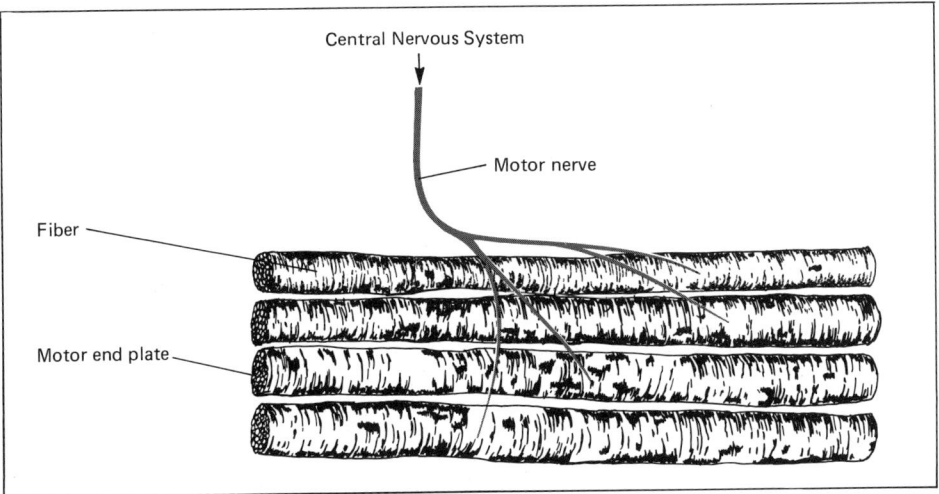

Figure 2–9. A motor unit of skeletal muscle. A single motor nerve from the central nervous system is shown supplying several muscle fibers through the motor endplates (neuromuscular junctions). (From The Physiological Basis of Physical Education and Athletics, third ed. by E. L. Fox and D. K. Mathews. Copyright © 1981 by CBS College Publishing. Reprinted by permission of CBS College Publishing.)

Fast-Twitch and Slow-Twitch Motor Units

There are at least two distinctly different types of motor units or muscle fibers in human skeletal muscle. The difference is in their energy or metabolic capabilities. For example, **slow-twitch (ST) fibers** are exceptionally well-equipped metabolically to perform low-intensity work over long periods of time. They get their name because they are slower to contract (Figure 2–10). As you might expect these fibers derive most of their energy from the oxygen system. **Fast-twitch (FT) fibers** are just the opposite; they are particularly suited for high-intensity work that can be sustained for only short periods of time. As you probably have already guessed, their name is derived from the faster contraction (Figure 2–10). Fast-twitch fibers rely largely on the anaerobic energy systems. In summary, when endurance-like activities are performed, the slow-twitch fibers are preferentially recruited to do the work; when sprintlike activities are performed, the fast-twitch fibers are preferred. In other words, slow-twitch fibers can be thought of as "endurance" fibers and fast-twitch fibers can be thought of as "sprint" fibers.

The percentage of slow-twitch and fast-twitch fibers found in your muscles is genetically determined; you are born with a certain ratio of slow-twitch

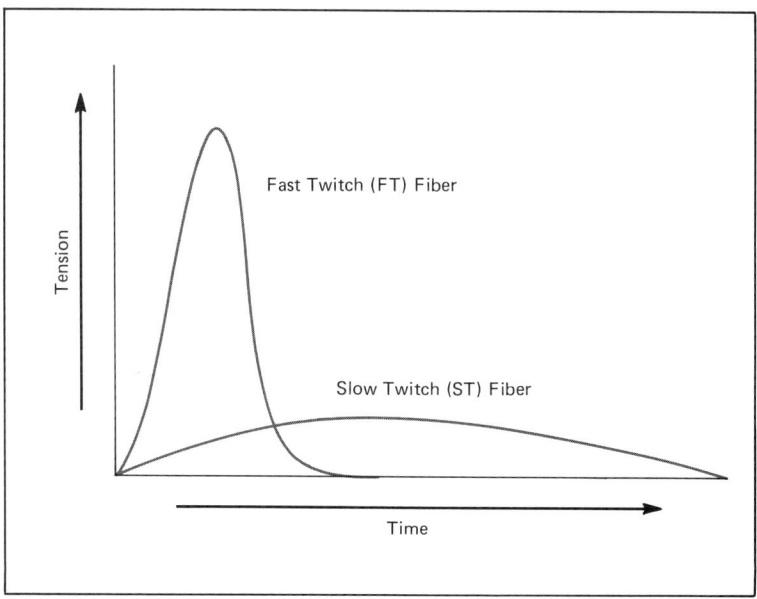

Figure 2–10. The time required by fast twitch fibers to generate maximal tension is about one third of that required by slow twitch fibers. (From Sports Physiology, *second ed. by E. L. Fox. Copyright © 1984 by CBS Publishing. Copyright 1979 by W. B. Saunders Co. Reprinted by permission of CBS College Publishing.)*

and fast-twitch fibers. This ratio is more or less fixed and cannot be changed by physical training. However, we will see later that there is selective **hypertrophy** (increased size) of the two fiber types depending upon the type of training and activity program used.

Joint Flexibility

As mentioned in Chapter 1, **flexibility** is the range of motion of a joint. Although flexibility is also sometimes referred to as static flexibility, we will use the simpler term flexibility. Flexibility involves the muscular system as well as the bones and joints.

Flexibility is limited by a number of structural components: (1) bone; (2) muscle; (3) ligaments and other structures associated with the joint capsule; (4) tendons and other connective tissues; and (5) skin. The shape and meeting surfaces of a joint determine the path of movement available to that joint. The flexibility of certain joints, such as a hinge-type joint (e.g., the elbow) is significantly limited by the bony structures. In contrast, the bony structure of a ball-and-socket joint (e.g., the shoulder) permits greater range of motion. In all joints, however, including hinge joints, the soft tissues provide the major limitation to the range of joint motion.

Several misconceptions about flexibility that need to be cleared-up are the notions of *double-jointed* and *muscle-bound*. Both of these terms are misnomers. A person is referred to as double-jointed if he or she possesses a high degree of flexibility in one or two joints. On the other hand, a muscle-bound person is one who has limited flexibility, again generally in only one or two joints. A high degree of flexibility in one joint but not necessarily in others demonstrates that flexibility is joint specific. Flexibility can be significantly improved with properly performed weight-resistance exercises and particularly with the stretching exercises discussed in Chapter 6.

The Cardiorespiratory System

Functionally, the **cardiorespiratory system**, i.e., the respiratory and circulatory systems, is responsible for the delivery of oxygen and nutrients to and the removal of carbon dioxide and waste products from the working muscles.

To better understand this system, let's follow the path taken by the oxygen found in the air we breathe on its journey to the muscle cell and the path taken by the carbon dioxide found in the muscle cell on its journey to the air in the environment.

The Lungs—Pulmonary Ventilation

The first step on our journey involves the movement of air into and out of the lungs. This process is called **pulmonary ventilation** or simply, **ventila-**

Figure 2–11. Representation of the tiny air sacs, called alveoli, *where gas exchange between the lungs and blood takes place.*

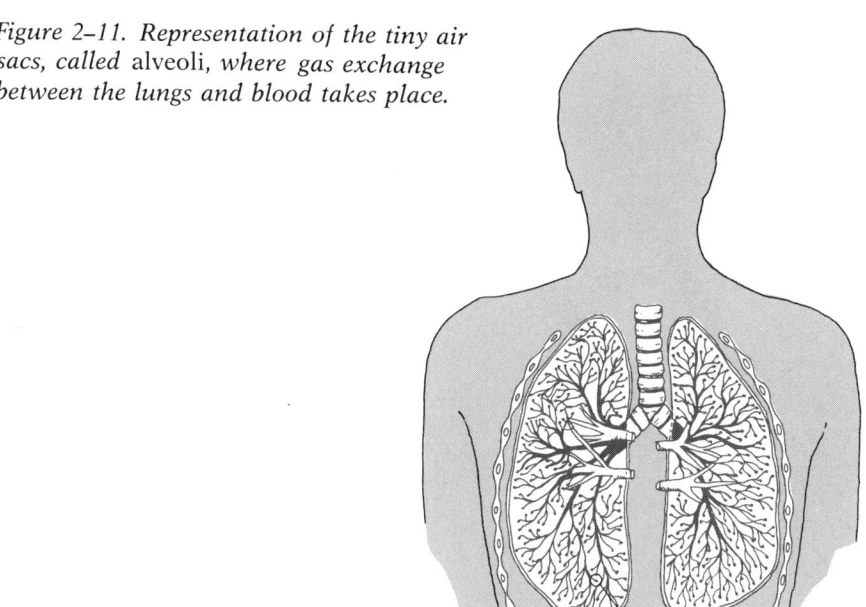

Alveolus

tion. In order for oxygen to eventually move from the air into the blood and for carbon dioxide to move from the blood into the air, a portion of the ventilated air must reach the **alveoli,** the tiny terminal air sacs found deep within the lungs (Figure 2–11). About 70 percent of the air ventilated reaches the alveoli. It is here and only here in the alveoli that the ventilated air comes in close contact with the blood. Contact between air and blood is necessary for **gas exchange** to take place. (This portion of ventilation is referred to as alveolar ventilation.)

When we exercise, the need for oxygen to maintain aerobic metabolism increases and so does the amount of air ventilated. The increase in pulmonary ventilation during exercise can be substantial. For example, at rest, we ventilate between 5 and 10 liters of air each minute (1 liter = 1.057 quarts). However, during maximal exercise, ventilation may reach values of 150 or even 200 liters each minute (Fox and Mathews, 1981). In a person with normal, healthy lungs, ventilation usually does not limit exercise performance. On the other hand, in a person with diseased lungs, exercise can be severely limited by an inability to bring in adequate amounts of oxygen via ventilation. Exercise programs specifically designed to improve lung function in diseased lungs have recently been shown to be effective in improving ventilatory capacity, which in turn significantly improves exercise tolerance.

Gas Exchange Between Air and Blood

The second step in our journey involves the exchange of oxygen and carbon dioxide between the air and the blood. Remember that in order for gas

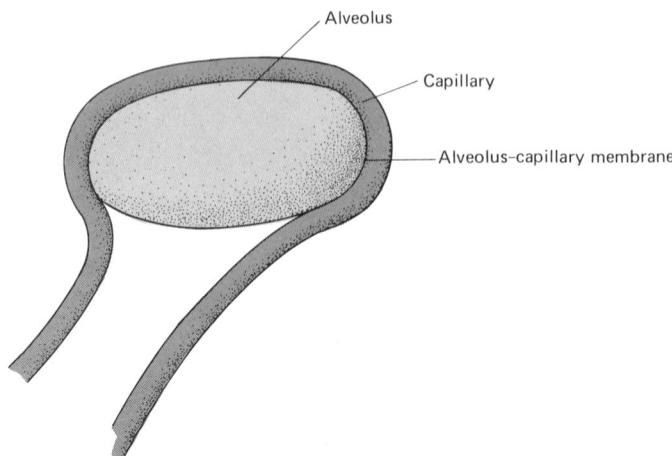

Figure 2–12. The relationship between a capillary and an alveolus.

exchange between air and blood to occur, the air has to be in intimate contact with the blood. This contact is made between the alveoli and the pulmonary capillaries. The pulmonary capillaries are tiny blood vessels that surround the alveoli as shown schematically in Figure 2–12. Note in the figure that the interface between the alveoli and the pulmonary capillaries is referred to as the **alveolocapillary membrane.**

Why does oxygen move from the air in the alveoli to the blood in the capillaries and why does carbon dioxide move in the opposite direction, i.e., from the blood to the air? The answer to these questions is **diffusion,** a physical process whereby molecules of gases move randomly because of their kinetic energy. When more molecules of gas occupy one side of a membrane compared with the other side, the side with the greater number of molecules has greater kinetic energy. As a result, there will be a net movement of gas molecules across the membrane toward the side with the lowest gas concentration until equilibrium is reached (Figure 2–13). In other words, gases always diffuse from an area of higher concentration to an area of lower concentration.

One more point about the diffusion of gases needs to be mentioned, that is, the concept of the **partial pressure** of a gas. When gases are in a mixture, such as air, the gas with the higher concentration also has a higher partial pressure. Partial pressure is the pressure exerted by a single gas in a gas mixture or in a liquid. Therefore, since gases diffuse from higher to lower concentrations, they also diffuse from higher to lower partial pressures. The partial pressure of oxygen is higher in the air in the alveoli than in the pulmonary capillary blood. By the same token, the partial pressure of carbon dioxide is higher in the blood than in the alveolar air.

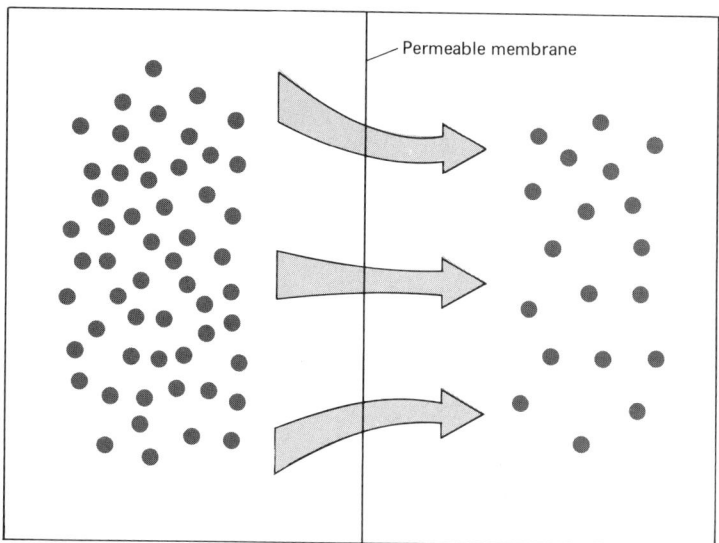

Figure 2–13. A net flow of gas molecules across a permeable membrane will occur in the direction of lowest gas concentration until equilibrium is reached.

Gas Transport by the Blood

Now that oxygen has diffused into the blood, the next step en route to the muscle cells is **gas transport** via the blood. How are the gases transported in the blood? Oxygen is carried as dissolved oxygen in the fluid portion of the blood, the **plasma,** and in chemical combination with **hemoglobin,** which is found in the red blood cells. About 98 to 99 percent of the oxygen is carried by hemoglobin with only 1 or 2 percent carried in solution by the plasma.

Hemoglobin is a complex compound made up of iron called *heme* and a protein called *globin.* The ability of hemoglobin to chemically combine with oxygen is the result of its iron or heme component. The chemical combination of oxygen to hemoglobin is referred to as oxyhemoglobin.

Carbon dioxide is also carried dissolved in the blood as well as in chemical combination. There are two major chemical forms of carbon dioxide that are carried in the blood. One of these, like oxygen, combines with hemoglobin. However, in the case of carbon dioxide, the chemically active site on the hemoglobin molecule is the protein or globin component and not the iron or heme component. This means that hemoglobin is capable of simultaneously combining with both oxygen and carbon dioxide. When carbon dioxide chemically combines with hemoglobin, it is referred to as a **carbamino-hemoglobin compound.** The globin component of hemoglobin is not the only protein that can combine with carbon dioxide. Carbon dioxide combines with other proteins found in the blood as well.

The second important form of carbon dioxide is the **bicarbonate ion.** Within the red blood cell, carbon dioxide readily combines with water to form carbonic acid. The reaction is as follows:

$$CO_2 \; + \; H_2O \; \rightarrow \; \overset{CA}{H_2CO_3}$$

(carbon dioxide)   (water)   (carbonic acid)

An enzyme found in the red cell called carbonic anhydrase (CA in the equation) facilitates or speeds up the reaction. As soon as the carbonic acid is formed, it dissociates or breaks up into a hydrogen ion (H^+) and a bicarbonate ion (HCO_3^-):

$$H_2CO_3 \; \rightarrow \; H^+ \; + \; HCO_3^-$$

(carbonic acid)   (hydrogen ion)   (bicarbonate ion)

Although the bicarbonate ions are formed within the red blood cell, they readily diffuse out of the red cell into the blood plasma. In this way, carbon dioxide is carried as bicarbonate ions in the blood.

The Heart and Blood Flow

Let's review for a moment. Fresh air, which is high in oxygen and low in carbon dioxide, is brought into the lungs, eventually reaching the alveoli. Oxygen diffuses across the alveolocapillary membrane into the capillary blood. At the same time carbon dioxide diffuses from the blood into the air in the alveoli. Most of the oxygen chemically combines with hemoglobin for transport to the muscle cells. Carbon dioxide also chemically combines with hemoglobin, but, in addition, forms bicarbonate ions for transport from the muscle cells to the alveolar air. This brings us to the next step in our journey—the transportation of the gases to and from the muscle cells. This job is the responsibility of the heart, the blood, and the blood vessels.

The heart is a muscular pump. As shown in Figure 2–14, it consists of four chambers, two on the left side and two on the right side. Because of this the heart is usually considered as two pumps, a left pump and a right pump. The right pump consists of the right **atrium** (upper chamber) and the right **ventricle** (lower chamber). The right heart pumps blood to the lungs where oxygen is picked up and carbon dioxide dumped off. Next, the left heart—the left atrium and left ventricle—pumps the blood, now rich in oxygen and poor in carbon dioxide, to all the tissues of the body, including the skeletal muscles.

The direction of the flow of blood through the heart is shown in Figure 2–14. Blood from the head and upper body tissues returns to the right atrium via the superior **vena cava,** whereas blood from the lower body tissues returns to the right atrium via the inferior vena cava. From the right atrium the blood is pumped into the right ventricle and from there to the lungs.

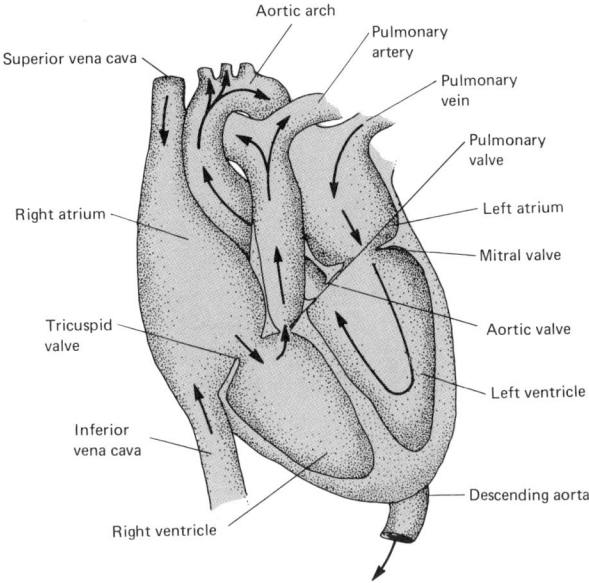

Figure 2–14. The major parts of the heart. Arrows indicate the direction of blood flow.

Aortic arch
Pulmonary artery
Superior vena cava
Pulmonary vein
Pulmonary valve
Right atrium
Left atrium
Mitral valve
Tricuspid valve
Aortic valve
Left ventricle
Inferior vena cava
Descending aorta
Right ventricle

As the right ventricle contracts, the tricuspid valve closes, preventing blood from flowing back into the right atrium. At the same time, the pulmonary valve opens, permitting the blood to flow into the **pulmonary arteries** toward the lungs.

After oxygen and carbon dioxide diffuse into and out of the pulmonary capillary blood, respectively, the freshly oxygenated blood returns to the left atrium via the pulmonary veins. The left atrium then pumps the blood into the left ventricle. As the left ventricle contracts, the mitral valve closes, preventing backflow into the left atrium, and the aortic valve opens, channeling the blood into the **aorta** on its way to all the tissues of the body.

When the blood reaches the body tissues, including the muscle cells, another exchange of gases takes place. In this case, it is between the blood (capillaries) and the tissues. Here the oxygen in the blood diffuses across the **tissue–capillary membrane** into the muscle cell, where it is used by the aerobic system in manufacturing ATP energy. Carbon dioxide, on the other hand, diffuses from the muscle cell into the venous blood. The blood, now low in oxygen and high in carbon dioxide, returns to the right heart where the cycle begins again.

Blood Supply to the Heart Muscle

The heart, being a muscle, also requires oxygen for use during the performance of its work. Contrary to popular belief, the blood that the heart pumps does not directly nourish or supply the heart muscle itself with oxygen. Instead, the heart has its own blood vessels and blood flow that supply it

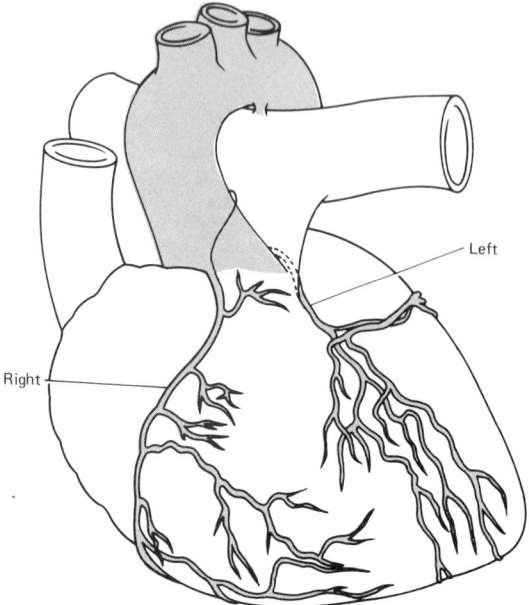

Figure 2–15. The major coronary arteries of the heart.

with oxygen and other nutrients and removes waste products such as carbon dioxide. As shown in Figure 2–15, the heart has two major coronary arteries (coronary = heart) that supply it with blood: the left **coronary artery** and its extensive branches supply the left side of the heart; the right coronary artery with its branches supply the right side of the heart. If one of these arteries or one of its branches is blocked so that blood flow through it is stopped, a **myocardial infarction** or heart attack occurs. More will be said about heart attacks in the next chapter.

Blood Pressure—Hypertension

Pressure is the force that moves the blood through the circulatory system. The **blood pressure** is highest in the arteries and lowest in the veins. The arterial pressure, however, fluctuates with the contraction and relaxation of the heart. During contraction, the arterial pressure reaches its highest level. Since contraction of the heart is referred to as **systole,** the blood pressure during this phase is called **systolic pressure.** Normally, it has a value of around 120 millimeters of mercury (mm Hg). This means that the pressure is great enough to raise a column of mercury 120 millimeters or just under 5 inches. Since mercury is 13.6 times denser than water, this means that the systolic pressure is great enough to raise a column of water 5 feet 7¾ inches. The blood pressure in the artery reaches its lowest level during diastole or the relaxation phase of the cardiac cycle. Diastolic pressure is normally about 80 mm Hg.

The reason why the blood pressure fluctuates in the arteries is because the walls of the arteries are elastic. When the heart contracts, dumping large volumes of blood into the arteries, the walls of each artery stretch or expand; during diastole the walls recoil. Thus, the blood in the arteries pulsates. You can feel this **pulse** by placing your fingers over the skin surface under which a major artery lies. The most common pulses are those of the radial artery in the wrist and of the carotid artery in the neck. Since each pulse represents one heart beat, we will learn in Chapter 4 how to take your pulse in order to determine what your heart rate is during your training or exercise sessions.

Hypertension means that the systolic and diastolic blood pressures are elevated. It is a very common cardiovascular disease in the United States. Although hypertension may be caused by a number of factors, most of which involve the kidneys, the most common form of high blood pressure is called *essential hypertension.* It has no known cause and therefore no known cure. One interesting fact, however, is that when people with hypertension participate in regular exercise programs, their blood pressure decreases toward normal values after several months. More will be said about this in the next chapter.

Exercise and the Heart

During exercise, particularly prolonged exercise, the muscles' need for oxygen increases. This need is met in three different ways: (1) by an increase in the **cardiac output** or the amount of blood pumped by the heart per minute; (2) by redirecting or shunting blood away from less active tissues to the muscles; and (3) by the muscle cells extracting more oxygen from the blood.

The increase in cardiac output during exercise can be substantial. For example, at rest, the cardiac output is about 5 or 6 liters/minute. However, during maximal exercise, it may reach 25 liters/minute in an untrained person or a value as high as 40 liters/minute in an endurance athlete. The relationship between cardiac output and exercise is shown in Figure 2–16. Notice that the two (cardiac output and exercise load expressed as oxygen consumption) are related in a linear fashion. This means that when the exercise gets harder or more intense, the muscles' need for oxygen and thus blood flow also increases and cardiac output increases proportionally.

Two factors that make up the cardiac output are (1) **heart rate** or the number of times the heart beats per minute; and (2) the **stroke volume** or the amount of blood pumped by the heart with each beat. Mathematically these two factors are related to cardiac output as follows:

$$CO = HR \times SV$$

(cardiac   (heart   (stroke
output)   rate)   volume)

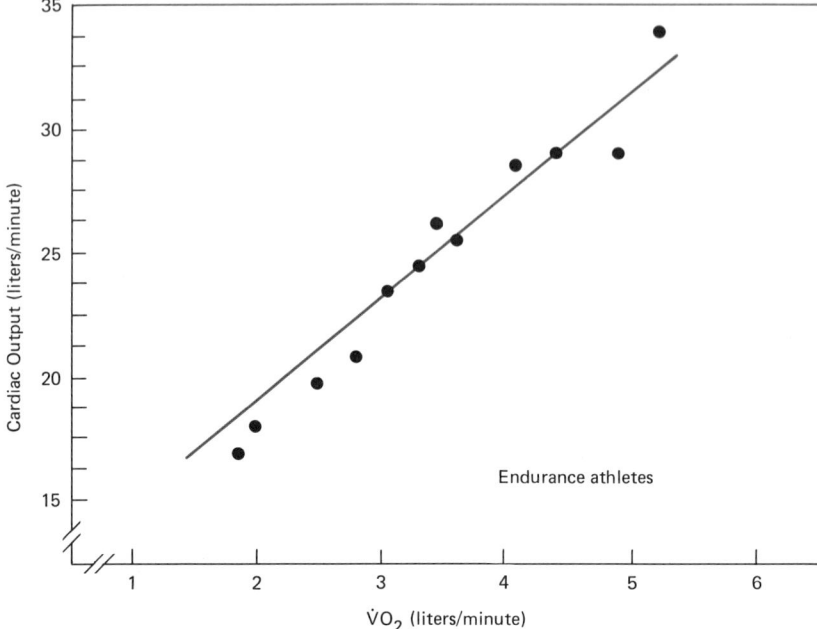

Figure 2–16. As exercise intensity ($\dot{V}O_2$) increases, cardiac output increases linearly. (From Sports Physiology, second ed. by E. L. Fox. Copyright © 1984 by CBS Publishing. Copyright 1979 by W. B. Saunders Co. Reprinted *by permission of CBS College Publishing.)*

For example, at rest the heart rate may be 75 beats per minute whereas the stroke volume may be 80 ml/beat (about 3 ounces of blood). Therefore, the cardiac output would be 75 × 80 = 6,000 ml or 6 liters/minute. During maximal exercise, the heart rate may reach 190 beats per minute whereas the stroke volume may be as high as 150 ml/beat for a cardiac output of 190 × 150 = 28,500 ml or 28.5 liters/minute.

From the preceding relationship, it is easy to see that cardiac output (CO) increases whenever heart rate (HR), stroke volume (SV), or both increase. Heart rate, like cardiac output, increases with exercise in a linear fashion as shown in Figure 2–17. Notice in Figure 2–17 that the maximum heart rate is close to 200 beats per minute. This value would be accurate for a young man (e.g., 20 years of age), since maximum heart rate declines with age and is slightly higher at any age for women. For example, for a 40-year-old man the maximum heart rate may be only 175 to 180 beats per minute. We will see in a later chapter that your maximum heart rate is a very important ingredient in your cardiorespiratory exercise prescription.

The stroke volume, i.e., the amount of blood pumped by the heart per beat, also increases with exercise but not in the same way as heart rate. Also shown in Figure 2–17, the stroke volume increases during the transition

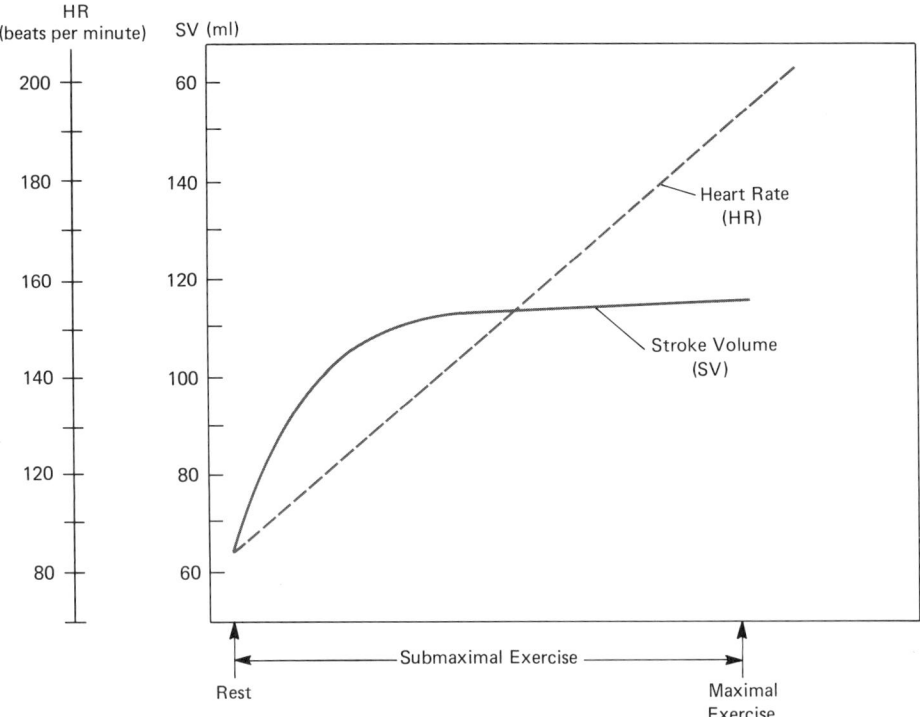

Figure 2–17. As exercise intensity increases, the heart rate increases linearly. Stroke volume will reach maximal limits at 40 to 50 percent of maximum. (From Lifetime Fitness *by E. L. Fox. Copyright © 1983 by CBS College Publishing. Reprinted by permission of Saunders College Publishing. CBS College Publishing.)*

from rest to exercise, but reaches its maximal value before the exercise load becomes maximal. This means that further increases in cardiac output once stroke volume reaches its maximum are caused entirely by an increase in heart rate.

The magnitude of the values for heart rate and stroke volume that make up a given cardiac output are important with regard to how much energy the heart must expend to do its work. For example, if the cardiac output is 6 liters/minute, the heart rate could be 75 beats per minute and the stroke volume 80 ml/beat (75 × 80 = 6,000 ml/beat or 6 liters) or the heart rate could be only 55 beats per minute and the stroke volume 109 ml/beat (55 × 109 ≈ 6 liters/minute). Even though the same amount of blood is being pumped per minute by the heart in both cases, the work of the heart would be less in the latter case where the heart rate is lower and the stroke volume higher. In other words, the heart pumps blood more efficiently with a relatively slower heart rate and a larger stroke volume. In Chapter 3, we will see that one of the benefits of endurance exercise training is a reduced heart

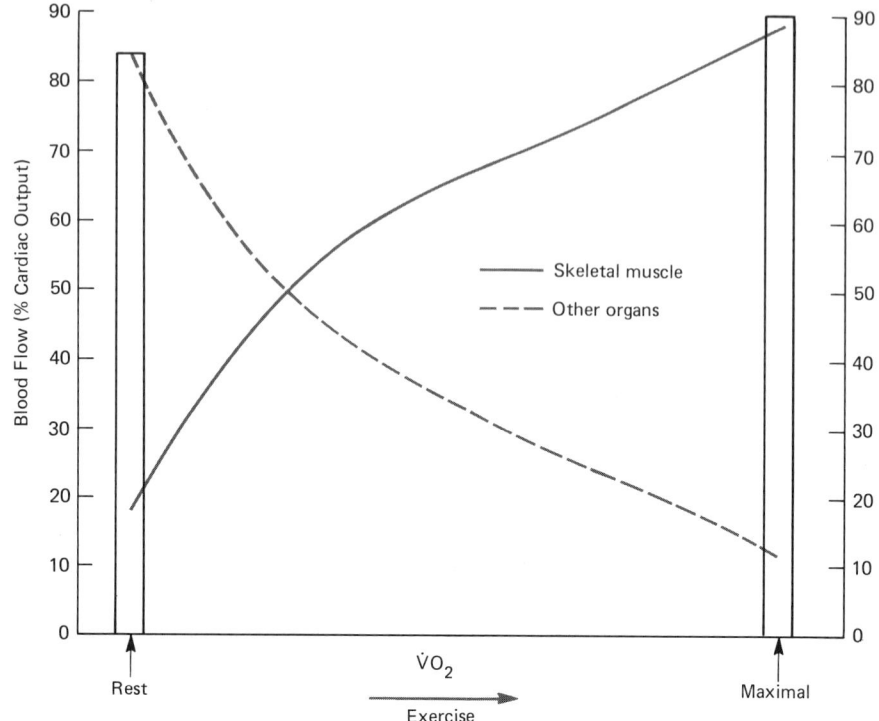

Figure 2–18. Distribution of blood (percent of cardiac output) to skeletal muscles and other organs during exercise. During maximal exercise, 80 to 90 percent of the cardiac output is distributed to the working muscles. (From The Physiological Basis of Physical Education and Athletics, third ed. *by E. L. Fox and D. K. Mathews. Copyright © 1981 by CBS College Publishing. Reprinted by permission of CBS College Publishing.)*

rate and an increased stroke volume at rest as well as during all levels of exercise.

Under resting conditions the skeletal muscles receive 20 percent of the blood pumped by the heart. This means that if the cardiac output were 6 liters/minute, then approximately 1.2 liters (6 × 0.2 = 1.2) of this would go to the skeletal muscles. During maximal exercise, the percentage is much greater, as much as 80 percent. In this case, if the cardiac output were 25 liters per minute, 20 liters would go to the muscles. The fact that a greater portion of blood is pumped to the muscles during exercise means that a smaller portion goes to the other tissues of the body, particularly the skin, the kidneys, and the gastrointestinal tract. This is shown in Figure 2–18.

The amount of oxygen extracted from the blood by the skeletal muscles varies. For example, under resting conditions only a small amount of oxygen is taken out of the blood and consumed by the muscle cells. Out of about 20 ml of oxygen sent to the muscles in each 100 ml of blood flow, only about 5 ml of oxygen are taken up or extracted by the muscles. In other words, at rest only about 25 percent of the oxygen delivered to the muscles is taken up and used. During exercise, however, much more oxygen is extracted from the blood by the muscle cells. During maximal exercise, for instance, as much as 90 percent of the oxygen delivered to the muscles is extracted (Figure 2–19).

Figure 2–19. Average changes in (A) cardiac output; (B) blood supply to working skeletal muscle; and (C) amount of oxygen extracted (arteriovenous difference).

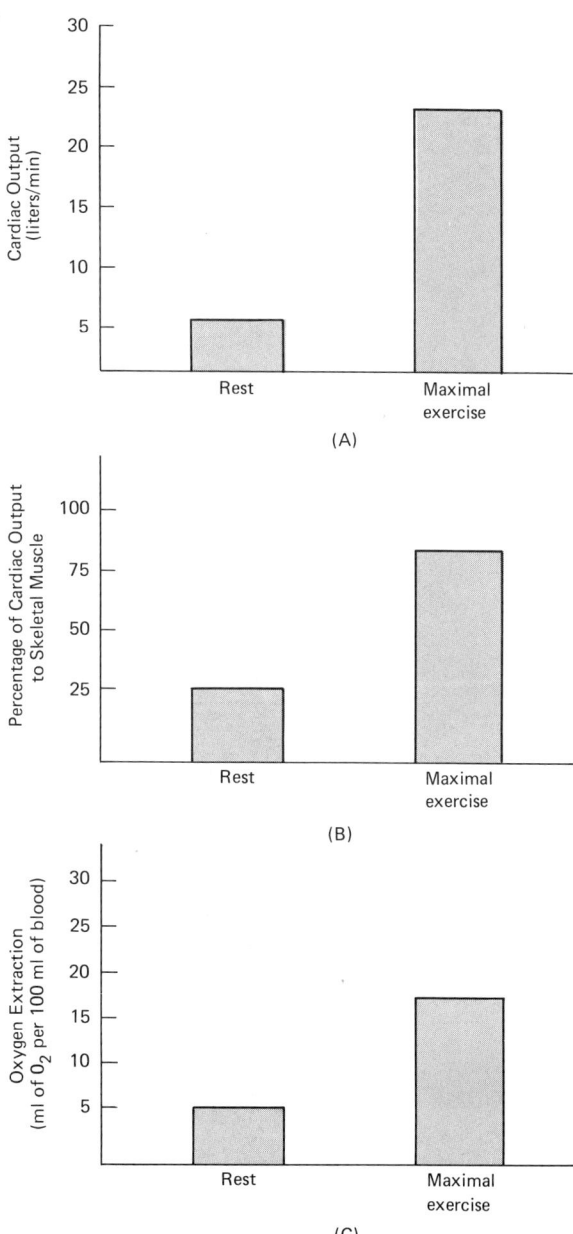

The Capacity of the Cardiorespiratory System— Maximal Oxygen Consumption

Because the main job of the cardiorespiratory system is to deliver oxygen to the body tissues, especially the working muscles, the capacity of this system can be measured by what is referred to as the **maximal oxygen consumption** test. Maximal oxygen consumption ($\dot{V}O_2$ max) is the amount of oxygen the body can consume or use, usually for one minute, during maximal exercise. The exercise test is usually performed either on a stationary bicycle (called a *bicycle ergometer*) or on a motor-driven treadmill (Figure 2–20). During the test the exercise load is slowly increased so that after 5 or 10 minutes the person is exhausted and can no longer exercise.

The actual determination of the amount of oxygen consumed involves measuring how much air and oxygen are taken in by the lungs and how much oxygen and carbon dioxide are exhaled. The idea is that if you know the amount of oxygen inspired and the amount expired, the difference between the two is how much was consumed or used. The measurements require expensive and complicated equipment and therefore only a

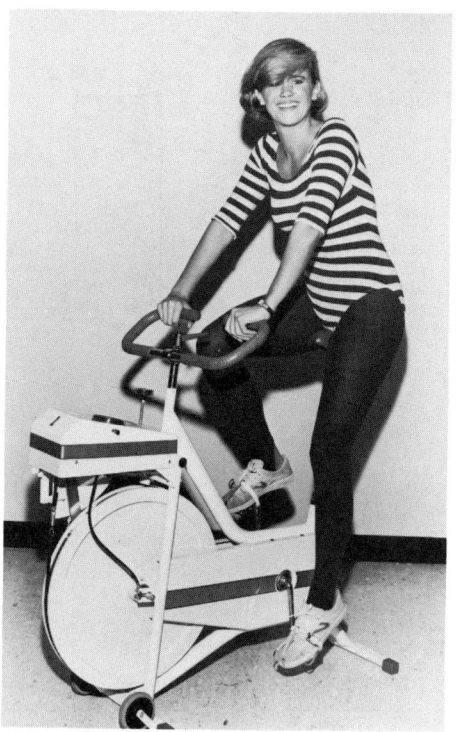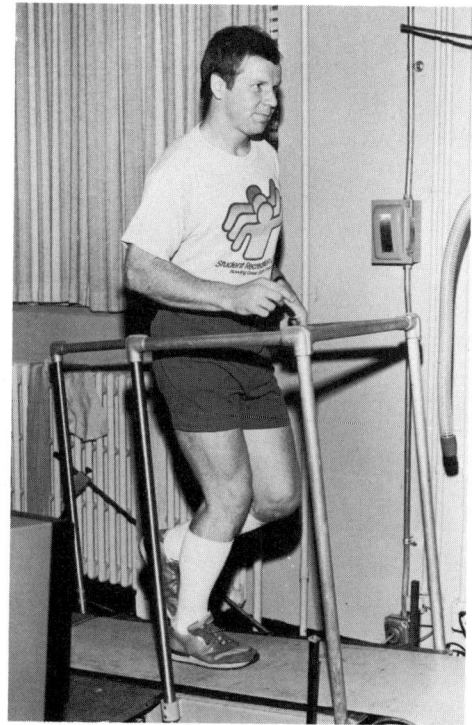

Figure 2–20. Modes of testing for maximal oxygen consumption.

few specialized laboratories are equipped to measure your maximal oxygen consumption (sometimes referred to as the **maximal aerobic power** or simply your **aerobic capacity**). Maximal oxygen consumption is the single most important physiological measure of the ability of your heart and lungs to deliver oxygen to the working muscles. Support for this statement lies in the fact that most of you who are out of shape can consume only about half as much oxygen maximally as can a marathon runner of the same age. More will be said about maximal oxygen consumption in Chapters 4 and 9.

SUMMARY

◊ Adenosine triphosphate (ATP) is the immediately usable form of energy in the human body. It is stored in small amounts in most tissues, particularly in muscle cells.

◊ There are three metabolic systems that supply ATP to the muscle cells: two are anaerobic (the ATP-PC system and the LA system) in that the chemical reactions involved do not require the oxygen we breathe, whereas the third (the oxygen or aerobic system) is aerobic and occurs only in the presence of abundant oxygen.

◊ The two anaerobic systems supply only limited amounts of ATP. Activities that are short in duration but high in intensity, such as sprinting, depend heavily on these two systems for ATP energy.

◊ The aerobic system supplies large amounts of ATP and thus is the major energy system used during long-duration, low-intensity activities, such as the 26-mile marathon.

◊ The scientific basis for nutritional fitness is related to metabolic energy production in two ways: (1) the foods we eat provide us with the chemical energy needed for the production of ATP; and (2) body weight control is determined by the balance of energy taken in as food versus energy expended through activity.

◊ Skeletal muscle consists of bundles of muscle fibers and their respective connective tissues.

◊ Each muscle cell or fiber contains thousands of myofibrils that are made up of two protein filaments, actin and myosin. When a muscle contracts, the actin filaments slide over the myosin filaments. This is called the sliding filament theory of muscular contraction.

◊ When a muscle contracts isotonically, it develops tension and shortens. When the shortening is done at a constant speed, the muscle is contracting isokinetically. In an isometric contraction, the muscle develops tension but does not change in length. In an eccentric or negative contraction, the muscle develops tension while lengthening.

◊ A motor unit is defined as a motor nerve and all of the muscle fibers it innervates. It is the basic functional unit of skeletal muscle.

◊ There are two basic types of motor units or muscle fibers in humans, slow-twitch (ST) and fast-twitch (FT). ST fibers are predominately used during long-duration or endurance activities whereas FT fibers are primarily recruited for short-term high-intensity efforts such as sprinting.

◊ Joint flexibility is defined as the range of motion of a joint. The terms double-jointed and muscle-bound are misnomers and refer to a large amount or very little flexibility, respectively.

◊ The cardiorespiratory system (respiration and circulation) is responsible for the delivery of oxygen to and the removal of carbon dioxide from the working muscles.

◊ Air taken into the lungs reaches the alveoli, where oxygen diffuses into the capillary blood pumped there by the right heart, and carbon dioxide diffuses from the blood into the air in the lungs. Oxygen is transported in the blood mainly by hemoglobin and is pumped by the left heart to all the tissues in the body including the skeletal muscles.

◊ The heart muscle is supplied with blood by two major arteries, the right coronary artery, which supplies the right side of the heart, and the left coronary artery, which supplies the left side. A heart attack occurs when the blood flow through one or both of these arteries is blocked.

◊ Pressure is the force that moves the blood through the circulatory system. The highest pressure in the artery is called systolic pressure; the lowest pressure is called diastolic pressure. Hypertension means high blood pressure.

◊ The amount of blood pumped by the heart, the cardiac output, is dependent upon two factors: (1) heart rate or the number of times the heart beats per minute; and (2) the stroke volume or the amount of blood pumped by the heart per beat. All three increase substantially during exercise.

◊ During prolonged exercise, the muscles' need for an increased amount of oxygen is met by increasing the cardiac output, by redirecting blood away from less active tissues to the muscles, and by the muscle cells increasing the amount of oxygen extracted from the blood.

◊ Maximal oxygen consumption refers to the amount of oxygen the body can use for any minute during maximal exercise. It is the single most important physiological measure of the ability of the heart and lungs to deliver oxygen to the working muscles.

STUDY QUESTIONS

1. Discuss the role of ATP in the use of energy in the human body.

2. Describe the energy systems and tell how they supply ATP to the muscle cells.

3. Discuss the relationship between the energy systems and the idea of an energy continuum.

4. Name the connective tissues of skeletal muscle and indicate with which part of the muscle they are associated.

5. Define the various ways a muscle can contract.

6. Define a motor unit. Why is it the basic functional unit of muscle?

7. What is meant by fast-twitch and slow-twitch muscle fibers?

8. Discuss how oxygen from the air we breathe ultimately reaches the muscle cells where it is consumed.

9. Why does the pressure in an artery fluctuate?

10. Discuss the two major factors that determine how much blood is pumped by the heart in one minute (cardiac output).

11. During prolonged exercise, how is the muscle's need for increased oxygen met?

12. Define maximal oxygen consumption and describe how it is measured.

REFERENCES AND SELECTED READINGS

Borhani, N. D.: Epidemiology of coronary heart disease. In E. A. Amsterdam, J. H. Wilmore, and A. N. de Maria (eds.): *Exercise in Cardiovascular Health and Disease.* New York: Yorke Medical Books, 1977.

Falls, H. B.; Baylor, A. M.; and Dishman, R. K.: *Essentials of Fitness.* Philadelphia: Saunders College Publishing, 1980, pp. 16–44.

Fox, E. L.: Energy sources during rest and exercise. In G. A. Stull (ed.): *Encyclopedia of Physical Education, Fitness, and Sports.* Salt Lake City: Brighton Publishing Co., 1980, pp. 251–258.

Fox, E. L.: *Sports Physiology,* second ed. Philadelphia: Saunders College Publishing, 1984, pp. 1–33, 82–119, 159, 191.

Fox, E. L.; and Mathews, D. K.: *Interval Training.* Philadelphia: W. B. Saunders, 1974, pp. 9–20.

Fox, E. L.; and Mathews, D. K.: *The Physiological Basis of Physical Education and Athletics,* 3rd ed. Philadelphia: Saunders College Publishing, 1981, pp. 11–32, 81–114, 183–255.

Wolff, O. H.: The pediatrician's responsibility for prevention of coronary heart disease. *Postgraduate Medical Journal,* 54:228–231, 1978.

Chapter 3
Cardiorespiratory (Endurance) Fitness

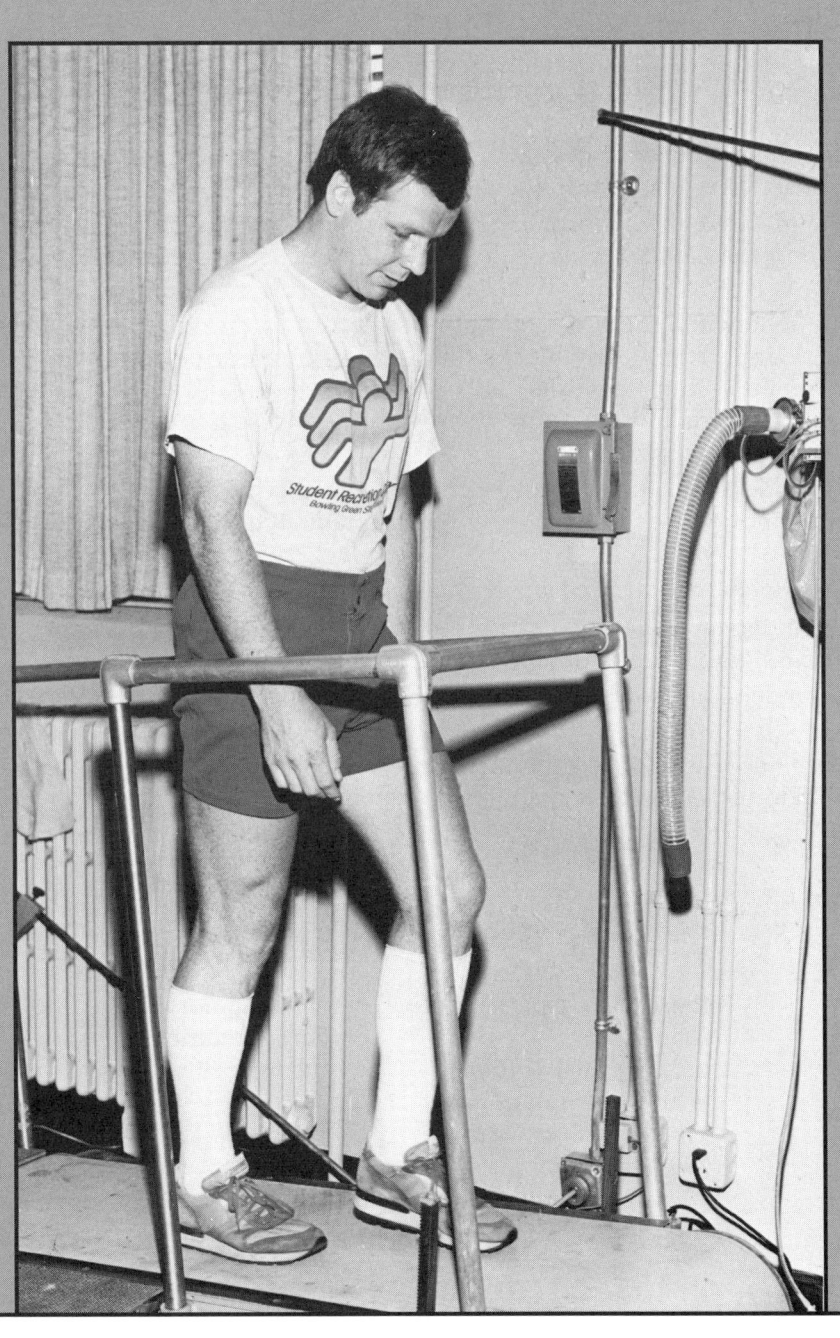

Chapter Outline

Learning Objectives

◇ To understand how regular exercise reduces the risk of coronary heart disease and other cardiovascular diseases.

◇ To understand that coronary heart disease is a disease of the heart muscle and of the blood vessels of the heart that can lead to death through heart attack (myocardial infarction).

◇ To understand the process of atherosclerosis, a disease that narrows and sometimes completely blocks the opening of an artery as a result of the build-up of fatty deposits. This process is the major cause of coronary heart disease and most other cardiovascular diseases such as stroke and high blood pressure.

◇ To understand that a stroke occurs when the blood supply to the brain is temporarily or permanently interrupted such as from a blood clot or burst artery.

◇ To understand and recognize the risk factors of coronary heart disease.

◇ To understand that the risk of and mortality (death) from coronary heart disease is much less in active persons than in inactive persons.

◇ To understand how chronic exercise training improves your cardiorespiratory fitness level and lowers your risk of coronary heart disease.

◇ To be able to identify the stressors in daily routines and to know how to deal with these sources of stress effectively.

Key Words and Phrases

atherosclerosis	cerebral hemorrhage
blood clot	cerebral thrombosis
cardiac dysrhythmias	circulatory efficiency
cardiorespiratory fitness	cholesterol
cardiovascular disease	coagulability
catecholamine	collateral circulation

coronary vasculature
coronary heart disease
endurance fitness
epidemiology
fibrinolysis
heart attack
high density lipoprotein (HDL)
low density lipoprotein (LDL)
maximal oxygen consumption

myocardial infarction
oxygen transport system
relaxation
risk factors
saturated fats
stress management
stress response
stroke

Introduction

T HIS chapter will focus on two aspects of **cardiorespiratory** or **endurance fitness:** (1) cardiorespiratory fitness and the risk of cardiovascular disease; and (2) the physiological changes and other changes that take place in improving cardiorespiratory fitness. It was mentioned earlier that the term *cardiorespiratory* refers to the heart and blood vessels whereas the terms *respiration* or *respiratory* refer to the exchange of oxygen and carbon dioxide between the air in the lungs and the blood and between the blood and the muscle cells. These basic functions were discussed in Chapter 2.

You will recall that cardiorespiratory fitness refers to the ability of the heart-lung system to deliver oxygen to and remove carbon dioxide from the working muscles during prolonged exercise activities. The greater this ability, the higher the cardiorespiratory fitness level or cardiovascular endurance.

Cardiorespiratory Fitness and the Risk of Cardiovascular Disease

Because cardiorespiratory fitness involves the circulatory system, it is not too surprising to find that one of the many cardiovascular disease risk factors is lack of regular exercise or a low level of cardiorespiratory fitness. Furthermore, there is little doubt that a regular exercise program leading to an increased cardiorespiratory fitness level is a significant factor in reducing the severity and perhaps even the number of cardiovascular diseases among the peoples of the world, particularly persons in the United States. For example, of all deaths in the United States, more than half are caused by cardiovascular diseases. As shown in Figure 3-1, cardiovascular diseases ranked ac-

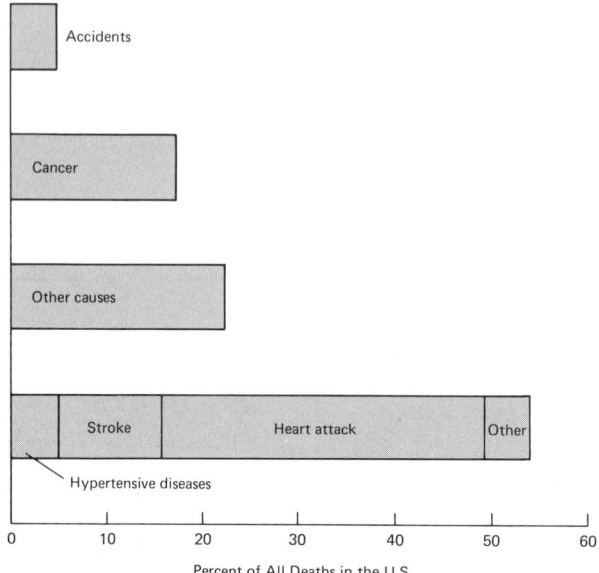

Figure 3–1. More than half of all deaths in the United States are due to cardiovascular diseases. (Adapted from The Physiological Basis of Physical Education and Athletics, third ed. *by E. L. Fox and D. K. Mathews. Copyright © 1981 by CBS College Publishing. Reprinted by permission of CBS College Publishing.)*

cording to their incidences in the United States are heart attack (34 percent), stroke (11 percent), hypertension (high blood pressure) (3 percent), and others (6 percent) (Borhani et al., 1977).

The Number One Killer—Coronary Heart Disease

What is coronary heart disease and what are the risk factors associated with it? These are the two major questions to be answered concerning coronary heart disease.

What Is Coronary Heart Disease? To begin to answer this question, it might be appropriate to give coronary heart disease a formal definition. **Coronary heart disease** is a **cardiovascular disease** that is concerned mainly with diseases of the heart muscle itself and of the blood vessels of the heart. It is the most severe of all the cardiovascular diseases since it directly affects the heart. As just mentioned, heart attacks caused by coronary heart disease account for 34 percent of all deaths in the United States.

The major cause of coronary heart disease is **atherosclerosis,** a disease that afflicts the blood vessels (arteries), including the coronary arteries that supply blood and oxygen to the heart muscle. In atherosclerosis, the lumen or opening of the artery (through which the blood flows) becomes narrowed as fatty deposits build up on the inside of the arterial walls. As shown in Figure 3–2, the build-up of fatty deposits may become so great that the flow of blood in that artery is completely blocked. When this happens, the portion of the heart muscle supplied by the artery looses its oxygen supply. As a

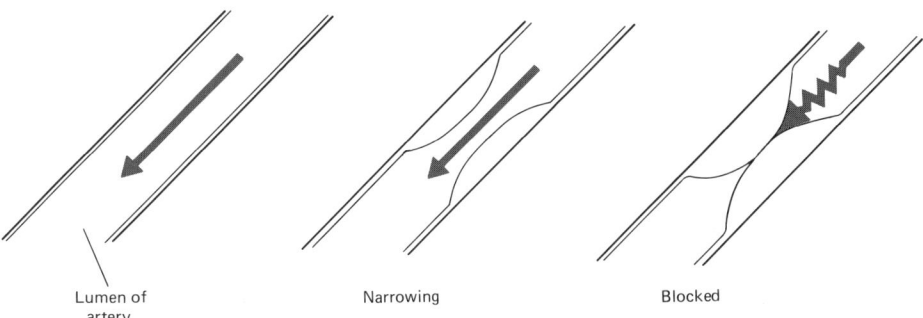

Lumen of artery   Narrowing   Blocked

Figure 3–2. The narrowing of the lumen of an artery by atherosclerosis is progressive. In an advanced stage, blood flow through the artery can be completely blocked. (From The Physiological Basis of Physical Education and Athletics, third ed. *by E. L. Fox and D. K. Mathews. Copyright © 1981 by CBS College Publishing. Reprinted by permission of CBS College Publishing.)*

result, a portion of the muscle tissue dies and a **heart attack** or **myocardial infarction** is said to have occurred.

A heart attack can occur even if the fatty deposits themselves do not completely block the artery. Blood flow through the artery may be blocked by the formation of a **blood clot** (see Figure 3–3). The irregular and rough surfaces on the inner walls of the arteries created by the fatty deposits easily trigger the blood clotting mechanism. Once the clot has formed it can lodge in the already narrowed lumen of an atherosclerotic artery, thus completely stopping the flow of blood. As before, a heart attack occurs.

The severity of any heart attack depends upon the location of the block along the artery.* For example, as shown in Figure 3–4, if the block occurs toward the beginning of the artery, then a large portion of heart muscle will be affected and the attack will be severe. If, however, the block occurs toward the end of the artery or at the end of one of its branches, only a

* For a review of the coronary arteries see Figure 2–15.

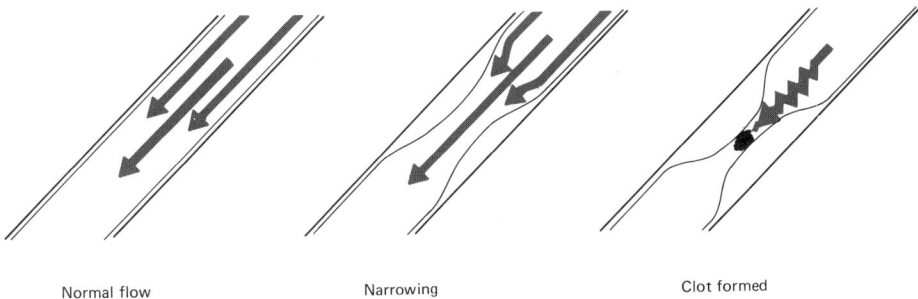

Normal flow   Narrowing   Clot formed

Figure 3–3. Blood flow through a narrowed vessel can be completely obstructed by a blood clot.

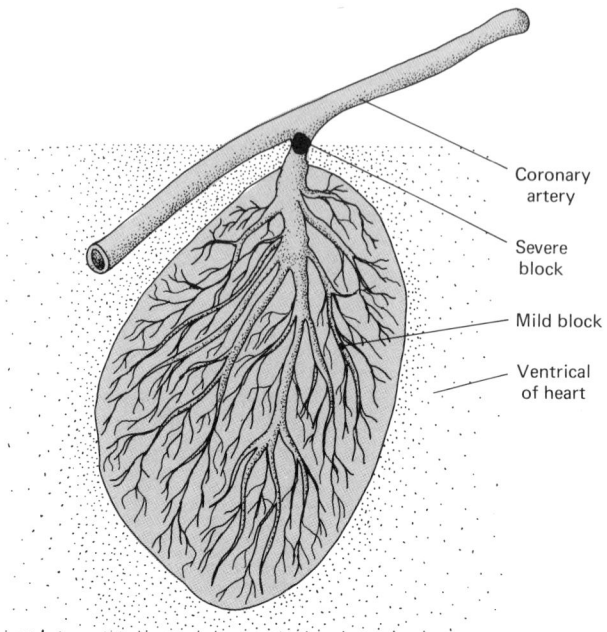

Figure 3–4. When a heart attack occurs, a large portion of ventricular muscle is affected if a large vessel is blocked near its origin. If the block occurs at the end of a branching vessel, the amount of muscle tissue affected is much less.

Coronary artery

Severe block

Mild block

Ventrical of heart

relatively small amount of heart tissue will be involved and the attack will be mild.

The build-up of fatty deposits on the inside of the walls of the arteries is caused by several factors, the most important being a high dietary intake of cholesterol and animal or saturated fats. Therefore, regulation of fat intake through the diet is an important step in reducing the risk of atherosclerosis and thus of coronary heart disease. It can even be a significant factor in reducing the risk of heart attack in those patients who already have athero-sclerosis. More on diet and fatty foods will be presented in Chapter 7.

Another factor commonly thought to be related to atherosclerosis is age. Generally, atherosclerosis is considered to be a disease of old age. While this is true, it is not always the case. For example, autopsies performed on young American soldiers killed during the Vietnam and Korean wars showed many of them to have moderate to severe stages of atherosclerosis (McNa-mara et al., 1971; Enos et al., 1953). Wolff (1978) has noted that more recent studies have shown that even children less than 5 years of age have the beginning stages of atherosclerosis.

Risk Factors of Coronary Heart Disease. As mentioned in the begin-ning of this chapter, lack of regular exercise or physical inactivity is one factor associated with an increased incidence of coronary heart disease. Such a **risk factor,** as you might have already guessed, is anything that increases the chances or probability of developing coronary heart disease sometime in your life. Two other coronary heart disease risk factors have

Table 3–1. Risk Factors Associated with Coronary Heart Disease.

Age
Sex
Heredity/family history
Tobacco smoking
Hypertension
Hyperlipidemia (blood cholesterol)
Lack of exercise
Obesity
Uncontrolled stress

already been mentioned: age and a high dietary intake of **cholesterol** and **saturated fats.**

All together, nine risk factors of coronary heart disease have so far been identified. These are given in Table 3–1. The first three risk factors—age, sex, and heredity—are beyond our direct control, that is, we can do nothing about them. However, all of the remaining risk factors are directly within our control. For example, we can stop smoking, or better yet, not start. We can regulate our food intake and exercise regularly to help avoid obesity and to increase our cardiorespiratory fitness level. We can regulate the dietary intake of salt to help lower our blood pressure, and of cholesterol, animal fats, and saturated fats to lower the chances of atherosclerosis. We can help control how much stress we are exposed to and how we respond to that stress. All of these controls and regulations can and do lead to a significant reduction in the risk of developing coronary heart disease.

The Three Big Risk Factors. While all the risk factors are important, three risk factors seem to be more important than the others. These are (1) cigarette smoking, (2) hypertension, and (3) high blood lipid levels (cholesterol). As shown in Figure 3–5, with none of these three risk factors, the relative risk of coronary heart disease is below average. If you are a smoker, then the relative risk increases to just above the average. If you are a smoker and you have high levels of blood cholesterol, then your risk of coronary heart disease is over twice that of the average and three times that if you have none of the three big risk factors. If all three risks are present, then your risk of coronary heart disease is five times that when none of the three are present. *Remember, the three big risk factors are directly under your own control; you can do something about them.*

What Is Your Risk of Coronary Heart Disease? A game-like test called RISKO, which can be used to estimate your present risk of coronary heart disease, has been published by the Michigan Heart Association. The test is presented in Table 3–2. The purpose of RISKO is to give you an estimate of your chances of suffering a heart attack. The game is played using Table

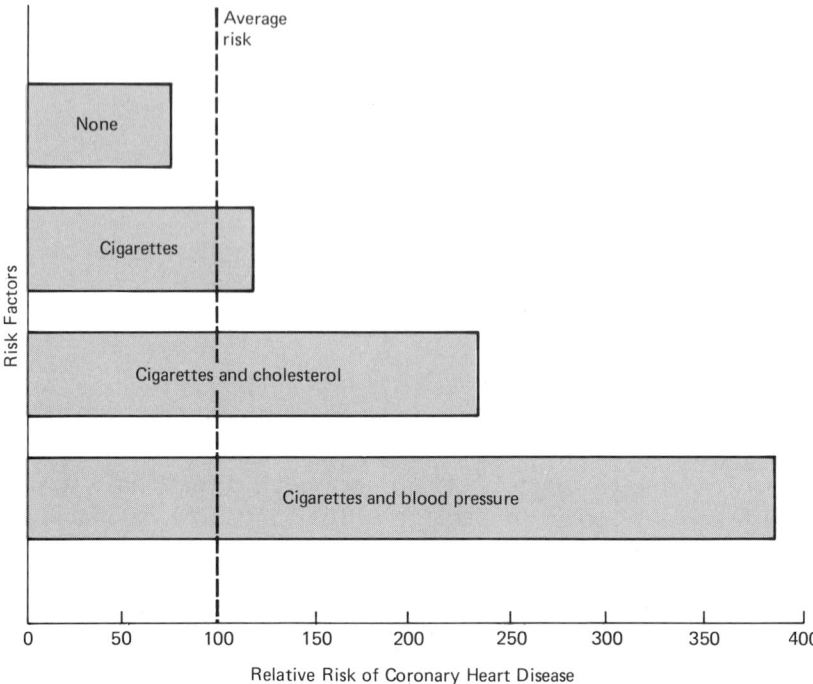

Figure 3–5. The relative risk of coronary heart disease in relation to the "big" three risk factors. If all three primary risk factors are present, the danger of a heart attack is five times that when none are present. (From Lifetime Fitness *by E. L. Fox. Copyright © 1983 by CBS College Publishing. Reprinted by permission of Saunders College Publishing. CBS College Publishing. Based on data from the American Heart Association.)*

3–2 by circling numbers, which from left to right represent an increase in your *risk factors.* These are medical conditions and habits associated with an increased danger of heart attack. Not all risk factors are measurable enough to be included in this game.

Study each risk factor and its row. (See p. 56 for explanations of some risk factors.) Find the number applicable to you and circle it. For example, if your age is 37, circle the number labeled "31 to 40." After checking out all the rows, add the circled numbers. This total—your score—is an estimate of your risk.

If you score:

> 6–11—Risk well below average.
> 12–17—Risk below average.
> 18–24—Risk generally average.
> 25–31—Risk moderate.
> 32–40—Risk at a dangerous level.
> 41–62—Danger urgent. See your doctor now.

Table 3–2. *RISKO: A Cardiac Risk Index.*

	10 to 20 1	21 to 30 2	31 to 40 3	41 to 50 4	51 to 60 6	61 to 70 8
1. Age	10 to 20 **1**	21 to 30 **2**	31 to 40 **3**	41 to 50 **4**	51 to 60 **6**	61 to 70 **8**
2. Heredity	No known history of cardiovascular disease **1**	One relative over 60 with cardiovascular disease **2**	Two relatives over 60 with cardiovascular disease **3**	One relative under 60 with cardiovascular disease **4**	Two relatives under 60 with cardiovascular disease **6**	Three relatives under 60 with cardiovascular disease **8**
3. Weight	More than 5 lbs below standard weight **0**	−5 to +5 lbs standard weight **1**	6–20 lbs overweight **2**	21–35 lbs overweight **3**	36–50 lbs overweight **5**	51–65 lbs overweight **7**
4. Tobacco smoking	Nonuser **0**	Cigar and/or pipe **1**	10 cigarettes or less a day **2**	20 cigarettes a day **4**	30 cigarettes a day **5**	40 cigarettes or more a day **10**
5. Exercise	Intensive occupational and recreational exertion **1**	Moderate occupational and recreational exertion **2**	Sedentary work and intense recreational exertion **3**	Sedentary work and moderate recreational exertion **5**	Sedentary work and light recreational exertion **6**	Complete lack of all exercise **8**
6. Cholesterol or % fat in diet	Cholesterol below 180 mg% **1**	Cholesterol 181–205 mg% **2**	Cholesterol 206–230 mg% **3**	Cholesterol 231–255 mg% **4**	Cholesterol 256–280 mg% **6**	Cholesterol 281–330 mg% **8**
	No animal or solid fats in diet **1**	10% animal or solid fat in diet **2**	20% animal or solid fat in diet **3**	30% animal or solid fat in diet **4**	40% animal or solid fat in diet **5**	50% animal or solid fat in diet **7**
7. Blood pressure	100 upper reading **1**	120 upper reading **2**	140 upper reading **3**	160 upper reading **4**	180 upper reading **6**	200 or over upper reading **8**
8. Sex	Female under 40 **1**	Female 40–50 **2**	Female over 50 **3**	Male **5**	Stocky male **6**	Bald stocky male **7**

Total score _____

RISKO is reprinted courtesy of the Michigan Heart Association. © Michigan Heart Association.

55

◇ *Heredity.* Count parents, grandparents, brothers, and sisters who have had heart attacks or strokes.

◇ *Tobacco Smoking.* If you inhale deeply and smoke a cigarette way down, add one to your classification. Do not subtract because you think you do not inhale or smoke only a half-inch on a cigarette.

◇ *Exercise.* Lower your score one point if you exercise regularly and frequently.

◇ *Cholesterol or Saturated Fat Intake Level.* A cholesterol blood level determination is best. If you can't get one from your doctor, then estimate honestly the percentage of solid fats you eat. These are usually of animal origin—lard, cream, butter, and beef and lamb fat. If you eat much of this, your cholesterol level probably will be high. The U.S. average, 40 percent, is too high for good health.

◇ *Blood Pressure.* If you have no recent reading but have passed an insurance or industrial examination, the chances are you have an upper reading of 140 or less.

◇ *Sex.* This line takes into account the fact that men have between six and ten times more heart attacks than women of childbearing age.

Risk of Other Cardiovascular Diseases

Many of the risk factors just mentioned are not only confined to coronary heart disease, but are also involved in the risk of other cardiovascular diseases such as stroke and high blood pressure or hypertension. As mentioned at the beginning of this chapter (see Figure 3–1), of all deaths in the United States, 11 percent are caused by stroke and 3 percent by hypertension.

A **stroke** occurs when the blood supply to the brain is either temporarily or permanently interrupted. Such interruptions can result from a blood clot that blocks one of the arteries in the brain or from the bursting of an artery. The former is referred to as a **cerebral thrombosis** (thrombosis = blood clot) and the latter as a **cerebral hemorrhage** (hemorrhage = bleeding). In cither case, the resultant stroke usually leads to variable degrees of paralysis and sometimes to death.

The usual causes of stroke are atherosclerosis and hypertension. Therefore, many of the same risk factors for coronary heart disease also apply to stroke and hypertension. These include exercise, since, according to Boyer and Kasch (1970), regular exercise has been shown to reduce blood pressure toward normal values in hypertensive subjects. Other important risk factors involved with stroke and hypertension are high blood cholesterol levels, tobacco smoking, and obesity.

Decreasing Your Risk of Coronary Heart Disease with Exercise

Earlier it was stated that sedentary living habits or the lack of regular exercise increase your risk of coronary heart disease. At least two important questions are raised by this statement. First, what evidence, particularly scientific evidence, is there that makes this statement true? And second, what physiological and other changes take place in your body to improve your cardiorespiratory fitness level and thus lessen your risk of coronary heart disease?

The Scientific Link Between Coronary Heart Disease and Physical Exercise

Over the past 30 years or so, hundreds of studies have been conducted in the hope of scientifically linking activity (exercise) level and the incidence of coronary heart disease. However, from an experimental or statistical aspect, a direct link between exercise and heart disease has not been established. The major reason for this is not because such a relationship does not exist, but because there are too many other risk factors (most of which have already been discussed) that cannot be precisely controlled, thereby preventing a totally clear scientific picture of the cause and effect relationship between inactivity and coronary heart disease.

How can we say then that regular exercise definitely reduces the risk of coronary heart disease? The answer is quite simple. Many studies have been conducted in which the incidence of coronary heart disease has been consistently shown to be much higher in persons who have inactive or sedentary occupations than in those who have active occupations.

One of the first of these studies was conducted by a group of British epidemiologists.* This group (Morris et al., 1953) studied the incidence of coronary heart disease in bus drivers, bus conductors, telephone operators (telephonists as they called them), and postmen. Both the bus drivers and telephone operators were considered to be in inactive or sedentary occupations since most of the work is performed while seated. On the other hand, both conductors and postmen have jobs that require considerable activity. In England, double-decker buses are popular or at least were popular during the early 1950s when the study was conducted. The bus conductor walks up and down the bus all day collecting tickets.

The incidence of coronary heart disease was found to be significantly

---

* **Epidemiology** is the study of the incidence, distribution, and control of a disease (coronary heart disease in this case) in a human community. A specific investigation is called an epidemiological study.

greater in the bus drivers and telephone operators than in the bus conductors and postmen. For example, of every 1,000 postmen, 1.85 had coronary heart disease, whereas of every 1,000 bus drivers, 3.2 had coronary heart disease. The researchers also found that coronary heart disease in the active workers seemed to appear later in life and was less severe than that experienced by the more sedentary workers.

The mortality (death) from coronary heart disease was also studied by these British researchers. The death rate from coronary heart disease found in sedentary workers was more than twice that of the active workers.

Throughout the years that followed the British group's original studies, several other populations were studied in the same way. Some of the populations studied include railroad employees, longshoremen, lumberjacks, civil service employees, and farmers. All of these epidemiological studies came to the same conclusion: *The risk of and mortality from coronary heart disease is much less in active persons than in inactive persons* (Paffenberger and Hale, 1975). Although mostly circumstantial, this is perhaps the best evidence now available that scientifically links physical activity to coronary heart disease.

What about cardiac rehabilitation programs? Can they give us a definitive answer concerning the relationship between exercise and coronary heart disease? A cardiac rehabilitation program, as the name implies, involves carefully prescribed and medically monitored exercise programs for selected patients who have had heart attacks. Therefore, they would appear to be able to give us some insight into coronary heart disease and physical activity. So far, however, this has not been the case. There are several reasons for this: (1) those patients selected to participate in a cardiac rehabilitation program have a low mortality rate; (2) most studies dealing with cardiac rehabilitation involve small numbers of patients; (3) there is a relatively high attrition (drop-out) rate in such programs; (4) the durations of the programs are relatively short; and (5) a large amount of money is necessary to conduct such studies. Unfortunately, with these drawbacks, studies evolving from cardiac rehabilitation programs cannot as yet supply us with the answers we are seeking.

Physiological and Other Changes that Improve Your Cardiorespiratory Fitness Levels

Why does regular physical activity or exercise lead to a reduction in the risk of coronary heart disease? Although the complete answer to this question is not known today, the following factors are thought to be involved.

Decreases in Other Coronary Risk Factors. Regular exercise programs, when properly prescribed,* usually lead to a reduction in the coronary risk factors of obesity, hypertension, and blood cholesterol levels.

---

* Exercise prescription will be covered in Chapter 4.

Obesity. Regular exercise generally leads to a reduction in total body weight. The subjects in one study were overweight college women (average age: 18.6 years). The exercise program they participated in consisted of walking/jogging 4½ to 5½ miles each day, six days per week for eight weeks. The caloric expenditure per exercise session was about 350 kcal. During the course of the eight-week exercise program, none of the women consciously limited her food intake. Therefore, the resulting changes in body composition were entirely the result of the exercise program. Here is what was found:

1. Total body weight was reduced by 2.4 kg (5.3 pounds) on the average. One subject lost as much as 4.3 kg or 9.5 pounds.
2. The percentage of body fat was reduced on the average by 10 percent with one subject decreasing her percentage of fat from 37.6 to 24.5 percent.
3. The total body fat was reduced by over 5 kg (over 10 pounds) on the average. One subject reduced her total body fat by 8.1 kg or nearly 18 pounds.
4. The fat-free weight, that is, the muscle mass or lean body mass* was maintained after the training program and in fact was slightly increased on the average.

Hypertension. As in the case of obesity, regular exercise training can lead to a decrease in both systolic and diastolic blood pressure. An example of this is shown in Figure 3–6. The subjects in this study were middle-aged men whose blood pressures were high enough for them to be classified as borderline hypertensives. The training program lasted for six months. Notice that after training, both systolic and diastolic pressures were lower at rest as well as during exercise (Boyer and Kasch, 1970).

Other information relating hypertension and exercise training includes the following:

1. Epidemiological surveys have found that people in physically active occupations have lower systolic and diastolic blood pressures than those in sedentary jobs.
2. Persons who are physically fit have lower blood pressures than those who are unfit.
3. The effects of exercise training on systolic and diastolic blood pressures of hypertensive persons are greater than those with blood pressures within the normal range.
4. Blood pressure may be reduced to a greater extent after exercise training when accompanied by a loss of body weight.
5. High blood pressure or hypertension has been shown to occur later in life and with less frequency in those who are physically active compared with those who are sedentary.

---

* More about fat-free weight is given in Chapter 8.

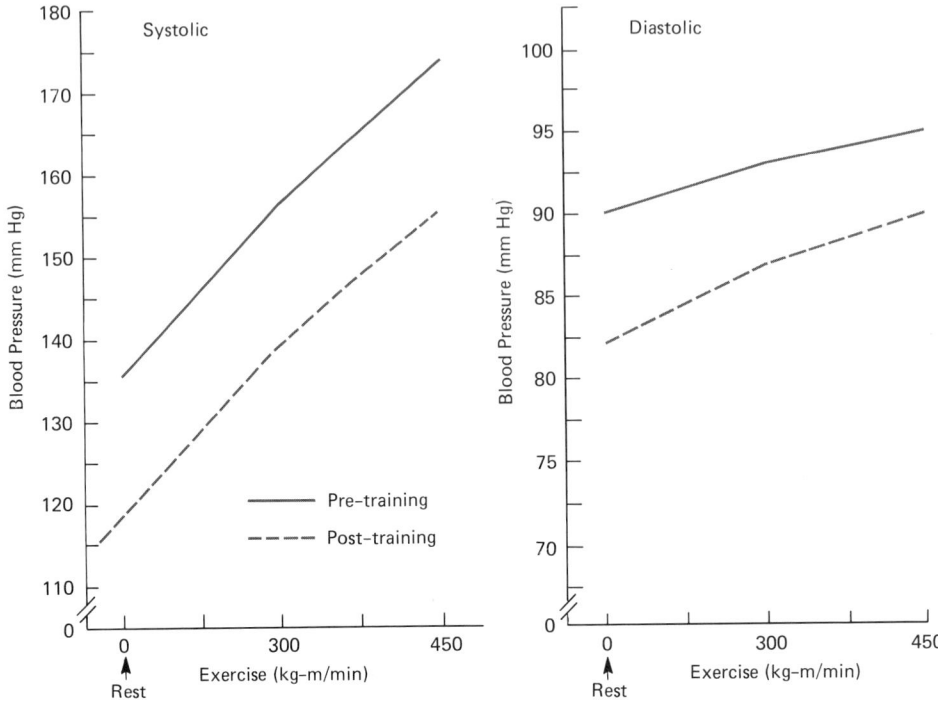

Figure 3–6. The typical change in blood pressure in a hypertensive person after a training program. (From Choquette, G. and Ferguson, R. J.: Blood pressure reduction in "Borderline" hypertensives following physical training. Can. Med. Assoc. J.: 108, 699–703. Reprinted from The Physiological Basis of Physical Education and Athletics, *third ed. by E. L. Fox and D. K. Mathews. Copyright © 1981 by CBS College Publishing. Reprinted by permission of CBS College Publishing.)*

Blood Cholesterol (Lipid) Levels.   Recent research has shown that regular exercise programs quite frequently lead to significant reductions in blood cholesterol levels. For example, as shown in Figure 3–7, based on the data of Wood et al. (1977) the blood cholesterol level in a group of middle-aged men (35 to 59 years) who averaged nearly 40 miles of jogging a week was significantly lower on the average than in a group of age-matched controls (the men who served as controls were the same age but did not exercise on a regular basis).

Later, in Chapter 7, we will also discover that regular exercise programs not only lower total blood cholesterol levels, but in addition, they lower the lipid fraction of cholesterol that is thought to contribute to the athero-sclerotic process and increase the lipid fraction that is protective against coronary heart disease. The blood lipid fraction of cholesterol that is thought to contribute to atherosclerosis is referred to as **low density lipoprotein** or **LDL** cholesterol whereas the blood lipid fraction that appears to be protec-

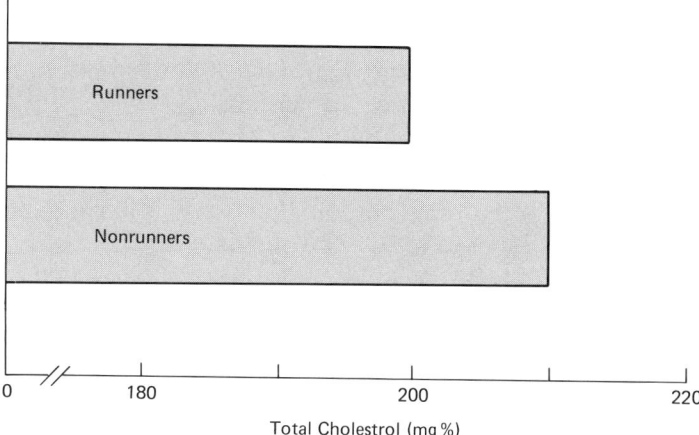

Figure 3–7. The effects of exercise training on levels of total cholesterol. (From Wood, P. D., et al.: The distribution of plasma lipoproteins in middle-aged male runners. Metabolism *25(11): 1249–1257, 1976.)*

tive against coronary heart disease is referred to as **high density lipoprotein** or **HDL** cholesterol. More about these lipoproteins is discussed in Chapter 7.

Physiological Changes with Exercise Training

Besides reducing the effect of several important coronary heart disease risk factors, regular exercise training leads to numerous physiological changes that are thought to contribute some protection against coronary heart disease. The most important changes are improvement in the oxygen transport system, increased circulatory efficiency, increased size and number of the blood vessels of the heart, reduced possibility of thrombosis, and reduced vulnerability to cardiac dysrhythmias.

Improvement in the Oxygen Transport System. Regular exercise training has been shown to improve the ability of the circulatory and respiratory systems (cardiorespiratory system) to deliver oxygen to and remove carbon dioxide from working muscles.

As pointed out in the last chapter, the single most valid physiological measure of the functional capacity of the **oxygen transport system** is the maximal aerobic power or the maximal amount of oxygen that can be consumed per minute during maximal exercise **(maximal oxygen consumption).** This measure has been extensively studied during exercise and it has been clearly demonstrated that training can lead to substantial improvements in its magnitude. The importance of this change is that the more oxygen you can consume, the better able you are to perform endurance activities. In other words, the higher your maximal oxygen consumption, the greater your cardiorespiratory or endurance fitness level.

The key alterations that lead to an improvement in maximal oxygen consumption after exercise training are:

1. An increase in the cardiac output, that is, in the amount of blood pumped by the heart per minute. The increase in cardiac output is almost entirely the result of an increase in the stroke volume, that is, in the amount of blood pumped by the heart with each beat. In turn, the increase in stroke volume is related to an increase in the size of the heart ventricle and to its ability to contract more forcefully.
2. An increase in the ability of the skeletal muscles to take up (from the blood) and use oxygen. These alterations are mainly the result of biochemical changes that occur within the muscle cells.

Increased Circulatory Efficiency. One of the most consistent and pronounced changes produced by chronic exercise training is a reduction in the heart rate. This is true at rest as well as during exercise. Endurance athletes such as long distance runners, for example, may have resting heart rates as low as 45 to 50 beats per minute, whereas their untrained contemporaries may have rates between 75 and 80 beats per minute. In addition, during maximal exercise, the athlete's maximal heart rate might be only 185 beats per minute whereas the untrained person's might be as high as 195 or even 200 beats per minute.

These changes in heart rate indicate that the heart has improved its pumping efficiency. What is pumping efficiency? Pumping efficiency is a measure of the stress placed on the heart when pumping a given amount of blood. In the last chapter it was explained that the amount of blood pumped by the heart in one minute (cardiac output) is determined by two factors: (1) how much blood is pumped with each beat (stroke volume); and (2) how many times the heart beats in one minute (heart rate). The relationship of these factors is:

$$\text{Cardiac Output} = \text{Heart Rate} \times \text{Stroke Volume}$$

Therefore, the same amount of blood can be pumped with a relatively high heart rate and a relatively low stroke volume or vice versa. For example, suppose a blood flow rate of 16 liters/minute was required while you were out jogging. This amount of blood can be pumped with a heart rate of 180 beats per minute and a stroke volume of 89 ml ($180 \times 89 = 16$ liters/minute) or with a heart rate of 140 beats per minute and a stroke volume of 114 ml ($140 \times 114 = 16$ liters/minute). However, the stress on the heart muscle itself is much less in the latter case. In other words, even though the heart is pumping the same amount of blood in each case, the heart muscle does not require as much oxygen when the rate is low and the stroke volume high. This is what is meant by improved **circulatory efficiency.**

Increased Blood Vessel Size and Capillarization of the Heart. Studies on rats have shown that the size of the **coronary vasculature** (the blood vessels of the heart) is increased by regular exercise training. The significance of such an increase is that it facilitates blood flow and consequently the delivery of oxygen to the heart muscle. No studies to date have demonstrated an increased vessel size in humans after exercise training. However, autopsy studies by Currens and White (1961) on the famous marathon runner Clarence DeMar showed his coronary vessels to be two to three times larger than normal. "Mr. Marathon," as he was called, regularly ran 26-mile marathon races until he was 69 years old. In this regard, it is tempting to attribute his large coronary vasculature to chronic exercise training; however, the fact that genetics may also have been involved cannot be completely ruled out.

Besides the possibility that regular or chronic exercise training leads to increased coronary vessel size, there is also the possibility that training leads to an increase in the number of vessels (capillaries) that supply the heart muscle. This change (sometimes referred to as an increase in **collateral circulation**), would also enhance blood flow and oxygen delivery to the heart.

An increase in collateral circulation is particularly important for those patients who have suffered heart attacks (that is, myocardial infarctions). As you will recall from Chapter 2, the left coronary artery and its branches supply blood to the left side of the heart and the right coronary artery and its branches to the right side of the heart. If a heart attack occurred because a branch of the right coronary artery became blocked, a portion of the right heart muscle would be without a blood supply and would die. However, exercise training might help protect that portion of heart muscle by causing an overlapping of collateral vessels.

Unfortunately, studies that directly confirm an increase in coronary collateral circulation with exercise training in humans are not numerous. In fact, most studies have been able to generate only indirect evidence for such an effect. For example, in a recent study on humans, only two of six patients with coronary heart disease showed some increased collateralization after exercise training (Leon and Blackburn, 1981). In addition, it could not be definitely determined whether these changes were the result of the exercise programs.

Reduced Possibility of Thrombosis (Blood Clot). As previously mentioned, a heart attack occurs when a blood clot (thrombus) lodges in a coronary artery or any of its branches and blocks the blood flow to a portion of the heart muscle. The rate of formation of the clot (called **coagulability**) is increased with acute exercise. This means, for example, that when you go out to exercise for 30 minutes or an hour, the tendency for clot formation is increased for that time period. Fortunately, this increased coagulability is counteracted by an increase in the rate at which a clot is dissolved (called **fibrinolysis**). It is believed that chronic exercise programs, that is, exercise training, decrease the increased tendency for blood to clot during acute

Table 3–3. Some Possible Effects of Chronic Exercise Training.

Fat percentage decreases
Blood pressure decreases (in hypertension)
Total cholesterol level decreases
HDL (high density lipoprotein) level increases
Oxygen consumption increases
Cardiac output increases
Incidence of strokes decreases
Oxygen extraction by muscle increases
Size of coronary vessels increases
Capillarization of heart increases
Risk of thrombosis decreases

exercise bouts. It also appears that training maintains the fibrinolytic system or the ability to dissolve clots. In this way, training appears to reduce the risk of thrombosis and the risk of serious cardiovascular accidents such as a heart attack.

Reduced Vulnerability to Cardiac Dysrhythmias. Disturbances in the rhythm (beating) of the heart **(cardiac dysrhythmias)** can lead to serious cardiac problems, including heart attack and death. It has been suggested that exercise training may reduce the susceptibility of the heart to such disturbances.

Other Effects of Exercise Training. Some other important effects of exercise training that have been reported include: (1) increases in red blood cell number and blood volume; (2) increase in thyroid function; (3) increase in growth hormone production; (4) improved tolerance to stress; and (5) a decrease in glucose intolerance.

Table 3–3 provides a summary of the effects of chronic exercise training.

Stress and Its Management

Each day we experience situations that evoke a **stress response.** These stressful situations that occur in day-to-day living are of themselves not problems if we are able to manage them properly. With learning and patience, **stress management** can be mastered and enable us to effectively deal with the everyday pressures we experience.

An inability to positively manage stress serves as an important risk factor for cardiovascular disease. Although the specific influence of stress on cardiovascular disease is not clear, that a relationship exists is well established. In addition, persons who are able to cope with stressors can more easily make or maintain life-style changes in the areas of smoking, eating, sleeping, and exercising.

Physical and Emotional Responses to Stress

Inappropriate reaction to a stressor has both physical and emotional results. Body chemistry is altered because of muscular contraction, which results in increased levels of lactic acid production, and there is a hormonal response that results in higher levels of **catecholamines,** which increase the heart rate and constrict peripheral blood vessels. This physiological response can trigger emotional changes as well, such as nervousness and irritability.

The most important effect of repeated unmanaged stress is that it contributes to high blood pressure, which is recognized as one of the three major causes of atherosclerosis. The proper management of stress can (1) avoid the contribution of stress to high blood pressure, decreasing the risk of heart attack; (2) help to improve eating, drinking, smoking, sleeping, and exercise habits; and (3) reduce nervousness and irritability.

Identifying Sources of Stress

In order to effectively deal with stress you must be able to identify the kinds of stressors to which you are exposed during your daily routine. Complete the chart found in Table 3–4. Have a friend or relative who knows your

Table 3–4. Self-Scoring Test for Stress Determination.*

Conduct	Often	Sometimes	Rarely
1. I experience unexplained headaches and backaches.	2	1	0
2. When I'm nervous I eat/drink/smoke.	2	1	0
3. When problems are not immediately solved I get worried.	2	1	0
4. I feel tired and restless.	2	1	0
5. I work at completion of tasks very close to the deadline.	2	1	0
6. My mood changes.	2	1	0
7. I'm too busy to allow time for physical activity.	2	1	0
8. I'm concerned on more than one problem and can't concentrate well.	2	1	0
9. People at work or home make me feel tense.	2	1	0
10. When people disagree with me I challenge them and feel as though I should not yield.	2	1	0

* Use the copy of this test and scoring form found in Appendix D.

Table 3–5. Evaluator Chart for Identifying Habits of a Close Friend or Relative.

Conduct	Often	Sometimes	Never
1. Seems to be in a hurry, moves and eats fast, hates to wait.	3	2	0
2. Talks very quickly, often interrupts.	3	2	0
3. Seems to worry about things of little consequence.	3	2	0
4. Unable to understand why so many others can't meet their responsibilities.	3	2	0
5. Loses patience quickly.	3	2	0
6. Seems to have a lot to do.	3	2	0

habits well complete the observer's chart found in Table 3–5. Scoring sheets for these are found in Appendix D. The combined scores from both these ratings are important in helping you to assess your present level of unmanaged stress and to assist you in identifying some of the specific sources of your stress.

Keeping a daily record of stressful situations with which you have difficulty is another useful means in specifically identifying sources of stress in need of management. Once you have noted your daily stress precipitators you have made significant progress toward reducing their abilities to affect you. The next stage is to employ stress management techniques.

Managing Stress

In developing a plan to reduce the negative effects of stress, you must develop skills that will help you to cope with stressful situations. **Relaxation** is a conscious release of muscular tension. To be able to relax you must be aware of the presence of tension and learn to reduce that tension. Various techniques have been used with success to promote relaxation. Benson (1975) has proposed the following technique:

1. Sit quietly in a comfortable position and close your eyes.
2. Beginning at the feet and progressing to the head, relax all your muscles.
3. Breathe through your nose. Each time you breathe out, silently say the word "one." Breathe easily and naturally.
4. Continue for 10 to 20 minutes. You may occasionally check the time, but do not use an alarm. When you finish, sit quietly for several minutes.
5. Maintain a positive attitude and permit relaxation to occur at its own pace. When distracting thoughts occur, try to ignore them by not dwelling upon them, and continue to repeat the word "one."

With practice you can be successful in attaining a relaxed state using this relatively simple technique. As the worksheet in Appendix D suggests, using this technique once or twice a day coupled with exercise and stressor awareness may have a positive influence on changes in habit and stress effects.

Role of Exercise in Stress

Physical exercise is itself a form of stress that produces some physiological changes similar to those associated with nonactivity-induced stress. The effects, however, are very different. Hans Selye (1956), a respected pioneer in the area of stress and its effects, recognized that exercise was a potent stressor. He suggested, however, that the trained person (that is, one who has reaped the benefits of repeated bouts of appropriate levels of exercise) should be better prepared to resist other kinds of "bad stressors" and that stressful situations are managed much better as a result of physical conditioning. Herbert A. DeVries (1975), an exercise physiologist, also concluded that rhythmic exercise, such as walking, running, swimming, or bicycling, when done at appropriate intensity and duration promoted significant relaxation in tense persons.

SUMMARY

◇ Regular exercise training reduces the risk of coronary heart disease and other cardiovascular diseases.

◇ Coronary heart disease is a cardiovascular disease that is concerned mainly with diseases of the heart muscle and of the blood vessels of the heart. It is the most severe of all the cardiovascular diseases.

◇ The major cause of coronary heart disease is atherosclerosis, a disease that afflicts the blood vessels (arteries) including the coronary arteries that supply blood and oxygen to the heart muscle.

◇ In atherosclerosis, the lumen or opening of the artery becomes narrowed as fatty deposits build up on its inside wall. This build-up may become so great that the flow of blood in the artery is completely blocked, leading to a heart attack (myocardial infarction). A heart attack can also occur when a blood clot lodges in an atherosclerotic artery that is narrowed but not occluded.

◇ There are nine known risk factors of coronary heart disease: (1) age; (2) sex; (3) heredity; (4) obesity; (5) tobacco smoking; (6) lack of exercise; (7) high blood lipid (cholesterol) level; (8) high blood pressure (hypertension); and (9) stress. The three big risk factors are (1) tobacco smoking; (2) high blood pressure; and (3) a high blood lipid (cholesterol) level.

◇ The risk factors for coronary heart disease are also related to other cardiovascular diseases such as stroke and high blood pressure. A stroke occurs when the blood supply to the brain is temporarily or permanently interrupted such as from a blood clot or a burst artery.

◇ A stroke caused by a blood clot is called a cerebral thrombosis whereas a stroke triggered by a burst artery is called a cerebral hemorrhage. Stroke is caused by atherosclerosis and high blood pressure.

◊ The best evidence now available that scientifically links physical activity to the incidence of coronary heart disease comes from epidemiological studies in which the relationships of the various factors that determine coronary heart disease in a human community are systematically investigated. The conclusion from these studies is that the risk of and mortality (death) from coronary heart disease is much less in active persons than in inactive persons.

◊ Physiological and other changes that improve your cardiorespiratory fitness level and reduce your overall risk of coronary heart disease include: (1) decreases in other coronary risk factors such as obesity, hypertension, and blood cholesterol levels; (2) improvement in the oxygen transport system; (3) increased circulatory efficiency; (4) increased blood vessel size and capillarization of the heart; (5) reduced possibility of thrombosis; (6) reduced vulnerability to cardiac dysrhythmias; and (7) other changes.

◊ Stress is an unavoidable factor of daily living. Our abilities to cope with stressful situations and to manage our responses to stress are important. To do these we should be able to identify sources of stress and employ relaxation techniques. Exercises that lead to a training effect can also have positive influences on our abilities to manage stress.

STUDY QUESTIONS

1. How many deaths are caused by cardiovascular diseases in the United States per year? Which of the cardiovascular diseases is the number one killer?
2. What is coronary heart disease?
3. What is atherosclerosis and how does it relate to cardiovascular diseases?
4. What is a heart attack and how does it occur?
5. List and discuss the risk factors of coronary heart disease.
6. What are the three major risk factors? Why?
7. What is your risk of coronary heart disease?
8. What is a stroke and what causes it?
9. Discuss the scientific link between coronary heart disease and physical activity.
10. Discuss the physiological and other changes that help improve your cardiorespiratory fitness level and lower your overall risk of coronary heart disease.
11. What factors can influence your ability to manage stress?

REFERENCES AND SELECTED READINGS

Benson, H.: *The Relaxation Response.* New York: William Morrow and Co., 1975.

Borhani, N. D.: Epidemiology of coronary heart disease. In E. A. Amsterdam, J. H. Wilmore, and A. N. DeMaria (eds.): *Exercise in Cardiovascular Health and Disease.* New York: Yorke Medical Books, 1977.

Boyer, J. C.; and Kasch, F. W.: Exercise therapy in hypertensive men. *Journal of the American Medical Association* 211:1668–1671, 1970.

Currens, J. H.; and White, P. D.: Half a century of running: Clinical, physiologic and autopsy findings in the case of Clarence DeMar (Mr. Marathon). *New England Journal of Medicine* 165:988–993, 1961.

DeVries, H. A.: Physical education, adult fitness programs: Does physical activity promote relaxation? *Journal of Health, Physical Education and Recreation* 46(7):53–54, 1975.

Enos, W. F.; Holmes, R. H.; and Beyer, J: Coronary disease among United States soldiers killed in action in Korea. *Journal of the American Medical Association* 152:1090–1093, 1953.

Falls, H. B.; Baylor, A. M.; and Dishman, R. K.: *Essentials of Fitness.* Philadelphia: Saunders College Publishing, 1980, pp. 45–59.

Fox, E. L.; and Mathews, D. K.: *The Physiological Basis of Physical Education and Athletics,* 3rd ed. Philadelphia: Saunders College Publishing, 1981, pp. 395–419.

Leon, A. S.; and Blackburn, H.: Physical inactivity and coronary heart disease. In N. M. Kaplan, and J. Stamler (eds.): *Preventive Cardiology.* Philadelphia: W. B. Saunders, 1981.

McNamara, J. J.; Molot, M. A.; Shenple, J. F.; and Culting, R. T.: Coronary artery disease in combat casualties in Vietnam. *Journal of the American Medical Association* 216:1185–1187, 1971.

Milvy, P.; Forbes, W. F.; and Brown, K. S.: A critical review of epidemiological studies of physical activity. In P. Milvy, (ed.): The Marathon: Physiological, Medical, Epidemiological and Psychological Studies. *Annals of the New York Academy of Sciences* 301:519–549, 1977.

Morris, J. N.; Heady, J. A.; Raffle, P. A. B.; Roberts, C. G.; and Parks, J. W.: Coronary heart disease and physical activity of work. *Lancet* 2:1053–1057; 1111–1120, 1953.

Paffenberger, R. S.; and Hale, W. E.: Work activity and coronary heart mortality. *New England Journal of Medicine* 292:545–550, 1975.

Pollock, M. L.; Wilmore, J. H.; and Fox, S. M., III: *Health and Fitness Through Physical Activity.* New York: John Wiley & Sons, 1978, pp. 1–21.

Selye, H.: *The Stress of Life.* New York: McGraw-Hill Book Co., 1956.

Wolff, O. H.: The pediatrician's responsibility for prevention of coronary heart disease. *Postgraduate Medical Journal* 54:228–231, 1978.

Wood, P. D.; Haskell, W. L.; Stern, M. P.; Lewis, S.; and Perry, C.: Plasma lipoprotein distributions in male and female runners. In P. Milvy (ed.): The Marathon: Physiological, Medical, Epidemiological and Psychological Studies. *Annals of the New York Academy of Sciences* 301:1977.

Chapter 4
Exercise Prescription for Cardiorespiratory Fitness Programs

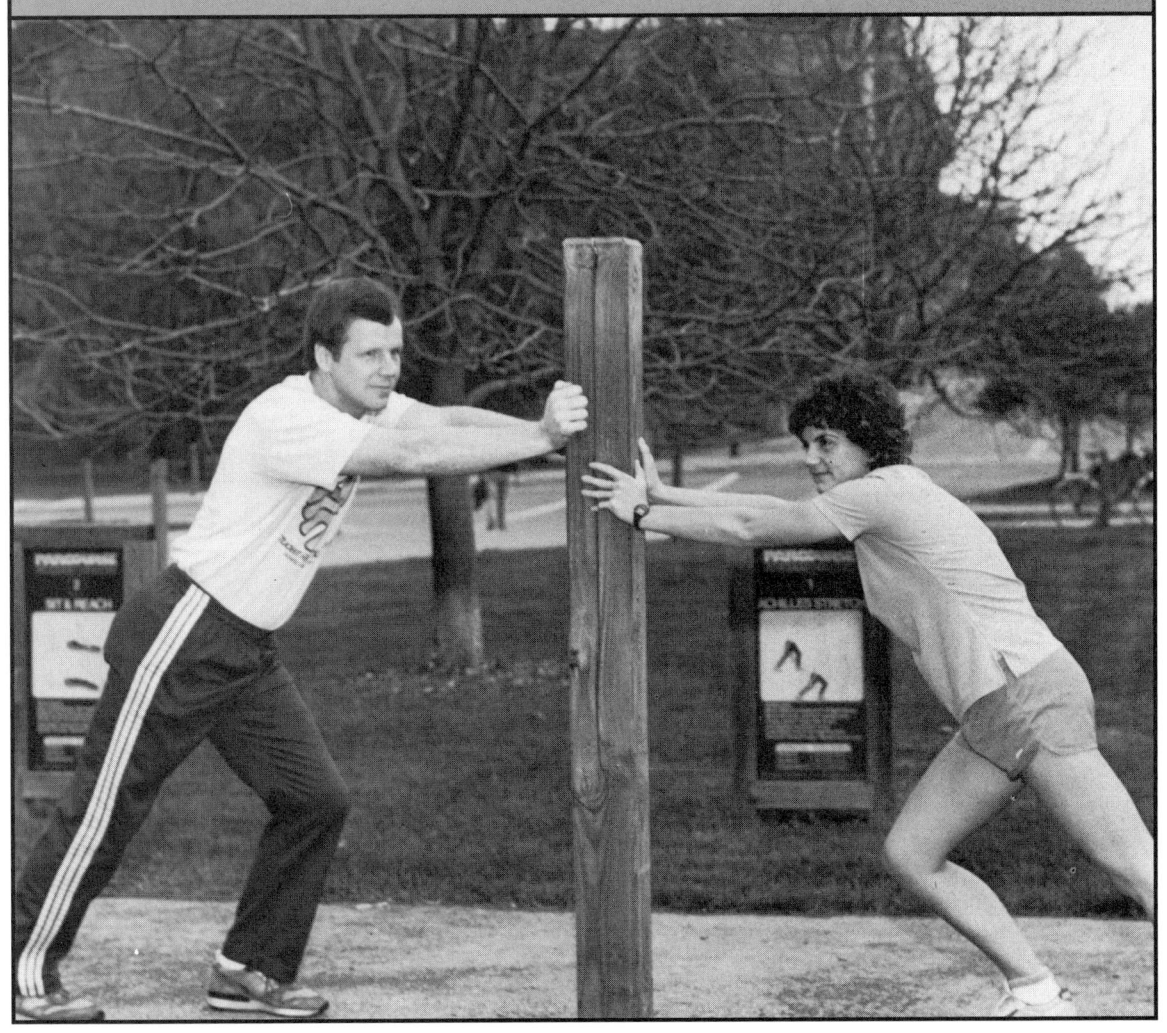

Chapter Outline

Learning Objectives

◇ To recognize the value of and necessity for an individualized exercise prescription.

◇ To understand the adaptive response to training and the effects of overload.

◇ To understand the influence that exercise intensity, frequency, duration, and mode have on the improvement of cardiovascular fitness.

◇ To understand the concept of METs and the use of METs in exercise prescription.

◇ To learn the skills necessary to develop an appropriate cardiovascular exercise program using walking/jogging, swimming, bicycling, or other appropriate forms of exercise.

◇ To understand the value of warming up before exercise and of gradually cooling down after exercise.

◇ To understand the effects of heat and humidity upon exercise response and to know how to appropriately adjust fluid intake under various environmental conditions.

Key Words and Phrases

acclimatization
adaptive response
Borg scale
cool-down
duration of exercise
exercise prescription
frequency of exercise
heart rate method
heart rate range
heart rate reserve
intensity of exercise

Karvonen's formula
maximal oxygen consumption
maximal heart rate
MET
mode of exercise
overload
perceived exertion
target heart rate
threshold for training
warm-up

Introduction

NOT all of the changes discussed in Chapter 3 will be realized in all exercise programs. Instead, there are specific guidelines that need to be followed in constructing an effective exercise program. The purpose of this chapter will be to familiarize you with the ingredients of a properly prescribed exercise training program that will improve your cardiorespiratory fitness level and at the same time lower your risk of developing coronary heart disease.

The Exercise Prescription

The **exercise prescription** is similar to a prescription given by a physician that designates a medicine to reduce or minimize symptoms caused by a disease. In our case, the "disease" is a low cardiorespiratory fitness level caused by a sedentary life-style; some of the "symptoms" are breathlessness upon exertion, chronic fatigue, overweight, and the gradual development of other risk factors. The correct prescription, of course, is regular participation in an exercise program involving activities that are carried out over prolonged periods of time and that sufficiently tax or stress the oxygen transport or the heart-lung system.

Factors Involved in the Exercise Prescription

What information is needed in order to write an exercise prescription? Basically information in two categories is necessary: (1) medical and physiological information; and (2) information about the quantity and quality of the exercise program itself.

The Medical Evaluation. Regardless of our age or intentions concerning a regular exercise program, each of us should certainly undergo periodic medical evaluation of our health status. A medical checkup becomes particularly important, however, when we are older or when we contemplate the initiation of an exercise training routine. This evaluation ensures that no condition exists that can be aggravated by regular exercise. Most experts involved in developing exercise programs will insist on a recent physical examination and a statement from a physician indicating the suitability of the person for participation in such a program.

The Physiological Assessment. It is essential to have accurate determinations of the levels of exercise that produce physiological and other benefits.

This assessment of individual capabilities provides information that permits the development of an exercise prescription. The specific variables to be measured and methods of testing are covered in Chapter 9. In this section we are more interested in the basic ingredients that constitute an appropriate cardiorespiratory training program.

Quantity and Quality of Exercise. The essence of a beneficial exercise training program is that it meets the established criteria to adequately stress the cardiorespiratory system. In order to provide sufficient amounts of stress, the **overload** principle must be used. This principle states that in order to obtain an **adaptive response** (i.e., an increase in capabilities) of a given system, demands must be put on that system that exceed those it normally encounters. A great deal of research has been done to determine the demands that must be placed on the cardiorespiratory system to result in adaptation. It has been concluded by the American College of Sports Medicine (1978) that in order to develop and maintain cardiorespiratory fitness four factors must be considered: (1) the **frequency of exercise;** (2) the **duration of** each **exercise** session; (3) the **intensity of exercise;** and (4) the **mode** or type **of exercise.** Because of their importance to an appropriate exercise program, let's look at each of these factors in more detail.

Frequency of Exercise. It has been determined that exercising three times per week is the minimum number of sessions required for cardiorespiratory improvement. It may be that four, five, or even six times per week will provide greater improvement, but the increase in cardiorespiratory adaptation is likely to be minimal (American College of Sports Medicine, 1980).

Duration of Exercise. The duration of the exercise period is the amount of time during each exercise session that the appropriate intensity (see following) must be continuously or nearly continuously maintained. The minimum time duration of each exercise session is 20 minutes. Duration and intensity of exercise will vary of course, one being dependent on the other. The duration of an exercise session may be optimal at 30 to 40 minutes if we choose an intensity level that is within the appropriate range noted below but at the lower end of that range.

Intensity of Exercise. The most individualized (i.e., dependent on the results of our physiological assessment) and critical criterion for determining an exercise prescription is the intensity of exercise or degree of difficulty imposed. A number of methods have been developed to determine the appropriate intensity levels. The first is the **heart rate (HR) method.** The heart rate response to exercise is very closely correlated with the exercise load. As such, heart rate can be used to determine when the work load is sufficient to overload the cardiorespiratory system. It is very popular to establish a **target heart rate** or a **heart rate range** that can be used to assess the intensity of the work being accomplished. This is an excellent and easily employed tool and can be measured by counting the pulse (HR) (Figure 4–1).

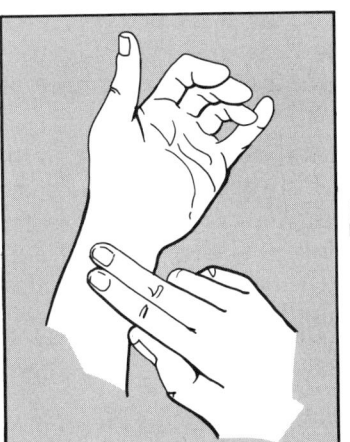

Press lightly
here

(A) Radial

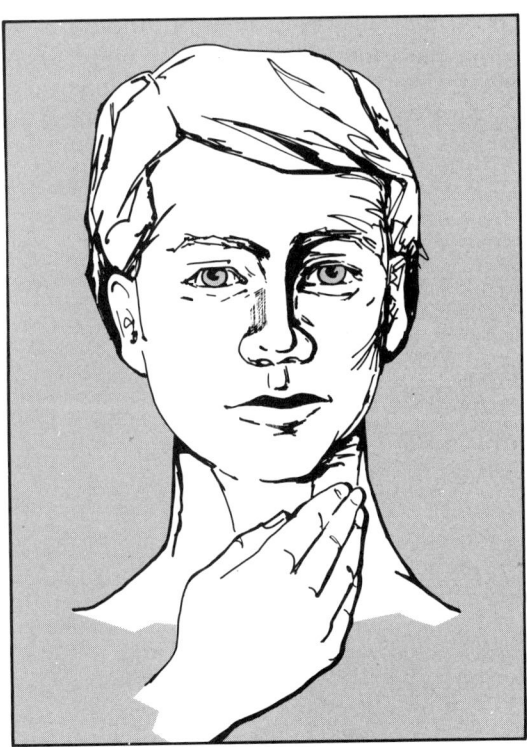

Press lightly

(B) Carotid

Figure 4–1. Sites at which the pulse can be palpated.

The results of a typical test on an untrained person demonstrate the relationship between heart rate and exercise load (Figure 4–2). As the exercise intensity increases, there are commensurate changes in heart rate.

Assessing Intensity.   Two methods are available to identify the heart rate level that must be maintained. Both are based in part on an accurate determination of **maximal heart rate.** First, maximal heart rate can be directly measured as part of the physiological assessment if a maximal exercise test has been included. Second, maximal heart rate can also be estimated based on your age using the following formula:

$$\text{Maximal Predicted HR} = 220 - \text{age}$$

For example, if your age is 21 years then your maximal predicted heart rate would be $220 - 21 = 199$ beats per minute. This formula, while very useful, may produce incorrect estimates because of individual variations. Such errors can be as great as ± 15 beats per minute and more.

The first method for determining an appropriate target heart rate range is a strict percentage of maximal heart rate. To find your target heart rate using this method, take your maximal heart rate (predicted or actual) and

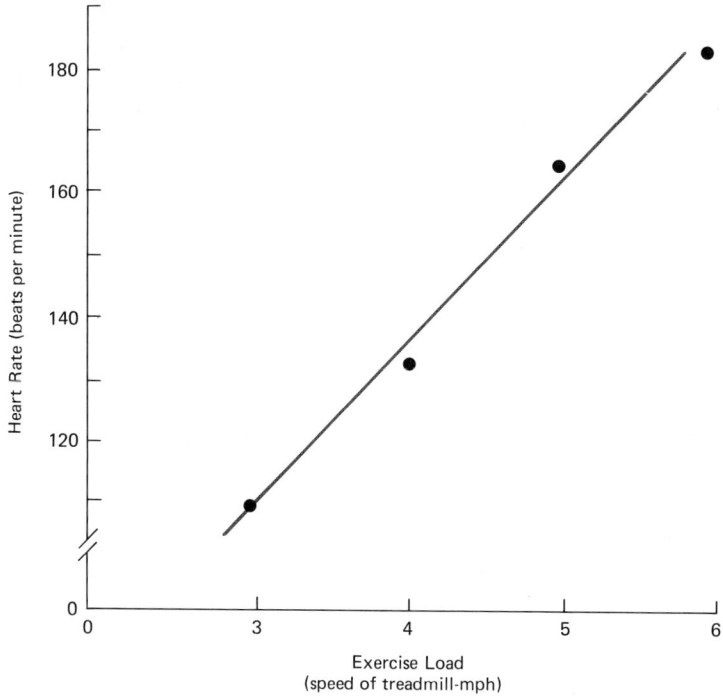

Figure 4–2. The linear relationship that exists between exercise load and heart rate.

multiply it by the appropriate percentage. The percentage to be used for this method is 75 to 90 percent of maximal heart rate. For our 21-year-old above, we would find:

1. $220 - 21 = 199$ predicted maximal heart rate
2. $199 \times .75 = 144$ lower end of heart rate range
   $199 \times .90 = 179$ upper end of heart rate range

A second method that is probably the more widely used of the two heart rate methods for determining appropriate exercise intensity is a determination of the **heart rate reserve.** This method is based on a formula developed by Karvonen et al. in the late 1950s. According to **Karvonen's formula,** the heart rate reserve (HRR) is the difference between maximal heart rate (max HR) and resting heart rate (rest HR).

$$HRR = max\ HR - rest\ HR$$

For example, with a max HR of 199 and a rest HR of 72, we find:

$$HRR = 199 - 72$$
$$HRR = 127\ beats\ per\ minute$$

In the study by Karvonen and co-workers (1957), it was found that an amount of stress sufficient to elicit an adaptive response or training effect was placed on the cardiorespiratory system if the person kept his or her heart rate at 60 percent of the HRR. This was called the **threshold for training,** and it serves as the minimum intensity or low end of the heart rate range when using this method. To establish a range for appropriate intensity, we use 85 percent as the upper end.

Once you have established the values for 60 and 85 percent of the HRR, these must each be added to the resting heart rate to find the exercise heart rate range. Karvonen's entire formula for the threshold heart rate would be:

$$Target\ heart\ rate = (max\ HR - rest\ HR) \times .60 + rest\ HR$$

For the 21-year-old with a resting heart rate of 72 (which is about average), the calculation would be:

$$HRR = max\ HR - rest\ HR$$
$$= 199 - 72$$
$$= 127\ beats\ per\ minute$$
$$60\ percent\ HRR = 127 \times .60$$
$$= 76.2\ beats\ per\ minute$$
$$lower\ end\ of\ range = rest\ HR + 60\ percent\ HRR$$
$$= 72 + 76.2$$
$$= 148\ beats\ per\ minute$$
$$85\ percent\ HRR = 127 \times .85$$
$$= 108\ beats\ per\ minute$$
$$upper\ end\ of\ range = rest\ HR + 85\ percent\ HRR$$
$$= 72 + 108$$
$$= 180\ beats\ per\ minute$$

Table 4–1. Calculated Values of Heart Rate for the Percentage of Maximal Heart Rate and Heart Rate Reserve Methods*

	Heart Rate	
Percentage	Max HR Method	HRR Method
60	119	148
65	129	155
70	139	161
75	149	167
80	159	174
85	169	180
90	179	186

* For a 21-year-old with a resting HR of 72 beats per minute and a predicted max HR of 199 beats per minute.

Using the same percentage values in the two different methods produces dissimilar results. Some of these differences are noted in Table 4–1.

The heart rate range for exercise established by either of these methods sets upper and lower limits appropriately based on the relative stress on the cardiovascular system. Those persons just beginning an exercise program should work within the lower part of the range in order to gradually adjust to the program and avoid overdoing it, which may result in overfatigue, possible injury, and disappointment. The well-conditioned person must be equally aware of not exceeding the upper limits of the range. There are no demonstrated cardiorespiratory benefits to be gained by exceeding the established maximum intensity. There is considerable information about the overstress and chronic fatigue that can result from training at an intensity that is too great.

Heart Rate Determination. Establishing a heart rate range is the most practical and most frequently used method to determine appropriate exercise intensity. There are at least two good reasons why this is true. First, it is fairly easy for most of us to learn to monitor our own heart rates. Figure 4–1 shows the two most common sites at which to palpate or feel your pulse. Press lightly with your first three fingers on the location noted. On the inside of your wrist (either the right or left—although right is illustrated) press down half way between the center of your arm and the thumb arch edge—about one to two inches up from where your hand and arm meet. You should feel pulsations in the radial artery. On your neck press lightly with three fingers half way between your chin and beginning of your neck about one inch to either side of the middle (the figure illustrates the left side). Here you should feel pulsations in the carotid artery. The best time to establish your resting heart rate is just after you wake up in the morning but before you get out of bed. Take your pulse for 15 seconds and multiply by 4 to find the beats per minute.

When exercising it is very difficult to monitor your pulse. Stop exercising first, and while cooling down (keep moving slowly—see Dos and Don'ts, Appendix A) take your pulse as soon as possible. Fifteen seconds after stopping, your heart rate begins to decline. If you wait too long after stopping you will lose accuracy in determining your heart rate during exercise. To ensure accuracy you can take your pulse for only 10 seconds after exercise and multiply by 6 to get beats per minute. This value, of course, should be within the range discussed previously.

A second reason for the wide use of heart rate range in determining appropriate exercise intensity is its continued value as an indicator as we progress in our fitness programs. As you will see, a pace per mile, for example, is another method for establishing appropriate intensity. As we adapt and our cardiorespiratory system improves we must continually increase our walking or running pace, thus rendering our original determination of appropriate pace useless. The heart rate range does not vary, however. Regardless of the progress we make the heart rate required to stimulate an adaptive response remains the same.

Perceived Exertion.   There are other valuable methods used to determine exercise intensity. Some people who exercise regularly never take their heart rates during or after exercise. They seem to make progress without becoming overstressed. You may feel then that the need for an indicator of your working level or degree of overload is not really necessary—just something to fill pages in a book. In fact, those people mentioned are using a technique

Table 4–2. Borg Scale for Perceived Exertion *

HR Expected (for 20-year-old)	Perceived Exertion Rating	Description
60	6	
70	7	very very light
80	8	
90	9	very light
100	10	
110	11	fairly light
120	12	
130	13	somewhat hard
140	14	
150	15	hard
160	16	
170	17	very hard
180	18	
190	19	very very hard
200	20	

* When using this scale the subject is asked to identify by the number listed how he or she perceives the work.

Reprinted with permission from Borg, G.: Subjective effort in relation to physical performance and working capacity. In Pick, H. L., editor: *Psychology: From Research to Practice.* New York: Plenum Publishing Co., 1978, pp. 333–361.

of which they may not even be aware; it's called **perceived exertion.** There is a formalized system for measuring perceived exertion developed by Borg (1982), which is sometimes called the **Borg Scale** (Table 4–2). It gives a quantitative identification of the feeling of fatigue. These feelings of fatigue are very highly correlated with heart rate—the basis upon which Borg built his scale—as can be noted in the table. The heart rates listed are for a 20-year-old person. For those persons beginning a regular exercise program it is difficult to associate a feeling of fatigue with the expected heart rate based on the scale. As conditioning improves and a person becomes accustomed to the exercise requirements, it is fairly easy to associate feelings of fatigue with heart rate, even if that person doesn't realize it.

When using perceived exertion to identify an appropriate level of exercise intensity, a range of 13 to 17 is usually established.

Oxygen Consumption. A third method used to determine appropriate exercise levels is a determination of maximal working capacity or **maximal oxygen consumption ($\dot{V}O_2$max).** $\dot{V}O_2$max is the amount of oxygen a person is able to use for energy production when working at his or her maximal capacity. This maximal working capacity can be determined directly through the use of a maximal exercise test, which is commonly done on a bicycle ergometer or treadmill. Maximal exercise testing requires special expertise depending upon the age and health status of the person to be tested. Also needed is specialized equipment to obtain the results necessary for the accurate determination of appropriate exercise. Maximal working capacity, or maximal oxygen consumption, can be estimated from standard submaximal work evaluation protocols as well. Maximal and submaximal testing methods will be discussed in Chapter 9.

By knowing the maximal capacity or $\dot{V}O_2$max, we can determine an appropriate exercise intensity. The relative intensity at which a person should work will depend upon that person's present state of fitness, conditioning background, and goals for the exercise program. The range for the percentage of $\dot{V}O_2$max that will result in cardiorespiratory adaptation is 55 to 85 percent. As a practical application we would expect a cardiac patient, cleared to exercise by a physician, to begin his or her program at 55 to 65 percent. A conditioned endurance performer, however, is likely to gain from an intensity of 75 to 85 percent $\dot{V}O_2$max. For example Jim Jogalot's $\dot{V}O_2$max was 50 ml of O_2 used per kilogram of body weight per minute (ml/kg-min, the standard method of expressing $\dot{V}O_2$). Since Jim is young and healthy, then:

$$\text{Exercise Intensity} = .65 \text{ to } .75 \ (\dot{V}O_2\text{max})$$
$$= .65 \text{ to } .75 \ (50 \text{ ml/kg-min})$$
$$= 32.5\text{–}37.5 \text{ ml/kg-min}$$

The concept of prescribing exercise based on maximal working capacity or $\dot{V}O_2$max is made easier to understand and implement by use of the **MET.** MET is an abbreviation for *metabolic equivalent,* which is the oxygen cost required for rest, or 3.5 ml of oxygen used per kilogram of body weight per minute (3.5 ml/kg-min). That is, on the average, we can expect every person to use 3.5 ml of O_2 per kilogram of body weight each minute while at complete rest, or 1 MET. As a person exercises the oxygen cost could increase, for example, to 35 ml/kg-min or 10 METs (35 ÷ 3.5 = 10). In the example given above for Mr. Jogalot, the same information could be expressed in METs:

$$\dot{V}O_2max = 50 \text{ ml/kg-min or } 14.3 \text{ METs}$$
$$\text{Exercise Intensity} = 32.5\text{--}37.5 \text{ ml/kg-min or } 9.3\text{--}10.7 \text{ METs}$$

The values we obtain using oxygen uptake or METs must be translated into a usable form. Many studies have been done to determine the efficiency with which we exercise. From this information it has been determined that in many activities we require a certain amount of oxygen in order to accomplish a given amount of work. Table 4–3 gives the MET value and oxygen uptake required for walking or running at the pace listed. If your exercise intensity is to be 10 METs, you would need to run at a pace of 10 minutes per mile and would use 35 ml of O_2 per kilogram of body weight per minute. In the example we used previously, Jim Jogalot's exercise prescription using the table would be:

Exercise Intensity: 32.5–37.5 ml/kg-min or 9.3–10.7 METs
Pace for 32.5 or 9.3: 10:50
Pace for 37.5 or 10.7: 9:15
Pace Range: 9:15–10:50 per mile

Table 4–3. Relationship Between Walking/Running Times on Level Ground and Oxygen Uptake or MET Equivalent

METs	Oxygen Uptake (ml/kg-min)	Time/Mile Walk	Run	
3.0	10.5	23:00		
4.0	14.0	15:55		
5.0	17.5			←(Since the efficiency with which we walk or run
6.0	21.0			at these levels differs considerably among indi-
7.0	24.5			viduals, we cannot relate a time to an oxygen
8.0	28.0			uptake or MET equivalent.)
9.0	31.5		11:20	
10.0	35.0		10:00	
11.0	38.5		9:00	
12.0	42.0		8:08	
13.0	45.5		7:22	
14.0	49.0		6:47	
15.0	52.5		6:33	

Notice that in Table 4–3 there is a boxed area or range of exercise intensity for which no times are given. This exists because it has been determined that the efficiency difference, or the rate at which we use oxygen, at the speeds within that range is variable. Although no precise determination of the O_2 requirement can be made, we must somehow determine what would be appropriate. Several examples of how we might make this determination follow. Jim Jogalot wants to jog (naturally) so his prescription assumes he will run. If Jim's training rate were within this boxed area, in order to develop an appropriate level of exercise he would have to assume that he would use oxygen at the same relative rate as expected for the speeds that are outside this area, although some error should be expected. This boxed area is between speeds of 100 and 134 meters per minute or 3.7 and 5.0 mph. To avoid what may be incorrect assumptions when you find that your appropriate MET or $\dot{V}O_2$ level is within this range, use your heart rate, which is associated with a given level of work during the evaluation of working capacity. Figure 4–3 provides an example of how this could be done. The line plotted represents the heart rate for J. Jogalot for the associated level of work during a maximal graded exercise test. The work requirement is

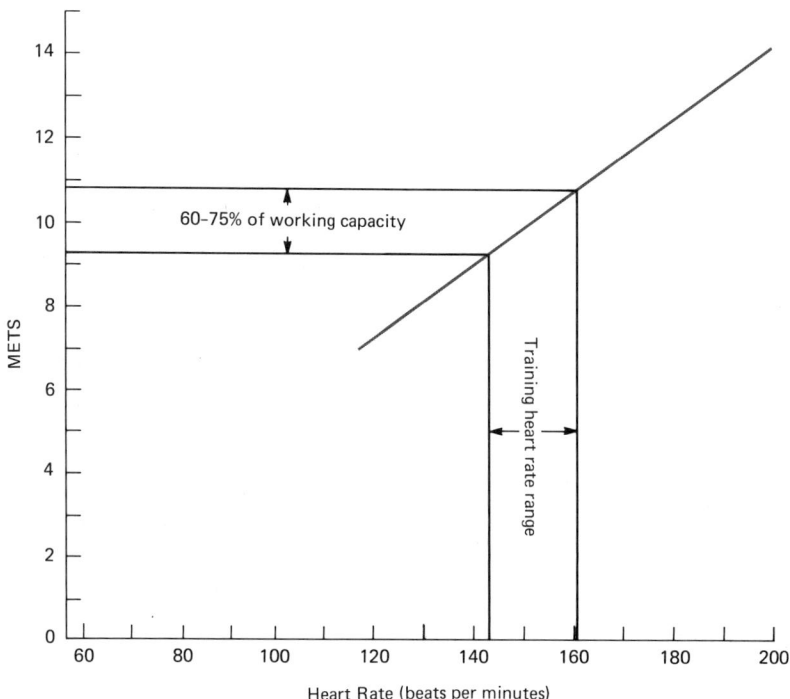

Figure 4–3. An example of the possible relationship between heart rate and MET level of work, and the method for determining heart rate range for exercise prescription.

expressed in METs in this graph but could be expressed in $\dot{V}O_2$ as well. At 9.3 METs (the previously determined intensity at the lower end of his training range), the associated heart rate was 143. At the upper end (10.7 METs), the heart rate was 160. This identifies the appropriate heart rate range in which Jim should train and is based on 65 to 75 percent of his maximal working capacity.

It is important to note that as you progress in your program of exercise training the initially established appropriate heart rate will remain valid as a criterion for assessing intensity. An initial pace (e.g., 2 miles in 24 minutes) will, of course, eventually become too easy to stimulate further cardiorespiratory adaptation and would need to be increased.

After three weeks of training following the guidelines provided, further changes in your cardiorespiratory system will be minimal. This means that you should increase either the intensity, duration, or frequency of exercise to make further improvement. No change in your pattern of exercise will mean that you will maintain your present level with little further improvement.

Modes of Exercise. In order for a type of exercise to provide cardiorespiratory adaptation it must involve large muscle groups, be rhythmical and continuous and at the same time provide an adequate but not too great intensity. Of no less importance is that the exercise activity be one that you can enjoy. The changes associated with training are short lived once that training has been discontinued. It is very important then to be able to choose a mode of exercise that you will look forward to continuing. In order to assist you in developing a program, we have listed a number of activities that can provide appropriate cardiorespiratory stimulation. A specific walk/jog program is provided first because of the relatively equal efficiency that we all have for this activity and because the requirements for special facilities and equipment are minimal. Methods of exercise training not included below are not likely to provide cardiorespiratory improvement unless the exercise can be done continuously for 20 to 30 minutes, during which time you maintain the appropriate exercise intensity.

Walk/Jog. A walking or jogging program provides an excellent means to obtain cardiovascular conditioning. Although many books have been written and entire courses are dedicated to enhancing our knowledge of running or jogging for fitness, the basic requirements are simple and the cardiovascular training effects unsurpassed. This is what makes these forms of cardiovascular conditioning the most popular and most highly recommended. You need appropriate clothes in which to run; this is discussed on p. 91 under environmental aspects. You will also need a pair of shoes (many types and brands are now available) that have been particularly designed for walking and jogging. Tennis shoes, comfortable street shoes, and the like can get you started, but in the long run (no pun intended) they may cause injury and frustration. A well-made pair of shoes of a reputable brand name is essential.

Although you can run just about anywhere, and many folks do, find a place where there is no traffic or at worst a minimum of cars passing you as you run. Popular running places include parks, bike paths, tracks, and streets and roads, although the latter pose a hazard of which you must be aware. Golf courses are popular running places too, although they pose at least one hazard.

While your efficiency, that is, the oxygen or energy cost, will vary slightly with different mechanics of walking or jogging, the differences are small. Adopt a comfortable style for jogging, being sure to land on the heel of your foot and to roll off the ball of your foot rather than running on your toes as a sprinter would. Relax your arms and breathe through your mouth and nose and you will probably be fine. Early in your program have an experienced runner, physical education teacher, or track coach take a look at your style so that any serious errors can be corrected.

Pages 85–88 include directions for a walk/jog program that has been designed to accommodate the novice as well as the well-trained participant. It provides you with progressive stages to follow as your conditioning improves.

You should start in the stage indicated by your actual or predicted maximal $\dot{V}O_2$. The chart provided in Table 4–4 indicates the appropriate stage in which to begin based on an assessment of $\dot{V}O_2$ max. This chart coincides with the values given in Table 9–2. Each stage has specific objectives that will serve as the exercise program for the participant. Remember to use HR range values to ensure appropriate intensity.

Within each stage the specific objectives are goals in themselves. Although he or she may not complete it at first, a participant should accomplish each

Table 4–4. Beginning Stages for a Walk/Run Program*

Age Range	Fitness Level				
	Superior	Excellent	Good	Fair	Poor
Men					
20–29	9	8	6	5	4
30–39	8	7	6	5	4
40–49	8	7	5	4	3
50–59	8	6	5	3	2
60+	7	5	3	2	1
Women					
20–29	7	7	6	5	3
30–39	7	6	5	5	3
40–49	6	6	4	2	2
50–59	6	4	3	2	1
60+	5	3	2	2	1

* Begin your program with the stage listed across from your age range and under your fitness level category.

objective successfully for three days before moving on to the next objective. Exceptions are the starred (*) objectives, which need only be done once. These starred objectives are self-assessment measures, which are ways of monitoring your progress. They may serve as specific indicators of your readiness to continue. It should be noted that each requires an effort that goes beyond the criteria necessary for training to occur. They might be considered similar to a track athlete's time trial, which is a practice race he or she runs to assess his or her present capability. Later stages provide many more of these self-assessment objectives. A person who can attain this level has a developed training program and needs a more comprehensive guide regarding the quality of his or her training. If you are unable to meet the time for a starred objective, go back one or two objectives and repeat them at a greater (faster) intensity, which should improve your capability of meeting the starred objective.

Progression through these stages should be gradual and slow. Pay careful attention to your training heart rate. Although a minimum of three repetitions of each nonstarred objective is required, three may not be optimal. Continue each objective until you feel comfortable in completing the task. Rest periods should be of sufficient length to allow you to become comfortable. Usually this will be about 3 to 5 minutes of slow walking. Walking periods in the upper stages may be eliminated, but do so with caution; they are included to provide a lower intensity needed by many.

Stage 1 Objectives:

 1. Walk for 10 minutes, rest 3 minutes, walk 10 minutes.
 2. Walk for 20 minutes.
 3. Walk 15 minutes, rest, walk ½ mile.
 4. Walk 1 mile, rest, walk 1 mile.
 *5. Walk ½ mile under 6:30 minutes, rest, walk 1 mile.
 6. Walk/run ¼ mile, walk 1 mile, walk/run ¼ mile.
 7. Walk 2 miles.
 8. Walk/run ½ mile, walk 1 mile, walk/run ½ mile.
 *9. Walk/run 1 mile (under 13:15 minutes), walk ½ mile, walk/run 1 mile.
   Go to Stage 2, Objective 3.

Stage 2 Objectives:

 1. Walk ½ mile, rest, walk ½ mile, rest, walk ½ mile.
 2. Walk 1 mile, rest, walk 1 mile.
 3. Run/walk 1¼ miles, rest, run/walk 1 mile.
 *4. Run/walk 1½ miles (under 20:15 minutes).
 5. Walk 2 miles.
 6. Run/walk 1 mile (under 12:00 minutes), walk 1 mile.
 *7. Run/walk 1½ miles (under 18:30 minutes).
   Go to Stage 3, Objective 3.

Stage 3 Objectives:

    1. Run/walk ½ mile, rest, run/walk ½ mile, rest, run/walk ½ mile.
    2. Run/walk 1 mile, rest, run/walk 1 mile.
    3. Run ½ mile (under 5:30 minutes), rest, run/walk 2 miles.
    4. Run/walk 2½ miles.
  5. Run/walk 2 miles (under 23:30 minutes).
    6. Run/walk 1 mile (under 11:00 minutes), rest, run walk 1½ miles.
  7. Run/walk 1½ miles (under 16:45 minutes).
      Go to Stage 4, Objective 3.

Stage 4 Objectives:

    1. Walk 1 mile, rest, run/walk ½ mile.
    2. Run ½ mile, walk ¼ mile, run ½ mile.
    3. Run ½ mile, walk ¼ mile, run ½ mile, walk ¼ mile, run ½ mile.
    4. Run/walk ¾ mile (under 8:00 minutes), rest, walk 1½ mile.
  5. Run/walk 1 mile (under 10:30 minutes), rest, walk 1½ mile.
    6. Run ¾ mile, walk ¼ mile, run ½ mile.
    7. Run 1 mile, rest, run/walk 1½ miles.
  8. Run/walk 1½ miles (under 16:00 minutes), rest, run/walk 1 mile.
      Go to Stage 5, Objective 3.

Stage 5 Objectives:

    1. Run/walk 1 mile, rest 10 minutes, run/walk 1 mile.
    2. Run ½ mile, walk ¼ mile, run ½ mile, walk ¼ mile, run ½ mile.
    3. Run ¾ mile, walk ¼ mile, run ¾ mile.
    4. Run ¾ mile (under 7:30 minutes), rest 10 minutes, run ½ mile.
    5. Run 1 mile, walk ½ mile, run ¾ mile.
  6. Run 1 mile (under 10:00 minutes), rest 10 minutes, run ½ mile.
    7. Run 1½ miles, walk ¼ mile, run ½ mile.
    8. Run 1¾ miles, walk ¼ mile, run ½ mile.
  9. Run 1½ miles (under 15 minutes), rest, celebrate and run ¾ mile.
      Go to Stage 6, Objective 2.

Stage 6 Objectives:

    1. Run 1 mile, walk ¼ mile, run 1 mile.
    2. Run 1½ miles, walk ¼ mile, run 1 mile.
    3. Run 1½ miles (under 14:30 minutes), rest 5–10 minutes, run 1 mile.
    4. Run 2 miles, walk ½ mile, run ½ mile.
    5. Run 2 miles (under 29 minutes), walk ¼ mile, run ½ mile.
    6. Run 2½ miles, rest 5–10 minutes, run ½ mile.
  7. Run 1½ miles (under 13:50 minutes), walk ¼ mile, run 1 mile.
    8. Run 2½ miles, walk ½ mile, run ¾ mile.
    9. Run 2 miles (under 18 minutes), walk ¼ mile, run 1 mile.
  10. Run 2 miles, walk ¼ mile, run 1 mile.

*11. Run 1½ miles (under 13:15 minutes), rest, celebrate and run 1½ miles.
Go to Stage 7, Objective 3.

Stage 7 Objectives:

1. Run 1½ miles, walk ¼ mile, run 1 mile.
2. Run 2 miles, walk ¼ mile, run 1 mile.
3. Run 2½ miles, walk ¼ mile, run 1½ miles.
4. Run 2 miles (under 17 minutes), walk ¼ mile, run 1½ miles.
5. Run 4 miles.
6. Run 1 mile (under 8 minutes), run 2 miles.
7. Run 4¼ miles.
*8. Run 1 mile (under 7:45 minutes), run 2 miles.
9. Run 4¾ miles.
*10. Run 1½ miles (under 12 minutes), run 2½ miles.
11. Run 5 miles, walk home.
12. Run 2 miles (under 16 minutes), run 2 miles.
*13. Run 1½ miles (under 11:30 minutes), walk ¼ mile, celebrate, run 2½ miles.
Go to Stage 8, Objective 4.

Stage 8 Objectives:

1. Run 2 miles, walk ¼ mile, run 1½ miles.
2. Run 2½ miles, walk ¼ mile, run 1½ miles.
3. Run 3 miles, walk ¼ mile, run 2 miles.
4. Run 2 miles (under 15:30 minutes), walk ¼ mile, run 2½ miles.
5. Run 5½ miles.
6. Run 1 mile (under 7:15 minutes), walk ¼ mile, run 3 miles.
7. Run 6 miles.
8. Run 3 miles (under 24:00 minutes), walk ¼ mile, run 2 miles.
9. Run 6½ miles.
*10. Run 1½ miles (under 10:15 minutes), walk ½ mile, run 3 miles.
11. Run 7 miles.
12. Run 2 miles (under 14:30 minutes), run 3 miles.
*13. Run 1½ miles (under 9:45 minutes), walk ¼ mile, run 4 miles.
Go to Stage 9, Objective 3.

Stage 9 Objectives:

1. Run 3 miles, walk ¼ mile, run 3 miles.
2. Run 4 miles, walk ¼ mile, run 2 miles.
3. Run 5 miles, walk ¼ mile, run 2 miles.
4. Run 4 miles (under 30:00 minutes), run 2 miles.
5. Run 6 miles.
6. Run 7 miles.
*7. Run 2 miles (under 13:30 minutes).

    8. Run 8 miles.
  *9. Run 5 miles (under 37:30 minutes).
 *10. Run 1 mile (under 6 minutes).
 *11. Run 2 miles (under 12 minutes).
 *12. Run 3 miles (under 20 minutes).
  13. Run 6 miles (under 44 minutes), run 2 miles.
 *14. Run 1½ miles (under 8:00 minutes).
        Go to Stage 10, Objective 2.

Stage 10 Objectives:

    1. Run 7 miles.
    2. Run 5 miles (under 35:00 minutes).
    3. Run 8 miles.
    4. Run 5 miles (under 33:00 minutes), run 3 miles.
  *5. Run 2 miles (under 11:00 minutes).
  *6. Run 3 miles (under 17:00 minutes).
    7. Run 6 miles (under 38:00 minutes), run 2 miles.
    8. Run a total of 90 miles in a 3-week period.
    9. Run a total of 45 miles in one week.
   10. Run a total of 60 miles in one week.
   11. Run a total of 75 miles in one week.

Swimming. The program for jogging could be adapted for swimming, although specific programs with general application are not usually given because of the varying efficiencies among swimmers. When we walk or jog, the efficiencies of different people remain approximately the same. That is to say, our use of oxygen to accomplish a given walking or jogging task is essentially the same. However, some people consider swimming survival in the water, while for others swimming seems to be a nearly effortless task. Since body weight is supported by the water, swimming places less stress on the hips, knees, and ankles. Because of this advantage, swimming can be used when minor injuries prevent you from running, walking, or cycling.

If you are a relatively good swimmer and would like to use the running program as a basis for your fitness program, then apply the 4:1 rule of thumb. The energy cost of swimming is about four times that of running so adjust the distance listed for running to ¼ and use the same time guidelines.

Bicycling. Cycling as a training mode has several advantages. It can be done outdoors or indoors on a stationary bicycle. Both have become very popular and are certainly appropriate means for producing cardiorespiratory endurance. Remember that putting in the time on your bike is not necessarily adequate. Therefore, you must meet the criteria established earlier with regard to frequency, duration, and, particularly, intensity. In order to adapt the training program provided for walking/jogging to cycling use the same times as a guide and multiply the distance by 2.5 times. Using this procedure, jogging 1 mile in 10:30 minutes (Stage 4, Objective 5) would translate into cycling 2½ miles in 10:30 minutes.

Safe, comfortable equipment is essential. The seat height should be adjusted so that your legs are fully extended (or nearly so) when the pedals reach the lowest point in their cycle. For beginners in particular a safe bicycle path is preferred to riding on the roads and competing for space with somewhat larger vehicles. Cycle clubs are becoming very popular. If there is a cycle club in your area contact it for information on places to ride, equipment shops, and planned trips or outings. Group activities are sometimes excellent motivations to continue your individual training program.

Stationary bicycles provide similar opportunities indoors, although the experience is considerably different. Some stationary bicycles have ergometers or "work meters," which are necessary for evaluation (see Chapter 9) but not for training. When using a stationary bicycle, it is wise to use your heart rate as a guide to determine if the intensity is correct. While pedaling rates on an outdoor bicycle for cardiorespiratory training usually fall between 70 and 90 revolutions per minute (rpm), keep your rate to 50 to 60 rpm on a stationary bicycle and adjust the wheel resistance to provide appropriate intensity.

Rope-Skipping. For the well-trained or highly accomplished person skipping rope may be a good cardiorespiratory exercise. It can also help with other variables of fitness and is used by many athletes who require coordination, agility, and balance to perform their sport well. The usefulness of rope-skipping as a general mode of cardiorespiratory exercise has not been established. It appears that those of us who have not used this method of training will find it of too great an intensity to be of cardiorespiratory value. For this reason, it is not recommended as an appropriate form of cardiorespiratory endurance training.

Aerobic Movement to Music. Choreographed dance routines that employ elements of ballet, jazz, and other dance forms in the gym or studio or in the water have understandably become very popular. Fitness criteria, particularly intensity, must be given special attention by exercise leaders in this area in order to avoid the pitfall of training at too little or too great an intensity. That the vigor of the routine can be adjusted to meet the needs of all participants and yet allow them to work together, that frequent short periods of low level exercise are used to assess heart rate response and then adjusted accordingly, along with the sheer fun make this a very desirable form of exercise training.

Other Modes of Exercise Training. Other successful training methods that have been used include cross-country skiing, circuit training, use of a parcourse, and walking or jogging on a miniature trampoline. Cross-country skiing may be the best form of cardiorespiratory training since it actively involves both the arms and legs in a rhythmical continuous manner. In order to use this mode of exercise, with its varying requirements (i.e., frequent changes in terrain, snow conditions, etc.) you would need to use your heart rate or perceived exertion as a means to adjust work intensity. Unfortunately, because of topographical and climatic conditions, this form of exercise can be used only to a limited extent in the United States.

Use of a parcourse is also becoming fairly popular and may be appropriate. Originally developed in Switzerland, a parcourse provides a course with stopping points at which are found directions for various exercise routines. There is considerable variation among those found in the United States and therefore it is difficult to assess their effectiveness. Many of the stations provide for improvement in other aspects of fitness rather than cardiorespiratory fitness. Because of the varying nature and the frequent stops, it is not recommended for the beginning exerciser as a sole source of cardiorespiratory training.

Walking or jogging in place on a miniature trampoline is another form of a cardiovascular training program. Although some questions about its effectiveness still exist, it appears to have the potential, if used properly, to elicit a training effect. As with any other means of cardiovascular conditioning, however, the minimum criteria for frequency, intensity, and duration of exercise must be met if a cardiovascular conditioning effect is to be expected. The "mini-tramp" or rebounder offers the advantages of needing only a small area, which makes it practical for use in the home, and eliminating much of the risk of injury associated with jogging or walking on a hard, unyielding surface.

Warm-up/Cool-down. Regardless of the mode of activity, your exercise prescription must include a period of reduced activity that will allow your body to get accustomed to the exercise you are about to do. A proper **warm-up** will provide you with the ability to tolerate the exercise session and assist in avoiding the negative attitude sometimes associated with training in its early stages. In addition, it has been shown that an appropriate warm-up will increase the temperature of your muscles, thus allowing them to stretch more easily and perform more efficiently. In order to be effective, the warm-up should include three kinds of activity: stretching exercises for flexibility; calisthenics to gradually increase the temperature of your muscles overall; and low level activity for 5 to 10 minutes of the specific type in which you will be engaged. Ordinarily a warm-up session should last approximately 15 minutes.

A **cool-down** period is also important after exercise. Never abruptly stop exercising. A low level of the activity just completed for about 5 minutes or longer will assist in the recovery from exercise and allow you to gradually return your cardiovascular system and working muscles to the pre-exercise state. Significant and dangerous sudden drops in blood pressure, for example, may occur after exercise if activity ceases without a gradual tapering.

Environmental Aspects. Appropriate exercise intensity as determined by the criteria previously noted in this chapter will need to be modified as the environmental conditions in which you exercise change. The precautions you must take are particularly important under the influence of high heat or humidity. You must decrease the intensity of your exercise, and perhaps the duration, when conditions are those to which you are unaccustomed. If you have established a given training intensity based on a time per distance covered, this will need to be modified. An established heart rate as an indicator of approximate intensity remains valid. This is because as we exercise in the heat the increased demand for cooling of the body is met by the circulatory system by increasing blood flow to the skin. In order to maintain sufficient blood flow to exercising muscles, our cardiac output must be increased commensurately. This adjustment in total cardiac output is attained by changes in heart rate. It is for this reason that heart rate will increase according to the effects of heat or humidity and can be used to ensure an appropriate training intensity.

Other precautions we can take to prevent various forms of heat illness include: (1) drinking about 15 ounces of water or a water preparation low in sugar content 30 minutes before exercise and about 5 ounces every 15 minutes during exercise; (2) limiting exercise intensity and duration for 5 to 9 days at the onset of changing environmental conditions (i.e., increased heat or humidity) to allow for acclimatization; and (3) wearing appropriate clothing to allow for maximal skin surface exposure (within the bounds of modesty, of course) to promote cooling.

Since exercise increases body temperature and those who exercise in cold weather wear adequate clothing for heat conservation, the effects of exposure to the cold are not generally of concern during exercise activities. Despite concern by some that exercise in very cold weather (below 15° Fahrenheit) will damage lung tissue, no evidence is available to support such a notion. Frostbite of exposed skin, particularly of the extremities, is a potential problem that requires appropriate protective clothing. Additional clothing will increase the cost of a given exercise task because of its additional weight and influence upon our mechanical efficiency. This means a somewhat decreased intensity of exercise will be necessary unless heart rate is the criterion being used to determine the appropriate intensity level. Failure to warm up properly before beginning exercise in the cold may also hinder your ability to maintain exercise intensity.

Some additional recommendations for cold weather exercisers, which are generally applicable and may increase your comfort on those cold days, would be to cover exposed skin on your face with petroleum jelly for protection, and head into the wind during the first half of exercise and go with the wind in the second half if you are unable to always keep the wind behind you. This reduces the chilling effect of wind on clothing that has become wet with sweat.

Exercise intensity must also be reduced as the altitude at which you exercise increases, particularly over 5,000 feet. The greater the altitude above this level, the more severe the limitation. As a general guide, you can expect your appropriate intensity for exercise to decrease about 3 percent for every 1,000 feet above 5,000 feet. Here again your heart rate response will change as the effects of altitude change and so heart rate as an indicator of intensity need not be adjusted. Although **acclimatization** will vary with the individual person and the altitude, it will require from 1 to 3 weeks.

SUMMARY

◇ The exercise prescription is an individualized plan to provide for adaptive changes in the cardiorespiratory system.

◇ The overload principle states that in order to obtain an adaptive response of the cardiovascular system we must make demands of this system that exceed those it normally encounters.

◇ The criteria for changes in cardiorespiratory fitness are frequency, intensity, duration, and mode of exercise.

◇ The minimum frequency of exercise is three days per week.

◇ The minimum intensity of exercise is 20 minutes per day.

◇ The appropriate intensity for exercise can be determined by: (1) heart rate range (relative to maximum heart rate) of 75 to 90 percent; (2) Karvonen's formula, which is target heart rate = (maximum heart rate − rest heart rate) × .60 + rest HR; (3) perceived exertion; and (4) an appropriate percentage, based on our conditioning level, of maximal working capacity.

◇ In order for the mode of exercise to be beneficial it must involve large muscle groups and be rhythmical and continuous. Included among the appropriate exercise modes are walking/jogging, swimming, cycling, and aerobic dance.

◇ When the three major forms of cardiovascular training are compared we find that when swimming for an equal amount of time as running one should go about ¼ the distance (4:1 rule of thumb) and when bicycling for an equal amount of time as running one should go about 2½ times the distance (1:2½ rule of thumb).

◇ A 10- to 15-minute moderate warm-up will improve performance and reduce the risk of injury.

◇ A cool-down after exercise will allow for a gradual return to resting levels and assist in recovery.

◇ The problems associated with exercising in a hot or humid environment can be reduced by: (1) drinking at 15-minute intervals; (2) allowing time for acclimatization; and (3) dressing appropriately.

STUDY QUESTIONS

1. What are the factors involved in the exercise prescription?

2. Discuss the overload principle as it applies to cardiorespiratory adaptation.

3. How is minimum intensity for exercise determined?

4. Why is there a maximum level for exercise intensity?

5. What is the recommended minimum frequency and duration of exercise?

6. Describe the relationship between heart rate and exercise load.

7. What is Karvonen's formula?
8. Discuss the use of heart rate range and perceived exertion as determinants of exercise intensity.
9. Design a program for yourself that would meet the criteria necessary to influence cardiorespiratory system adaptation.
10. Give the equivalent distances for bicycling and swimming for a 6-mile run.
11. List five activities that will produce cardiorespiratory adaptation.

REFERENCES AND SELECTED READINGS

American College of Sports Medicine: Guidelines for *Exercise Prescription and Training*, 2nd edition. Philadelphia: Lea & Febiger, 1980.

American College of Sports Medicine: Position Statement on the Quality and Quantity of Exercise. *Medicine and Science in Sports* 10:7, 1978.

Amsterdam, E. A.; Wilmore, J. H.; and DeMaria, A. N.: *Exercise in Cardiovascular Health and Disease.* New York: Yorke Medical Books, 1977.

Borg, G. A. V.: Psychophysical bases of perceived exertion. *Medicine and Science in Sports and Exercise* 14:377–381, 1982.

Fox, E. L.; Mathews, D. K.; and Barstow, J.: *Interval Training for Lifetime Fitness.* New York: Dial Press, 1980.

Fox, E. L.; and Mathews, D. K.: *The Physiological Basis of Physical Education and Athletics*, 3rd edition. Philadelphia: Saunders College Publishing, 1981, pp. 293–413.

Karvonen, M.; Kentala, E.; and Mustala, O.: The effects of training on heart rate. A longitudinal study. *Annales Medicinal Experimentales Biologial Fennial* 35:307–315, 1957.

Chapter 5
Muscular Strength and Endurance Fitness—Weight Training Programs

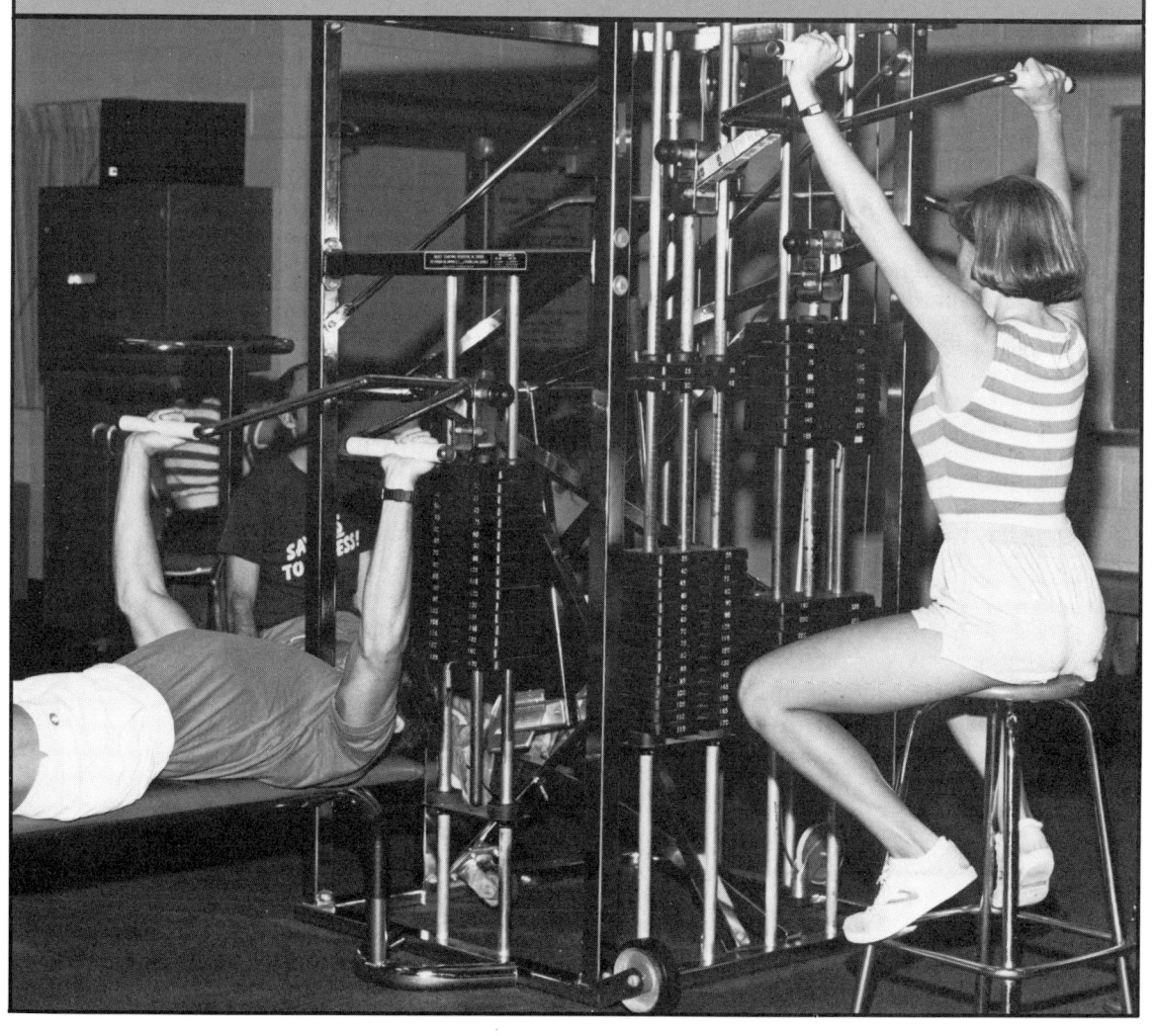

Chapter Outline

Learning Objectives

◇ To understand the principles basic to the development of a weight training program.

◇ To know the safety considerations important to the conduct of a weight resistance program.

◇ To distinguish between the types of muscular contraction and the effects of isotonic, isometric, and isokinetic training methods.

◇ To be able to develop a weight resistance program to meet your specific needs.

◇ To identify a series of weight resistance exercises that will provide a well-rounded program.

◇ To understand the unique potential value of circuit training as a muscular strength and endurance conditioning exercise.

◇ To understand the physiological changes that are associated with a regular weight resistance program.

◇ To understand the similarities and differences of response in men and women involved in weight training programs.

◇ To become aware of the different theories of the cause of delayed muscle soreness.

Key Words and Phrases

accommodating resistance
arrangement of exercises
circuit training
concentric contraction
delayed muscle soreness
eccentric contraction
fiber splitting
hypertrophy
isokinetic contraction
isometric contraction

isotonic contraction
mitochondria
overload
phosphagens
progressive resistance
repetition maximum
sets
specificity of training
testosterone
Valsalva maneuver

Introduction

T HE increasing number of facilities that provide weight training equipment and programs are testimony to the popularity of the use of weight resistance exercise. As you will see in this chapter, there are many beneficial effects from properly conducted weight training exercise programs, but some misconceptions also exist with respect to these programs. The myth still exists that as a result of a strength training program, men become muscle-bound or inflexible and women lose their feminine characteristics.

While the study of the implementation procedures and effects of weight training programs is an ongoing process, we have learned a great deal particularly from information gathered during the last 20 years. The purpose of this chapter is to provide a description of the principles and effects of weight resistance programs.

Guidelines for Program Implementation

There are a number of basic principles that must be considered when developing a weight training program (Table 5–1). You cannot proceed with a training program without remembering the basic concept that the results obtained from any program are dependent upon the specific nature of the training regimen. Any random program that involves lifting weights will not be adequate. As in any other form of exercise training, the product is dependent upon the process. As such, you should be particularly mindful of the following principles.

Overload Principle

Increases in strength are dependent upon placing a demand on a muscle that is greater than that which it normally encounters. Increases in strength are a result of the physiological adaptation of the muscle to a stress. In order for the various adaptive mechanisms of the muscle to respond, the stress applied must represent an **overload.** To realize an increase in strength then, whether a beginner to strength training or a seasoned veteran, you must impose a resistance greater than that to which the muscle has been accustomed. Not increasing resistance as the training program progresses will mean that you will maintain a given level of strength but will not increase your strength.

Table 5-1. Principles to Be Considered When Developing Weight Training Programs.

Basic Principles of Weight Training Program Implementation
Overload
Progressive resistance
Specificity
Arrangement of exercises
Frequency
Duration
Safety

Progressive Resistance Principle

In order to put the overload principle into effect, you should follow a progressive program. These two principles are closely related. **Progressive resistance** refers to a gradual increase in the resistance (overload) applied. Once the muscle adapts to the original load, the load cannot effect further progress. Progressive loads serve as appropriate stimuli for further adaptive increases in strength. The techniques described in this chapter under "Implementing Isotonic Weight Training Programs" are designed to assist you in developing a program that incorporates the principles of overload and progressive resistance.

Specificity Principle

The adaptation of the muscle to a weight training program can vary in many ways. The changes in strength will be different depending on several factors: the speed at which the exercise is done; the angle of the joint and whether or not the exercise is done throughout its full range of motion; the particular muscle or muscle groups that contribute to the movement; and, perhaps, the degree to which neural factors influence the exercise. These are important specific criteria to be considered, since they will influence the resulting muscle performance.

In order to meet the principle of **specificity of training,** a weight resistance program generally should include exercise patterns and speeds of movements that resemble as closely as possible those of the activity for which the person is training. For example, a shot putter (track and field) should do an incline bench press at approximately 45° rather than the more common bench press at 90° (see Figure 5–3) in order to produce movement patterns that resemble those of putting the shot. While it would be difficult to perform this exercise at speeds equal to or greater than those achieved in an actual shot put event, a shot putter may get speed specificity and perhaps improve technique and delivery by using an underweight shot (e.g., 10-pound shot for a high school shot putter). Studies with isokinetic testing equipment indicate that training isokinetically will improve strength at the speed at which the person trained and at lower speeds as well. Whether this concept can be applied to other modes of strength training is questionable, but attention should be paid to including in your program opportunities to challenge all of the principles outlined. While the principle of specificity also applies to a person with a general interest in achieving the benefits of weight training, the implications are different. As such, a highly speed- and muscle-specific program may not be needed.

Very few of the activities in which we are involved require strength at only a single joint angle. Most weight resistance exercises thus are done throughout the full range of motion of a joint. Doing so not only increases strength at all angles of the joint but also helps to maintain flexibility. This is one reason why isometric resistance training is limited in its application.

Arrangement of Exercises Principle

In order to obtain maximum benefit from a training session and to ensure consistency from day to day, it is wise to properly order your exercise routine. This generally means that exercises should be arranged so that those mainly involving the largest muscle groups are done first. This principle also refers to alternating upper and lower body exercises.

According to the **arrangement of exercises** half squats or leg presses would be done first, for example, then bench presses followed by toe raisers and wrist curls. This limited routine alternates upper and lower body exercises and proceeds from larger to smaller muscle groups.

Frequency

Sufficient evidence has been found to indicate that for most persons involved in a weight resistance program, and particularly for someone just beginning, a frequency of three times per week or every other day is optimum (O'Shea, 1976). It appears that muscles respond optimally to a day of relative rest between weight resistance exercise bouts. Those dedicated persons who train every day usually follow a pattern of upper body exercises on one day followed by lower body exercises the next.

Duration

The duration of resistance exercise training sessions will vary with the type and purpose of the program. Duration is not as important a principle here as it is with cardiovascular conditioning. Nevertheless, certain types of programs discussed in this chapter do have time restrictions that should be followed.

Safety

Safety is certainly an important consideration when participating in any program, and particularly in one that involves the lifting of weight greater than normally encountered. The following list of appropriate procedures will assist you in enjoying a safe weight resistance exercise program.

1. Always consult your physician before beginning a weight training program. There are some limitations or contraindications to weight training that may apply to you.
2. Never use weight training as a means of self-treatment. Any weakness or abnormal condition or injury should be properly diagnosed and treated by a professional trained in that area of medicine.
3. Proper clothing is essential. Wear loosely fitted clothes to avoid chafing and to reduce the risk of being snagged. Shorts and T-shirts are appropriate for general lifting. High top shoes with a rigid slip-free sole are best for footwear. Weight belts to maintain support of the lower back are useful but may not be a necessity for the beginning lifter. They are not a substitute for proper technique and will not protect the unwise lifter who ventures beyond reasonable limits.
4. Learn the proper technique for each exercise from a qualified instructor and follow that advice regardless of the influence of weight-room "experts."
5. Always warm up before each training session. Warm-up should include a general warm-up, e.g. stretching exercises and running in place for 10 to 15 minutes, and a specific warm-up. Before each exercise do three to five repetitions with a light weight for a specific warm-up.
6. In order to avoid inordinate changes in blood pressure associated with the **Valsalva maneuver*** maintain a constant breathing pattern. Do not hold your breath. The basic pattern most lifters follow is to exhale as the weight is moved away from the body (usually first phase of exercise) and to inhale as the weight is moved toward the body.
7. Starting a program should involve a break-in period of a week or two. During this period, use light loads to learn the technique well and to gradually introduce your muscles to this new experience. Gradual application of overload resistance will help in reducing the delayed soreness associated with beginning a weight training program.
8. Have a program of exercises planned daily and don't succumb to the lure of competition, which is often unspoken but always present in a weight room.
9. When using free weights be sure spotters are available, collars are fastened tightly, the weights are balanced properly, and chalk is used to ensure proper grip and reduce the chance of slipping.

* Valsalva maneuver: A forced expiration or pressure on the thorax with the glottis (trachea) closed.

Types of Weight Resistance Exercises

Weight resistance programs vary in their use of three basic types of muscle movements: **isotonic contraction, isometric contraction,** and **isokinetic contraction.** Each has effects that influence adaptive changes in the muscle in somewhat different ways. Each type has both positive and negative aspects to be considered. The following descriptions should be helpful in determining which particular type to use for your purposes. Note that although there is considerable information regarding the methods of implementation and effects of various programs, many unanswered questions still exist.

Isotonic Programs

Isotonic means the "same resistance." Free weight exercising is a popular method of isotonic exercise (e.g., barbells). Closely associated with this term and ordinarily considered to be part of this general heading is a weight training method called **accommodating resistance.** In this method the resistance varies throughout the range of motion but is dependent upon a fixed accommodation that cannot be tailored to meet individual force production capabilities. Weight training machines such as Universal Gym and Nautilus employ accommodating resistance. Whether the resistance is variable (Universal, Nautilus) or fixed (free weights), the tension developed is not maximum over the full range of motion. For example, when lifting a constant load the tension developed by the knee extenders varies according to the joint angle (Figure 5–1); the greatest potential to produce tension is at approximately 120° of flexion. While the accommodating resistance machines attempt to reflect this changing potential it is impossible to assess and provide for each person's tension-producing capabilities. Free weights are limited in that the amount of weight used must represent the most inefficient angle of pull.

Isotonic muscular contractions can be further classified as concentric and eccentric. A **concentric contraction** is one in which the muscle shortens while tension is developed. An example is lifting a load in your hand from a position in which your elbow is at 180° or straight and the load is at your side while you are in a standing position (Figure 5–2A). An **eccentric contraction** is one in which the muscle lengthens while tension is developed; this is sometimes referred to as negative work. The return of the load (Figure 5–2B) to the resting position is an eccentric contraction.

Implementing Isotonic Weight Training Programs. Weight resistance programs of isotonic exercises have varying designs but usually rely on repetitions of a given exercise, which are done in groups or **sets.** Early

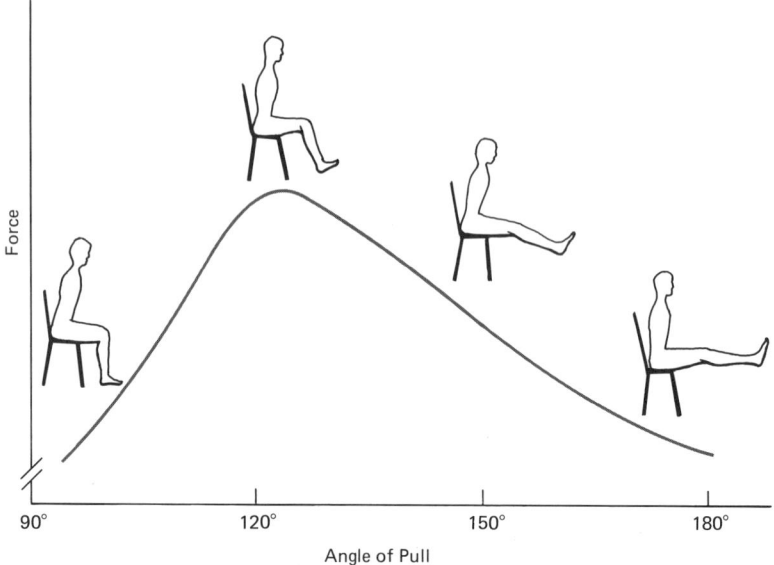

Figure 5–1. Force production or torque curve for the muscles of the thigh (quadriceps) that extend the leg.

studies of isotonic exercises for weight resistance training established the concept of repetition maximum or RM in order to employ the overload and progressive resistance principles. Today nearly everyone using free weights or variable resistance machines as a means for weight training uses

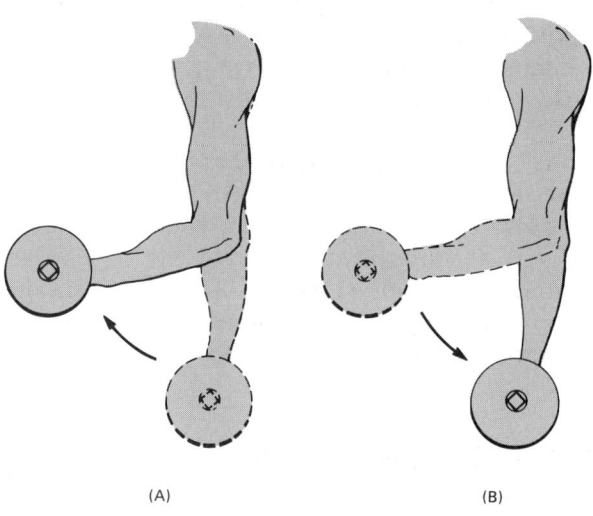

Figure 5–2. A contraction is: (A) concentric when the muscle responsible for the action (the biceps in this case) shortens during work; and (B) eccentric when the muscle lengthens.

(A) (B)

this concept of repetition maximum. A **repetition maximum** (RM) is the maximum load a muscle or muscle group can lift a weight a given number of times before fatiguing and thus be unable to continue. For example, if a person can repetitively lift a weight ten times and no more before fatiguing, then that weight is his or her 10 RM. All isotonic training programs use the RM concept; however, they vary in the number of repetitions used and in the number of sets to be accomplished. For example, the two basic programs that follow are used by two different weight training coaches.

College A	*College B*
Set 1—10 RM	Set 1—8 RM
Set 2—8 RM	Set 2—8 RM
Set 3—6 RM	Set 3—8 RM
Set 4—4 RM	

Of course, the weight that represents an RM for each person will vary and the weight each person uses will vary from exercise to exercise, but the basic program remains the same. At College A, the weight for each person will change as the number of repetitions decreases with each set. At College B the weight used would be the same for each set of eight repetitions.

The reason for the difference of opinion is that evidence gathered through controlled investigations does not provide a clear indication of the effects obtained from any given program. At one time it was generally believed, although very little supportive evidence existed, that three sets were optimum and that varying the weight directly influenced the changes in muscular adaptation; that is, 2 to 4 RM loads resulted in strength gains while 8 to 12 RM loads were generally used to improve muscular endurance. Strength was measured by a person's ability to perform a single RM, while many investigators measured endurance by the total time subjects were able to sustain an exercise with a fairly light load at a given frequency of repetitions (e.g., 40 repetitions per minute).

Since that time, research results have led to the conclusion that significant strength gains in an isotonic program may be made by using from one to six sets with loads that vary the repetitions from 2 RM to 10 RM. Since time is a factor for many general conditioning programs, it is suggested that one set of 10 RM be used. An example of a basic free weight isotonic weight training program requiring a single set is found in Table 5–2 (see p. 104). A complete description of each exercise listed in Table 5–2 is provided in Figures 5–3 to 5–11.

For those persons with more time who wish to have a well-rounded program, we suggest doing three sets and within those three sets a total of 24 repetitions. Each set would use the same load with an undefined number of repetitions (i.e., do as many as possible in each set) taking 1½ minutes rest between sets. If the total number of repetitions exceeds 24, then on

Table 5–2. Basic Isotonic Exercise Program Starting Loads.

Exercise	Beginning Load	Repetitions
Bench press	50 percent maximum	10
Lateral raises, lying (dumbbells)	5–10 pounds each	10
Lateral raises, standing (dumbbells)	5–10 pounds each	10
Standing press	30 percent maximum	10
Arm curl	25 percent maximum	10
Triceps extension	25 percent maximum	10
Side bend (dumbbells)	10–20 pounds each	10
Leg press/half squat	50 percent maximum	10
Toe raises	50 percent maximum	10
Sit-ups (bent knee)	Incline then weight held on chest	20

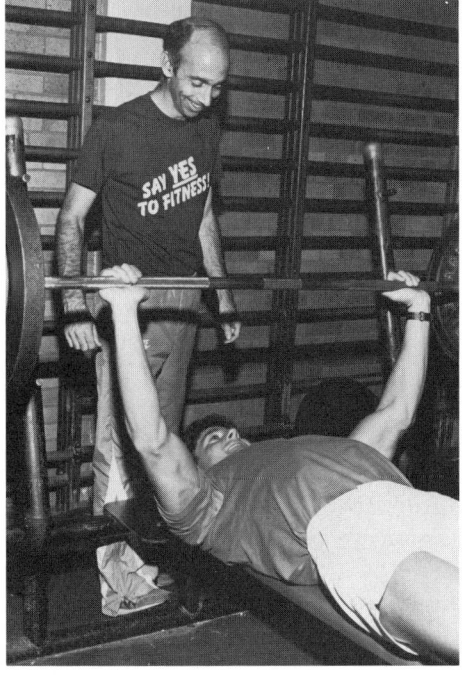 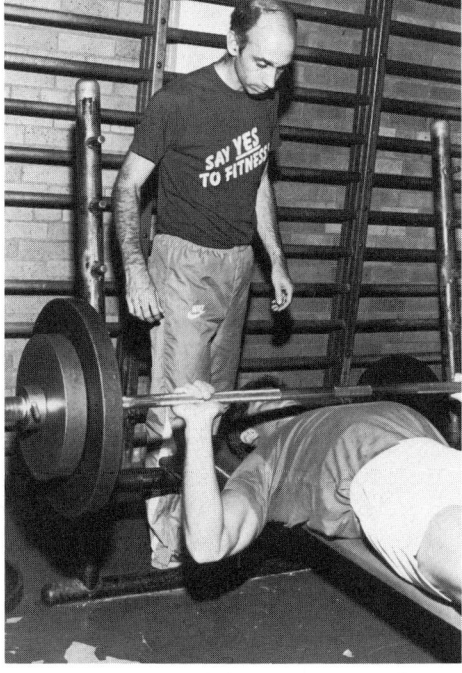

(A)   (B)

Figure 5–3. Bench press. (A) Lie on your back on a bench, holding the barbell over your chest with your arms extended, shoulder-width apart, and your hands in a pronated (overhand) grip. (B) Lower the barbell to your chest and return. Return to start and repeat. Exercises the anterior chest and posterior upper arm.

your next exercise day the load should be increased. The exercises listed in Table 5–2 provide an appropriate well-rounded program. In any program using more than one set, the recommended time period between sets is usually 1 to 3 minutes.

Figure 5–4. Lateral raises (lying). (A) Lie on your back on a bench holding a dumbbell in each hand. (B) With arms straight, but not locked, raise the dumbbells from the floor to touch above your chest. Return to start and repeat. Exercises the anterior chest.

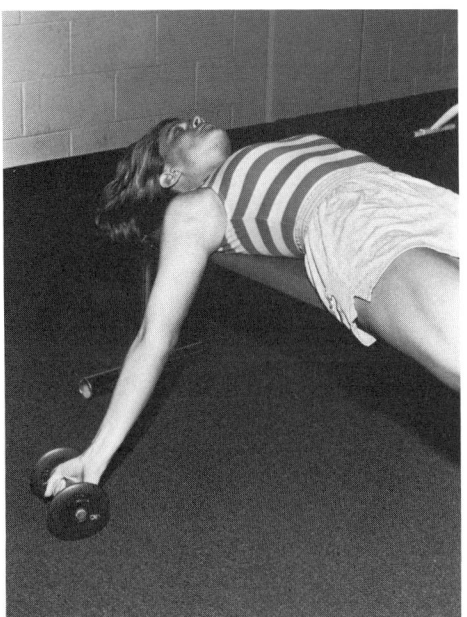

(A)

(B)

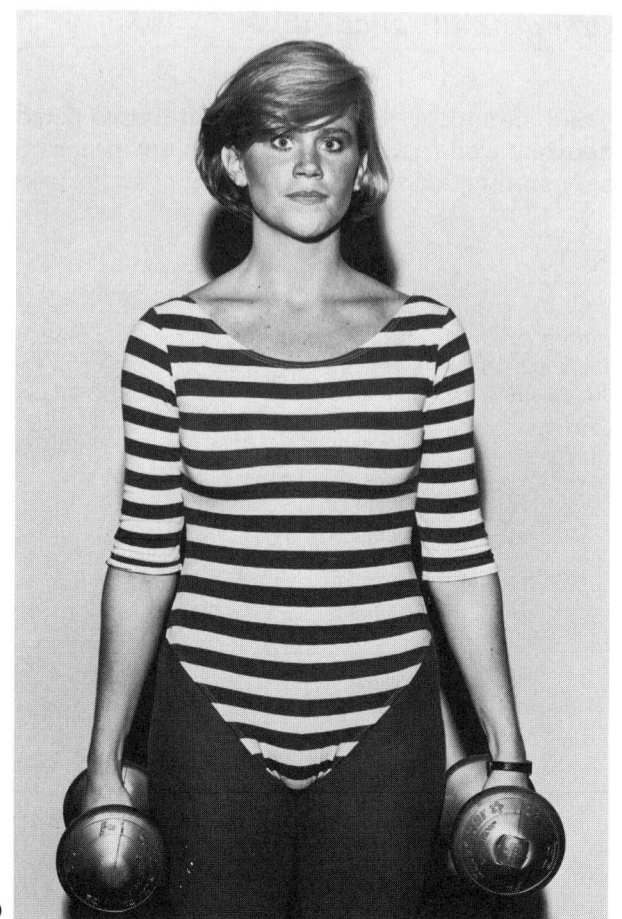

(A)

Figure 5–5. Lateral raises (standing). (A) Stand erect with arms at your sides and dumbbells in each hand. (B) Raise the dumbbells laterally with your arms straight to about shoulder level. Return to starting position and repeat. Exercises the superior shoulder.

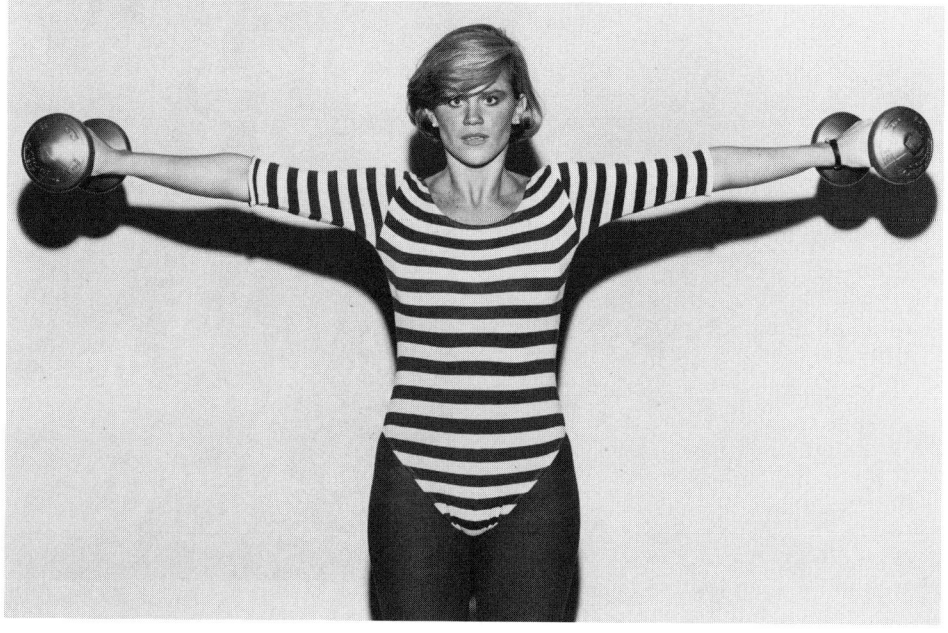

(B)

106

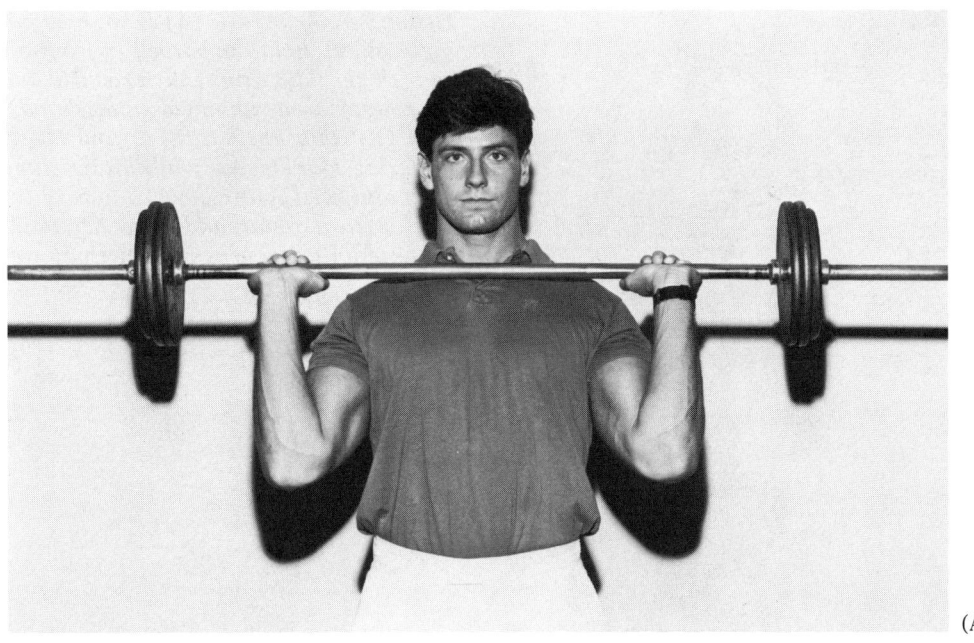

Figure 5–6. Standing press. (A) Stand erect and hold the barbell in front of your chest in a pronated (overhand) grip with the hands about shoulder-width apart. (B) Raise the weight overhead by fully extending the arms, then return. Keep your back straight and do not bend your knees. Exercises the posterior upper arm and superior shoulder.

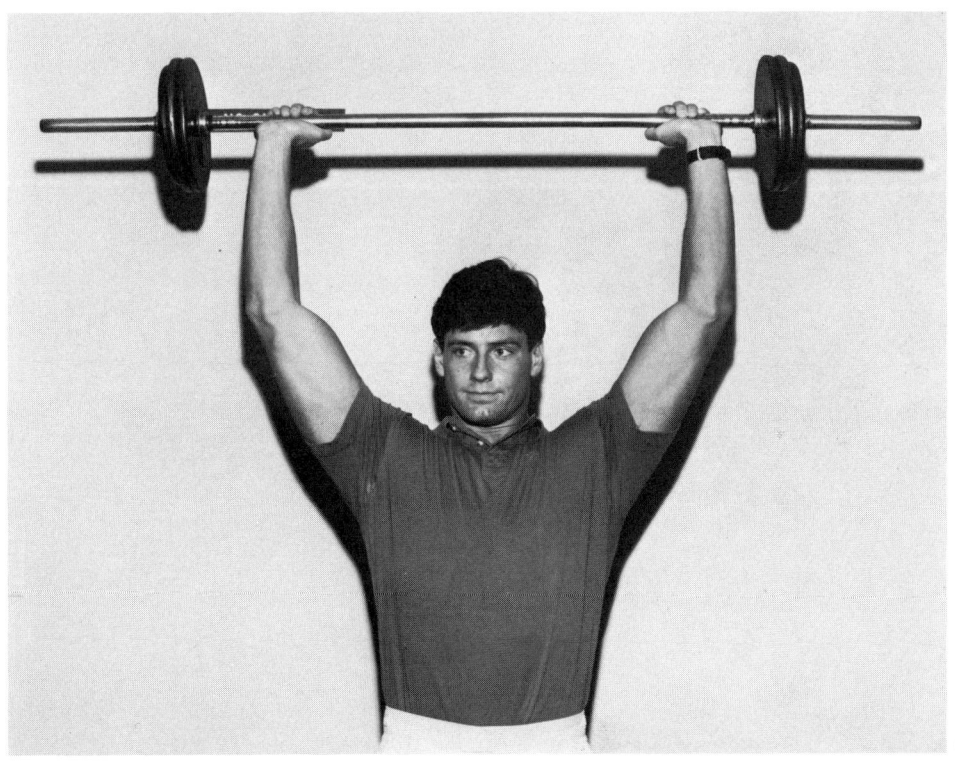

(B)

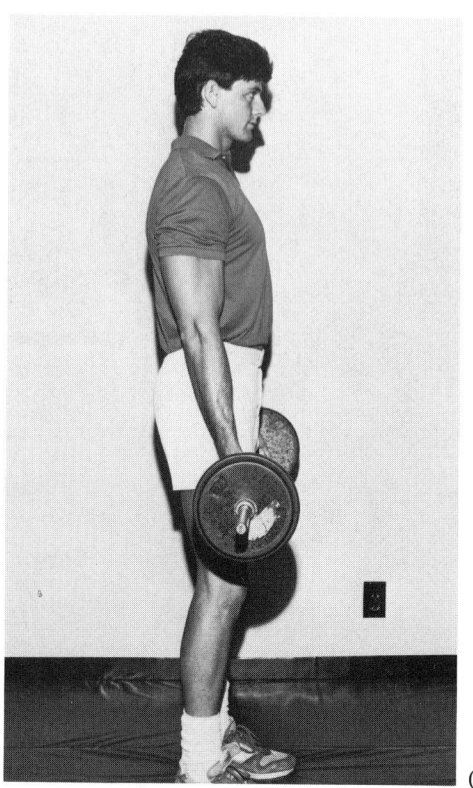

Figure 5–7. Arm curl. (A) From a standing position, hold the barbell in front of your thighs with arms fully extended and your hands in a supinated (underhand) grip. (B) Raise the barbell to your chest by flexing your elbows. While lifting, stand erect and keep your elbows in toward the sides. Return to start and repeat. Exercises the anterior upper arm and anterior lower arm.

(A)

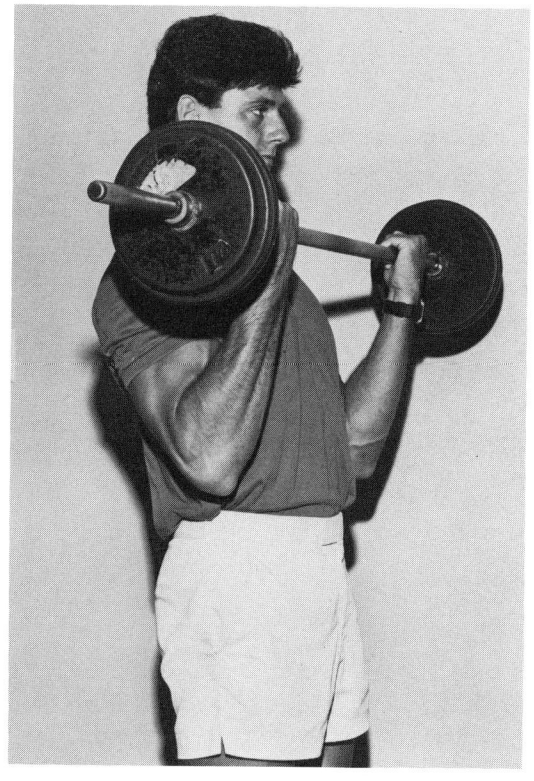

(B)

Figure 5–8. Triceps extension. (A) Lie on your back on a bench holding the barbell with a pronated (overhand) grip, resting the bar on the bench behind your head. (B) Raise the bar directly above your chest, arms extended. Return to start and repeat. Exercises the posterior upper arm and anterior shoulder.

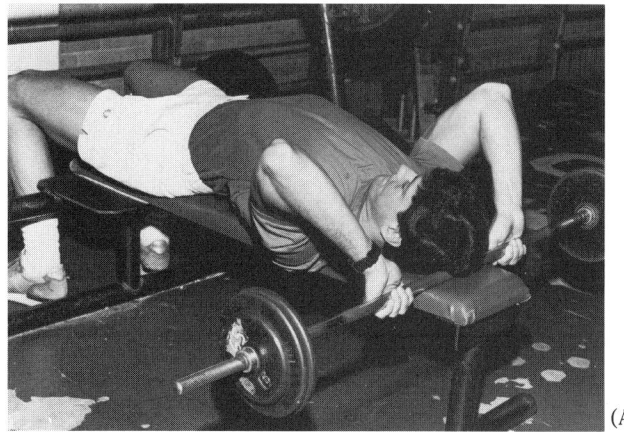

(A)

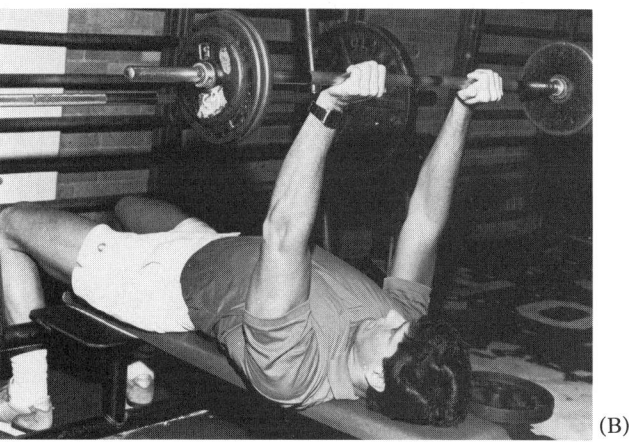

(B)

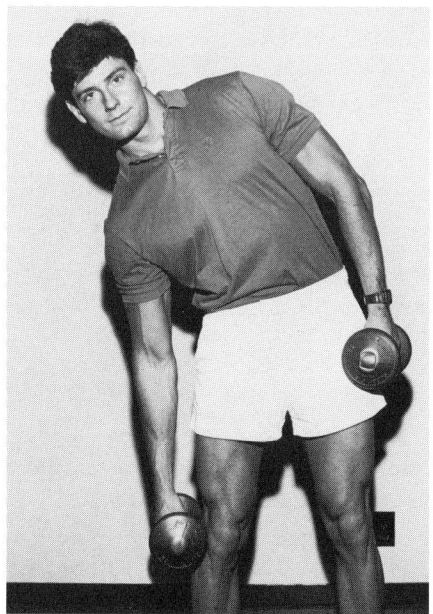

Figure 5–9. Side bend. Standing with a dumbbell in each hand and without bending forward, lean to each side alternately. Repeat. Exercises the lateral trunk.

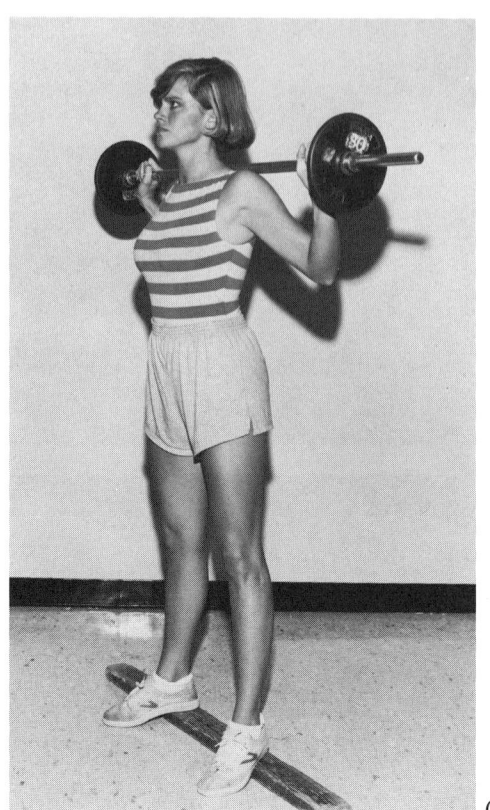

Figure 5–10. Half squat. (A) Standing erect, place the barbell on your shoulders behind your neck. Your hands should be in a pronated grip and far apart. (B) Keeping your back straight, lower the weight by flexing your knees to a 90-degree angle and return. Repeat. Exercises the back and anterior upper leg.

(A)

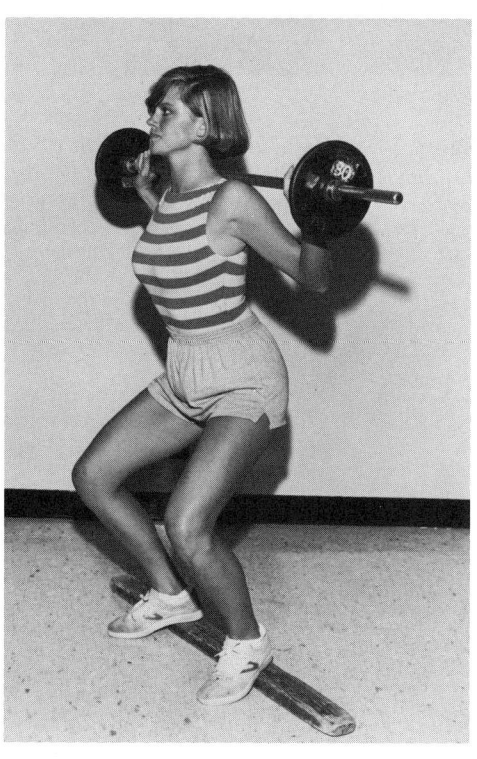

(B)

110

Figure 5–11. Toe raises. (A) Standing with your feet 8 inches apart and the balls of your feet elevated on a 2-inch board, place the barbell behind your neck and across your shoulders. (B) Rise up on your toes to full extension. Return to start and repeat. Exercises the posterior lower leg.

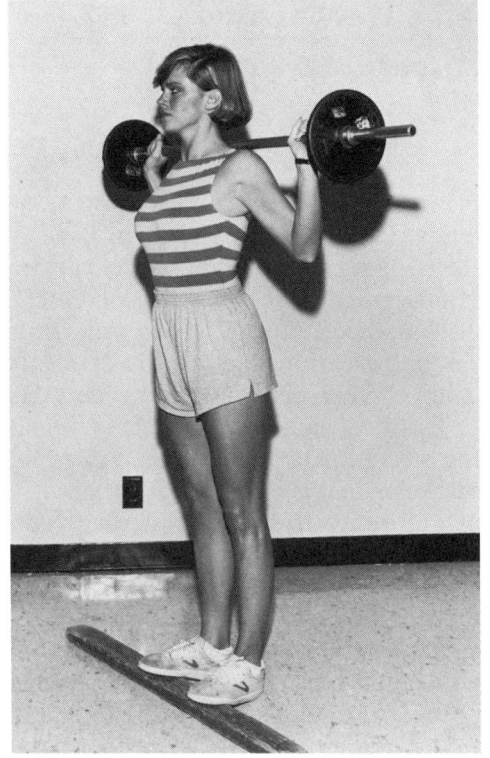

(A)

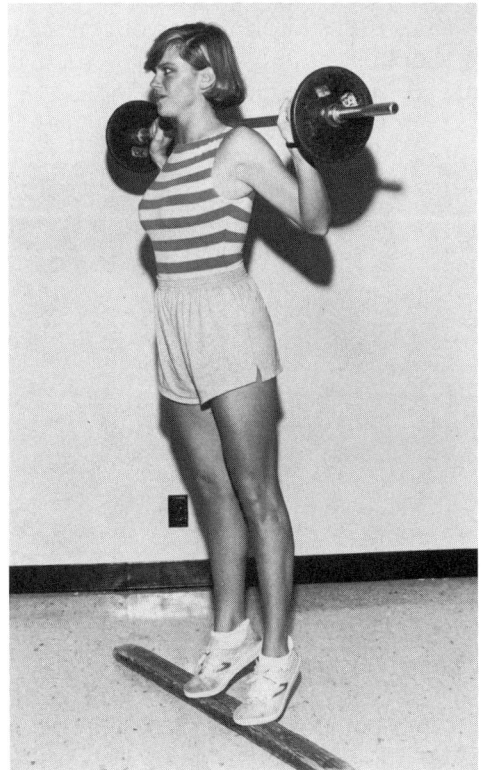

(B)

111

Isometric Programs

Isometric muscular contractions are performed against an immovable resistance (Figure 5–12). The term itself means "same length" and refers to the unchanging length of the muscle during contraction. There has been a considerable amount of investigation into the appropriate number and intensity of isometric contractions in order to determine the most effective program. The information gathered is certainly not conclusive, but some aspects of isometric exercise have been identified.

The most significant aspect is the lack of effect isometrics have on improving strength throughout the range of motion. As you might expect, based on the principle of specificity there is very little increase in strength at angles of pull other than the angle at which the isometric training has occurred. Perhaps the most practical application of isometrics would involve contractions at four or five different angles across the full range of motion of a joint. In any case, a 5- to 10-second maximal contraction repeated five times appears to be the optimum procedure to obtain maximum effectiveness from an isometric program. Using a program such as this, the strength gains seen at the angle used for isometric training are significant.

It should be noted that isometric exertion is more stressful to the cardiovascular system than dynamic work. Isometric exercise results in larger increases in systolic and diastolic blood pressure and requires a greater amount of work by the left ventricle. As such, isometric exercise may not be appropriate for some people.

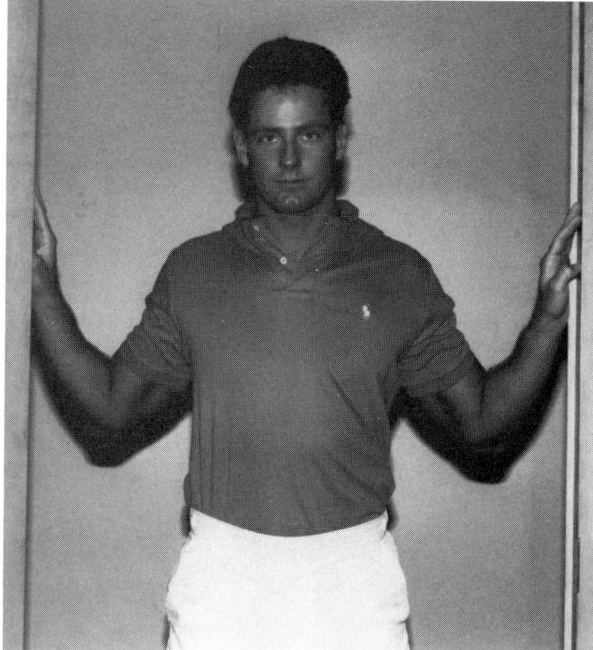

Figure 5–12. An example of isometric contractions.

Isokinetic Programs

The use of isokinetic contractions is a relative newcomer to the field of resistance exercise and seems to be the most effective for many purposes. The term means "same movement," indicating that an **isokinetic contraction** is one in which maximal tension is developed throughout the full range of joint motion by having the speed of movement fixed. The principle behind a fixed speed is based on the relationship between velocity of movement and force generation capability (force–velocity relationship). Simply stated, the faster the speed of movement, the less force one is able to produce. For example, a feather can be pushed across a room very quickly but little force is required to do so. If, however, you were to push an automobile (even a subcompact) across a room, you would move it much more slowly than the feather and expend a large amount of force in the process. To maintain a constant speed of contraction requires specialized and relatively expensive equipment, which makes the use of this mode of resistance training prohibitive for most. Isokinetic equipment has provided a much more controlled method of assessing the effectiveness of resistance training programs,

Figure 5–13. Isokinetic contraction assessment using the Cybex II dynamometer.

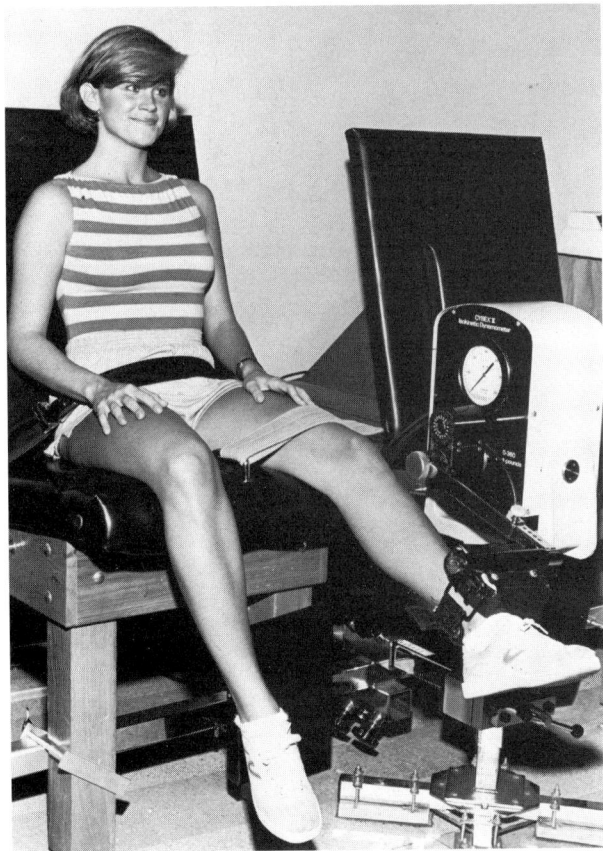

Table 5–3. Comparison Evaluation and Ranking of the Types of Resistance Training Programs.*

Type of Program	Range of Motion	Speed/ Force Production Specificity	Rate of Strength Gain	Safety Factors	Cost of Equipment	Use By Groups of 10 or More	Ease of Use for Beginner	Soreness Level Associated
Isotonic								
Free weights	3	3	3	3	2	2	4	4
Variable resistance	2	2	2	2	3	3	1	3
Isometric	4	4	4	4	1	1	2	2
Isokinetic	1	1	1	1	4	4	3	1

* Each mode is evaluated and ranked in comparison with the others listed based on its potential. A score of 1 = most desirable, 4 = least desirable.

114

as well as a valuable diagnostic tool for determining muscle function variables (Figure 5–13). Maximally stressing a muscle at every angle of pull and providing specificity with regard to speed of movement meet principles that are difficult if not impossible to attain with other forms of weight resistance exercise. The movement patterns used in training should simulate as closely as possible the movements of the athlete's event. The training speed should be as fast or faster than that required for performance. Studies using isokinetic equipment have indicated that strength gains occur at the speed used for training as well as at slower speeds (Fox, 1983). The number of repetitions, which are always maximal contractions, should be between eight and fifteen, with three sets of each exercise.

A ranking of each of the methods for weight resistance training according to some variables of concern is provided in Table 5–3. Each mode has strengths and weaknesses but the type of muscular training that is ranked the highest is isokinetic training.

Circuit Training

Circuit training consists of stations that include different weight resistance exercises and possibly cardiovascular conditioning exercises done in sequence with little rest between each exercise. Circuit training has become popular for a number of reasons. The development of weight training apparatuses that have multiple stations (e.g., Universal Gym) and do not require the handling of plates, as is the case with barbells, has provided an effective way to deal with a group of people and allow for short periods of exercise and rest. The numbers of people involved in group classes at weight training facilities of schools and colleges have made this form of weight resistance training desirable. Add to this the opportunity this method provides to vary the exercise, and we can see that such a program would have considerable appeal to an instructor of a group, regardless of the requirements of the group. Recent research has indicated that circuit training done properly and including stations that potentially improve the cardiovascular system may increase muscular strength, endurance, and cardiovascular endurance.

Although there is considerable variety among the various circuit training programs, most follow these general guidelines.

1. As with other weight resistance programs, the frequency of training should be three times per week or every other day.
2. Usually the circuit should be completed two to three times per session.
3. Six to fifteen stations should be included in the circuit.
4. The load for each weight resistance exercise should be 40 to 55 percent of a single RM.
5. The number of repetitions accomplished at each station should be 75 to 100 percent of the maximum number attainable in the work period.
6. The work period should be 15 to 30 seconds long and the rest period (time to change stations) 15 to 60 seconds long.

Table 5–4. Example of a Circuit Training Program.

Frequency:	Three times per week
Circuits per session:	Two
Load:	50 percent of 1 RM load
Number of repetitions:	Maximum possible in 30 seconds
Work/Rest ratio:	30 seconds/30 seconds

Station	*Exercise*
1 2 3	3 minutes continuous pedaling on stationary bike
4	Bench press
5	Leg press
6 7 8	3 minutes continuous rope skipping
9	Bent knee sit up
10	Standing press
11 12 13	3 minutes continuous jogging in place on mini-tramp
14	Arm curl
15	Pull down (lat machine)

When implementing a program of circuit training, keep in mind that as you adapt with increases in strength and endurance, the makeup of the program must vary as well in order to follow the principle of progressive resistance. For example, more stations must be added, or the load or number of repetitions increased in order to create overload.

An example of a typical circuit training program can be found in Table 5–4. The program presented here is designed as an overall conditioning program that provides opportunities for increases in strength in the major muscle groups and possible improvements in cardiovascular conditioning. Remember, as with any weight resistance exercise program, circuit training should be preceded by an appropriate warm-up period including flexibility exercises.

Effects of Weight Resistance Programs

The most notable change that occurs with resistance training is an increase in muscle size; this is called **hypertrophy.** There is little question that the strength of a given muscle or muscle group is very closely related to the cross-sectional area. Training will increase the diameter of the individual muscle fiber by increasing the number of myofibrils per fiber, increasing the total protein, and increasing the size of connective tissue of the muscle.

There has been some information published recently that supports the idea that hypertrophy of a muscle may be caused by an increase in the number of fibers as well as the changes mentioned above. The increase in fiber number is the result of a process called **fiber splitting** in which some fibers split longitudinally to become two functionally separate fibers. This evidence has come only from studies in animal populations, and discussion over those results continues. It is difficult to say that such a change occurs in humans but it is possible (Fox, 1983).

It should be noted that much of the increased muscle size that occurs with training is the result of selective hypertrophy of fast twitch (FT) motor units, which were discussed in Chapter 2. Since these motor units are the ones called upon to perform the work, for the most part, it is understandable why most of the change would occur here. No evidence has yet been presented to indicate that the ratio (by number) of FT fibers to slow twitch (ST) fibers is changed. The characteristics of myofibrils of a motor unit are determined by the nerve that innervates them. Since the dominating characteristics of the nerve are unchanged by the training program, no interconversion of fiber types occurs. Resistance training also produces some important biochemical changes in the muscle. The concentration of **phosphagens** (ATP/PC), which are, of course, highly responsible for energy production during weight training, may increase. Little or no changes have been found in enzymes associated with the anaerobic systems, however.

The conclusion that can be drawn based on the above changes is that improvement in muscle function is the result of hypertrophy and perhaps of associated adaptations of the nervous system, such as changes in fiber recruitment patterns, synchronization of motor units, and the overcoming of nervous inhibition factors.

Another biochemical change that takes place in muscle is a decrease in the density of **mitochondria** when muscle fiber diameters are increased without an appropriate stimulus to increase the capacity of the aerobic system (Fox, 1983). This results in a decreased ability to do aerobic work. It is for this reason that it is recommended that persons involved in a weight resistance program maintain an appropriate aerobically stimulating program as well.

Certainly body composition changes are expected as a result of a weight resistance program. Lean body weight, particularly muscle mass, will increase and there will be a reduction in body fat as well. For some, this may mean no change in total weight or an increase in weight. Weight resistance exercise is an excellent method to increase lean weight and total weight. For a more detailed discussion of body composition and weight change, see Chapter 8.

In principle, women respond to a weight training program essentially the same as men. Women do have less hypertrophy than men largely because change in muscle size is mediated by the hormone **testosterone,** which is present in much lower levels in women.

Delayed muscle soreness is an effect of some modes of weight training, particularly for a beginner or when a new overload has been added. Delayed muscle soreness is the pain that peaks about 24 to 48 hours after the exercise. The cause of this soreness is still a subject of study but three theories have been advanced (Abraham, 1977):

1. Direct damage to muscle fiber tissue may be the cause of soreness.
2. Spasms of the muscle, which cause ischemia (reduced blood flow), result in pain and precipitate a cycle of spasm-pain-spasm.
3. Damage to the connective tissue that runs throughout the muscle may be responsible.

The connective tissue damage theory seems to have the most support from recent studies, but none of the theories has provided a clear answer to a painful problem.

There are a couple of interesting notes about resistance training and soreness. Its onset for the beginner is usually inevitable, greatest following eccentric exercise, and virtually nonexistent following isokinetic exercise. Some reports suggest that a program of light exercise, particularly gradual stretching of the affected muscle groups, will help to alleviate the soreness.

SUMMARY

◇ In order to ensure the effectiveness of a weight resistance program we must implement the principles of overload, progressive resistance, specificity, arrangement of exercises, frequency and duration.

◇ Safety considerations important in weight training are: (1) be sure you have no medical limitations; (2) seek professional help for injuries; (3) wear appropriate loose fitting exercise clothes; (4) learn proper techniques; (5) warm up; (6) do not hold your breath; (7) start gradually; and (8) have a planned program.

◇ Weight training programs may use isotonic, isometric, or isokinetic types of contraction.

◇ Isotonic programs involve concentric and eccentric contractions and utilize the concept of repetition maximum (RM) and sets. RM is the maximum load that can be lifted a given number of times before the muscle or muscle group becomes fatigued.

◇ Isometric programs involve force production against an immovable resistance.

◇ Isokinetic programs require expensive equipment but provide the best results by maintaining a speed of contraction while allowing for maximal resistance at all angles of pull. No eccentric or negative work is done.

◇ Circuit training can accommodate large groups safely and provides a cardiovascular benefit.

◇ Weight training increases muscle fiber diameter and connective tissue size with a suggested possibility of increasing fiber number or fiber splitting. Other changes with a weight resistance program include an increased concentration of phosphagens, enhanced effect of nervous influence, and an increase in lean body weight.

◊ Delayed muscle soreness, which peaks 24 to 48 hours after exercise to which we are unaccustomed, may be caused by damage to muscle fibers, connective tissue damage, or muscle spasm.

STUDY QUESTIONS

1. List the basic principles underlying the development of a weight training program.
2. What is specificity as applied to weight training?
3. Give three examples of how you might employ the principle of specificity for a shot putter.
4. Discuss the safety principles to be followed particularly when starting a weight training program.
5. Define isometric, isotonic, and isokinetic muscular contraction.
6. Choose a method of weight training (isotonic, isometric, or isokinetic) and explain why it is the best to use.
7. What is the difference between muscular strength and endurance?
8. How can circuit training have an effect on cardiovascular endurance?
9. List the expected changes resulting from a weight training program.
10. Why are the strength capabilities of women, on the average, less than those of men?
11. List the three theories of delayed muscle soreness.
12. List ten weight training exercises that provide good overall improvement in strength and endurance.

REFERENCES AND SELECTED READINGS

Abraham, W.: Factors in delayed muscle soreness. *Medicine and Science in Sports* 9:11–20, 1977.

Falls, H. G.; Baylor, A. M.; and Dishman, R. K.: *Essentials of Fitness.* Philadelphia: Saunders College Publishing, 1980.

Fox, E. L.: *Sports Physiology*, 2nd edition. Philadelphia: Saunders College Publishing, 1983, pp. 123–161.

Kearney, J. T.: Resistance Training: Development of Muscular Strength and Endurance. In E. J. Burke (ed.): *Toward an Understanding of Human Performance.* Ithaca, NY: Monument Publications, 1980.

Laubach, L.: Comparative muscular strength of men and women: A review of the literature. *Aviation Space and Environmental Medicine* 47:534–542, 1976.

O'Shea, J. P.: *Scientific Principles and Methods of Strength Fitness*, 2nd edition. Reading, MA: Addison-Wesley Publishing Co., 1976.

Vitale, F.: *Individualized Fitness Programs.* Englewood Cliffs, NJ: Prentice-Hall, 1973.

Westcott, W.: *Strength Fitness.* Boston: Allyn & Bacon Inc., 1982.

Chapter 6
Muscular and Joint Flexibility

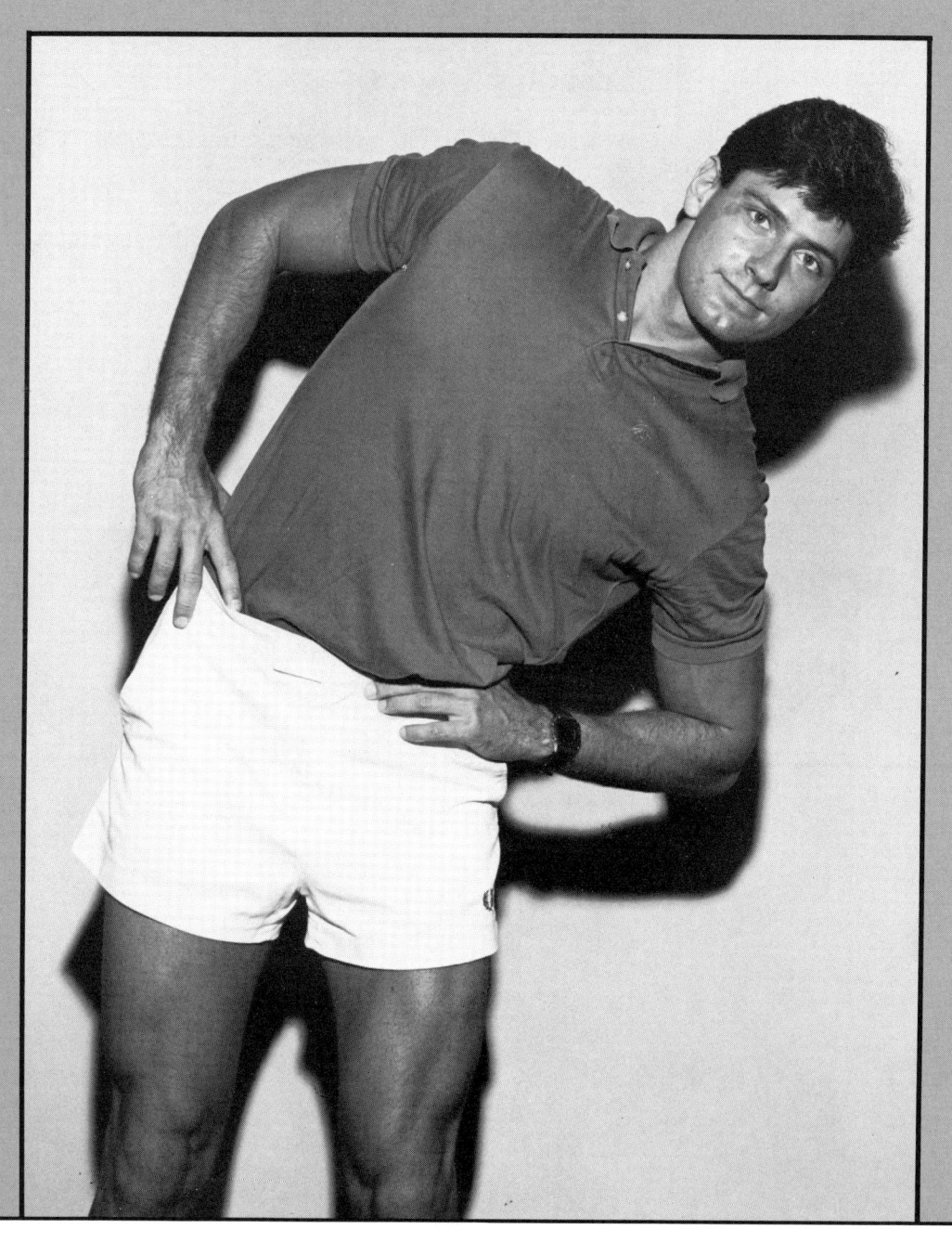

Chapter Outline

Learning Objectives

◇ To understand the importance of developing and maintaining optimal flexibility.

◇ To understand the factors that may inhibit flexibility.

◇ To understand the possible relationship between nonspecific low back pain and poor hip flexibility.

◇ To learn stretching exercises that will maintain optimal flexibility.

◇ To learn the appropriate procedures to follow to implement a safe and effective stretching program.

Key Words and Phrases

antagonist muscle groups
ballistic stretching
dynamic flexibility
elasticity
flexibility

Golgi tendon organs
muscle spindle
range of motion
static flexibility
static stretching

Introduction

S TRENGTH and endurance are not the only properties of a muscle that have implications for performance and fitness. Flexibility is also an important component of fitness. It may be that the lack of flexibility contributes to many of the nonspecific orthopedic and muscular problems we associate with growing old as well as to many injury problems of the young. Of interest regarding flexibility are the following factors: (1) the normal **range of motion;** (2) the causes of restricted motion; and (3) methods that can increase the range of motion. Of interest to us as well is the importance of maintaining an optimum range of motion. Keep in mind that, just as is the case for muscular strength and endurance, the potential for flexibility varies from person to person and from joint to joint.

Definitions

Flexibility is simply defined as the range of motion of a joint. This is technically the definition for **static flexibility** as opposed to **dynamic flexibility,** which is the opposition or resistance of a joint to motion. Dynamic flexibility is an interesting concept but of little concern to us in our discussion of flexibility. A term sometimes confused with flexibility is **elasticity,** which is the quality of the property of muscle and connective tissue (or any other material) to immediately return to its original size or shape. It is possible to become too flexible and to negatively influence the elastic property of muscles or connective tissue and thereby become vulnerable to injury.

Limitations to Flexibility

There are a number of factors that decrease flexibility. The structural limits to flexibility as mentioned previously differ among people but are generally the result of the combined effects of bone (the potential range depends on joint type), muscle, connective tissue, ligaments, and other structures associated with the joint capsule, and skin. Of course, each of these factors contributes to the inhibition of flexibility differently. Disregarding the limits imposed by bony structures, we find that the soft tissue associated with the joint capsule and the muscle belly provides nearly 90 percent of the resistance of a joint to flexion. The contribution of the tendon to this resistance is at the extremes of the range of motion. These soft tissues (muscle, joint capsule structures, and tendon) will respond to stretching exercises, and their limitations can thus be improved.

It poses no problem for a 4-year-old boy or girl to sit on the floor, legs straight in front, and place his or her head between the knees and on the floor. Since very few adults can still achieve that feat does age effect our flexibility? As we grow older our joints probably do inherently lose some of their capabilities to move through the full range of motion, but most of the problem lies not with our age but our failure to maintain a stress on the factors that influence range of motion. Just as we have seen in other areas, failure to challenge a structure results in atrophy—in this case inflexibility. The muscles, joint capsule structures, and tendons will adapt to imposed demands at any age.

Other factors that can contribute to decreased flexibility include joint disorders and injury. In most of these cases a series of appropriate stretching exercises prescribed by a physician will improve the limited range of motion. In some cases appropriate stretching exercises are essential for normal function.

We sometimes hear that weight training causes you to be muscle-bound and decreases your flexibility. This is not the case. A properly conducted weight training program that includes moving the resistance through a full range of motion will in fact improve flexibility. The combination of strength and flexibility in well-trained gymnasts is an example. Just as in the case of any training program, it is useful for the weight trainer to spend a certain amount of time specifically on flexibility exercises.

Importance of Flexibility and Stretching Exercises

Optimal flexibility has been shown, through research, to have many significant benefits. It not only enhances our ability to perform certain skills but recent developments in physical medicine and various forms of rehabilitation indicate that regular programs of stretching may enhance our general health and physical fitness. Regular stretching exercises are an essential part of every serious athlete's training program in that they will help an athlete to perform up to his or her capability and reduce the risk of muscular injury.

Some **antagonist muscle groups** (i.e., muscles that work in opposition to each other) have an inherent imbalance; one group is responsible for extension and the other is responsible for flexion. This circumstance exists, for example, in the muscle groups that flex and extend the lower leg. The quadriceps muscle group responsible for knee extension is able to produce approximately 60 percent more force than the hamstring group, which flexes the knee. This can create a potentially dangerous situation in high power activities such as sprinting. The performer who has not taken care to ensure optimal flexibility of both muscle groups, particularly the hamstrings, increases the risk of injury. Add to this the efficiency of movement demon-

Table 6–1. AAHPERD Health Related Physical Fitness Test Components.

Cardiorespiratory function
  Mile run or 9-minute run
  A 1½ mile run or 12-minute run are optional for students
    13 years of age or older
Body composition (leanness/fatness)
  Sum of triceps and subscapular skinfold
Abdominal and low-back hamstring musculoskeletal function
  Modified, timed sit-ups
  Sit and reach

strated by the flexible athlete versus the inflexible athlete and sufficient evidence is present to encourage those who train regularly to include stretching exercises as part of their routines.

There is some evidence that delayed muscle soreness, which was discussed in Chapter 5, may be relieved by a regular stretching program during the period of soreness and may be lessened by a stretching program before the activity that causes the muscle soreness to occur (Fox, 1981).

The American Alliance for Health, Physical Education, Recreation, and Dance (AAHPERD) has developed a health related fitness test (Table 6–1). You will find that one of the variables measured is hip and back flexibility. The reason such a test has been included is the strong relationship that exists between nonspecific lower back pain and poor hip joint flexibility. Chronic low back pain must be evaluated by a physician before any attempt can be made to alleviate the problem. Often an increased use of stretching exercises along with weight control and strengthening of the abdominal musculature will alleviate the pain. The AAHPERD has recognized the problem and the solution and has attempted to provide an assessment for elementary and secondary school pupils to teach them the usefulness of stretching and to encourage them to maintain good flexibility throughout life.

Flexibility or Stretching Exercises

Stretching exercises have been developed to improve the range of motion of all the pertinent joints in the body. The reason so many different exercises have been developed is the specific influence of each exercise. A good stretching program should be one that includes a wide variety of exercises to gain or maintain an optimum range of motion overall. Figures 6–1 through 6–17 describe stretching exercises that provide a good overall flexibility program. Each of these exercises when done properly will improve the flexibility of a given muscle group and associated joint structures. Each of the exercises must be done to improve overall flexibility.

What is the proper procedure to follow when implementing a stretching program? There are two methods that can be used to do these stretching exercises. One is **static stretching,** which involves a gradual lengthening of the muscle group to be stretched and then holding the final stretched position for a period of time. The other method is **ballistic stretching,** which involves quick forceful action to increase the stretch of the muscle and an immediate return to resting or near resting length. Ballistic stretching is sometimes characterized as having a "bobbing" motion. Both methods seem to improve flexibility although the extent to which each causes improvement is not clear. It is clear that the static stretching method is preferred and recommended. The reasons for using static stretching are (1) there is less chance for injury since the momentum of the movement is negligible and it will not overcome built-in protective mechanisms in muscle tissue; and (2) less soreness results from this type of stretching. Static stretching appropriately challenges muscle sense organs by stretching the **Golgi tendon organs,** which are located within the tendon of the muscle. This results in the inhibition of contraction or a relaxation of the muscle group being stretched. When ballistic stretching is used another muscle sense organ, the **muscle spindle,** which is within the belly of the muscle, is activated and causes a contraction response of the muscles being stretched. This is counter-productive.

Static stretching should be done so that the movement is done very slowly and gradually until the maximum position is attained. This position should be held for 10 to 15 seconds. Do not hold your breath during this time, but maintain a normal breathing pattern. Each exercise can be repeated two or three times and the entire group of exercises repeated 3 to 5 days per week. It is helpful during each exercise if you concentrate on relaxing the muscle group being stretched. Some of the exercises in Figures 6–1 to 6–17 use gravity to assist in the stretching phase. A possibility for lengthening the degree of stretch is the use of a "buddy" system (Figure 6–18). Your buddy must be fully aware of your limits so as not to cause overstretching of the muscle. You are advised to use this system with extreme caution since it has the potential for injury.

Flexibility exercises can be most productive and least stressful if they are preceded by a light warm-up. Such a warm-up might include 5 to 8 minutes of brisk walking before beginning your stretching routine and then stretching through 60 to 80 percent of the range of motion before each exercise.

There has been considerable discussion over the proper time to do stretching exercises. Some feel that stretching is best done before another activity, for example, before your daily run. Others believe that stretching is most effective after the activity. If your activity will be done at a high level, for example, interval sprinting or a race or competitive event where you will be called upon to work throughout your full range of motion, then stretching before the event may be useful as a part of the warm-up. To generally increase overall flexibility, however, it makes little difference when your stretching exercises are done.

Figure 6–1. Neck rotation. Move your head in a circular pattern, first to one side and hold, then to the front and hold (chin down), then the other side and hold, and then back and hold.

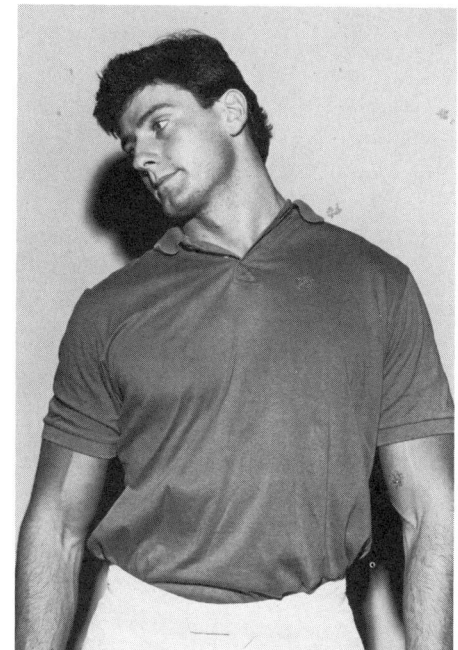

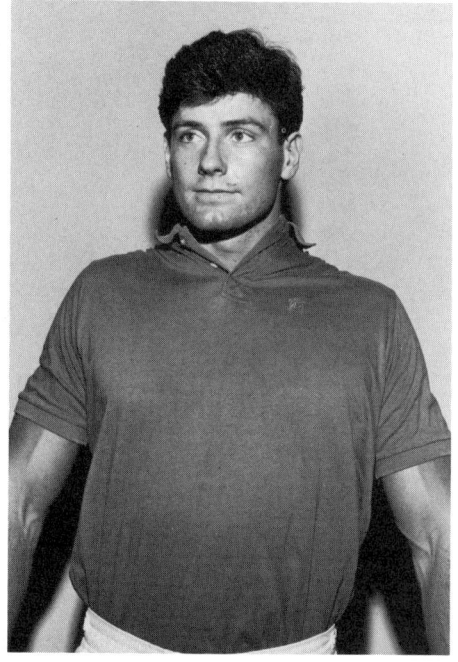

Figure 6–2. Shoulder girdle rotation. Move your shoulders back and hold, then up and hold and then forward and hold.

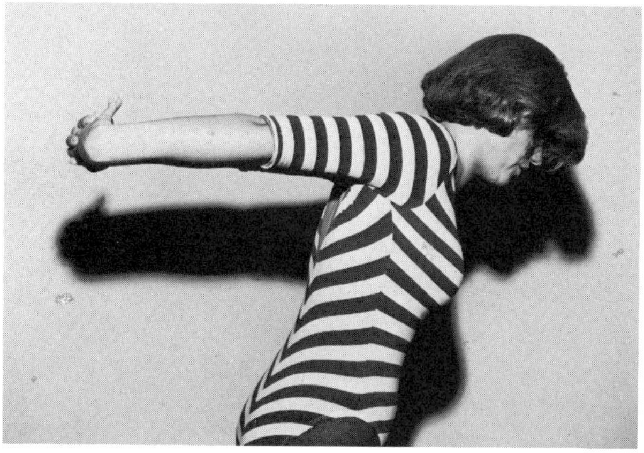

Figure 6–3. Behind back arm raise. With a towel or your hands clasped (if you are flexible enough) raise your hands up behind you. Remain standing erect.

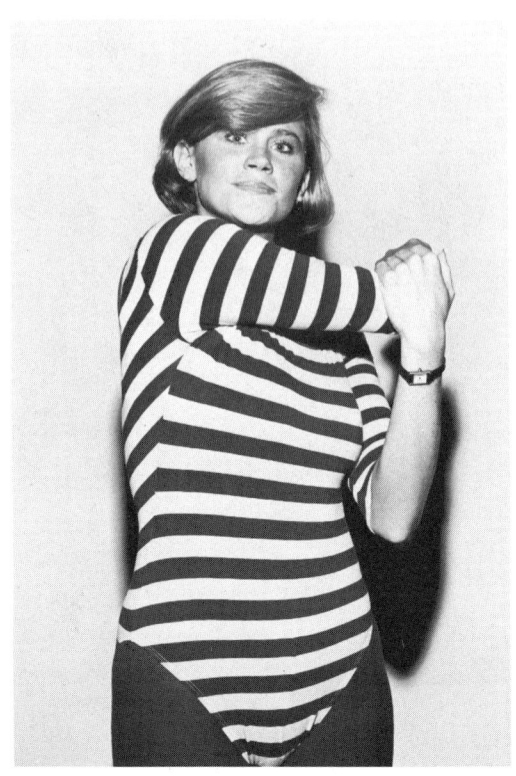

Figure 6–4. Shoulder girdle stretch. Grasp your elbow with the opposite hand and pull gently to the opposite shoulder.

Figure 6–5. Lateral flexion. Flex the trunk first to one side and hold, then repeat to the other side and hold. Do not twist the spine.

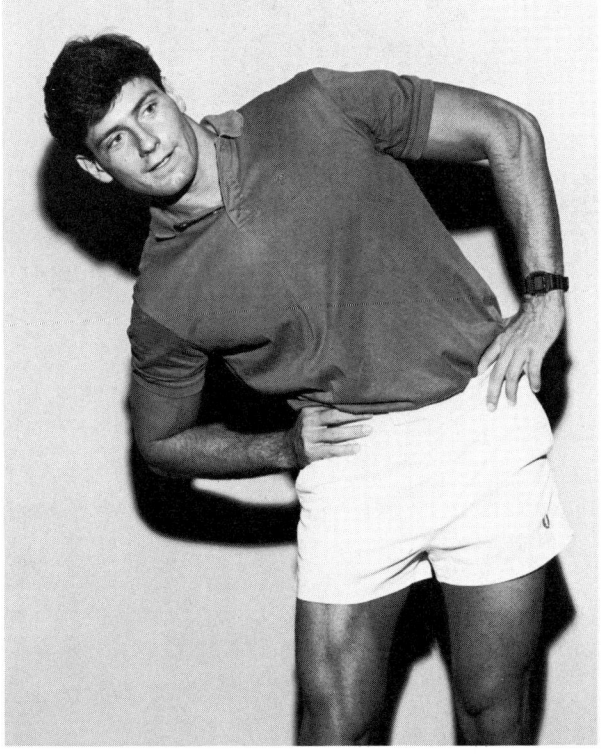

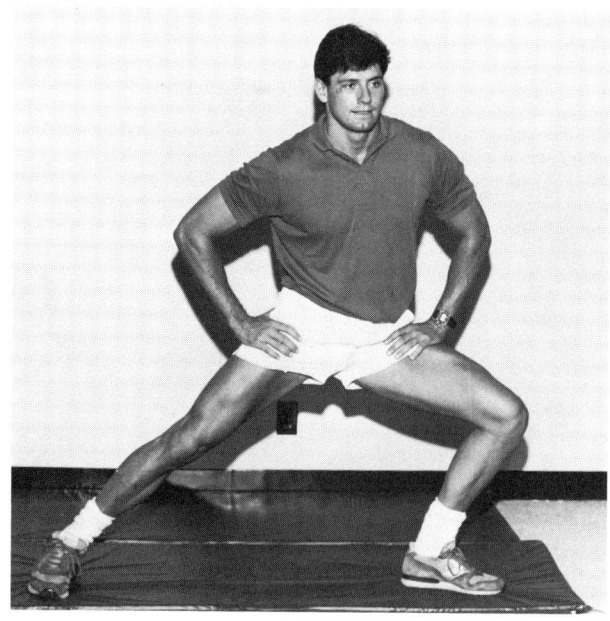

Figure 6–6. Side lunge. With your feet spread wide, turn one foot perpendicular and shift your weight in that direction and hold; then repeat to the other side and hold. Keep your hips facing forward.

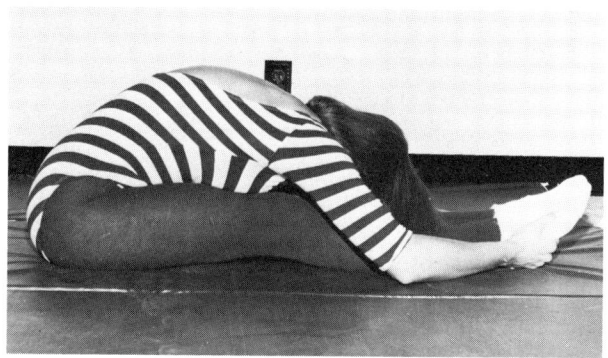

Figure 6–7. Sitting toe touch. Keep your knees straight but not locked. Reach toward your feet. Keep your back rounded, not flat.

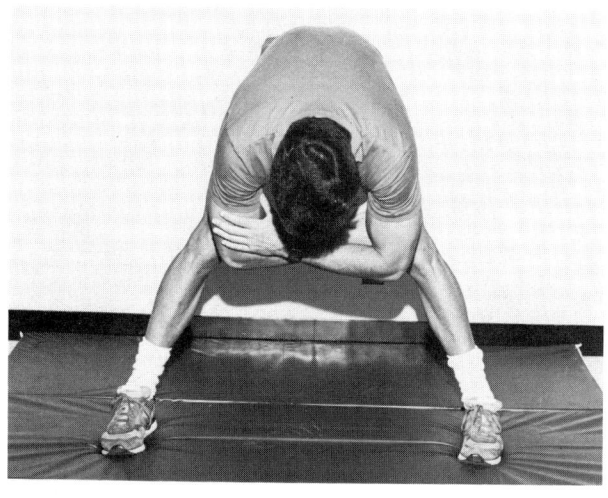

Figure 6–8. Straddle stretch. With your feet spread wide and your arms folded, bend at the hips, keeping your knees straight but not locked, and reach toward the floor with your elbows.

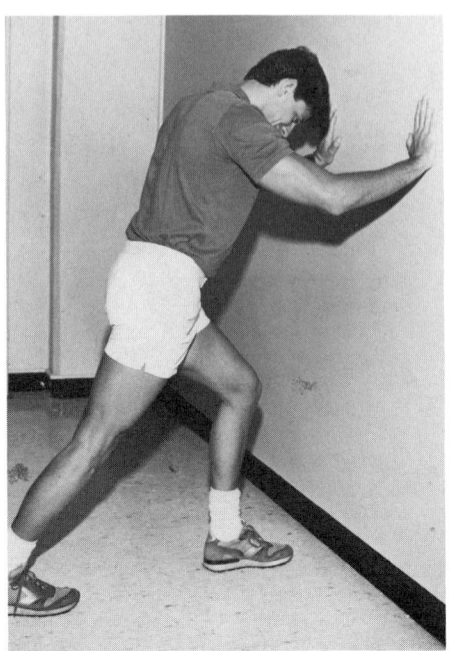

Figure 6–9. Lower leg stretch. Lean against the wall with your trunk and knees straight. Keep your heels on the floor and gently lean closer to the wall by bending your elbows.

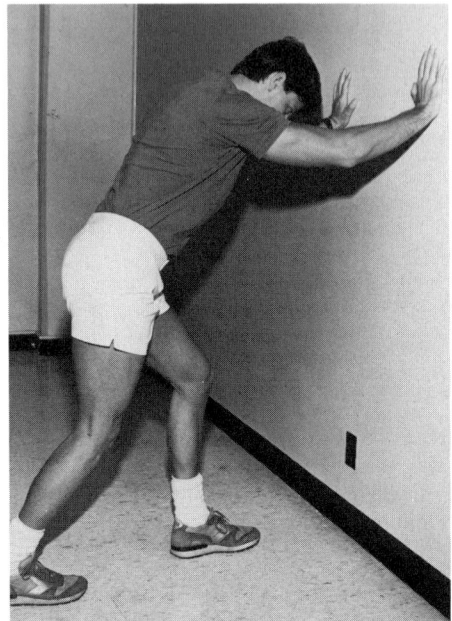

Figure 6–10. Achilles stretch. Assume the same position as in Figure 6–9 but bend your knees toward the wall, keeping your heels on the floor.

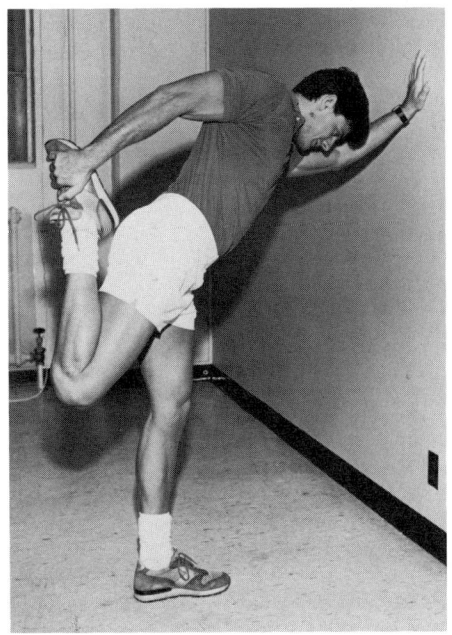

Figure 6–11. Anterior thigh stretch. Grasp your foot, with the hand on the same side behind your body. Gently pull up on the leg while remaining as erect as possible. Use the opposite hand for balance against a wall. Be sure to keep your hip joints fully extended. Repeat on the other side.

130

Figure 6–12. Sit and reach. With your feet together and your knees kept straight reach forward toward your toes. If your toes can be reached, gently pull back toward your chest. If this exercise poses little challenge, lift your heels off the floor.

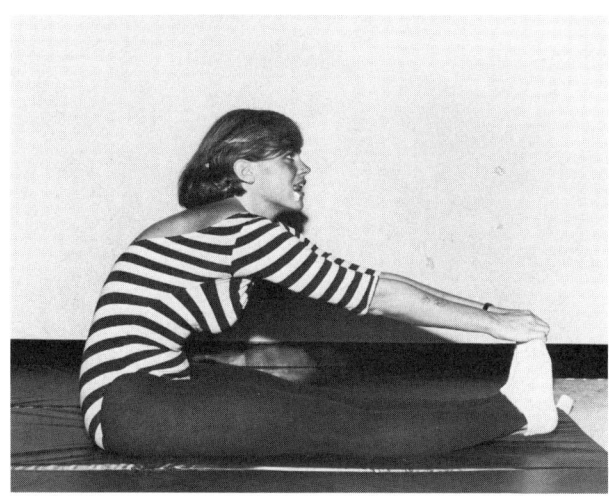

Figure 6–13. Modified hurdler stretch. In a sitting position, place the sole of one foot against the inside of the opposite knee. Reach forward with your hand toward the extended foot. Keep both knees on the floor.

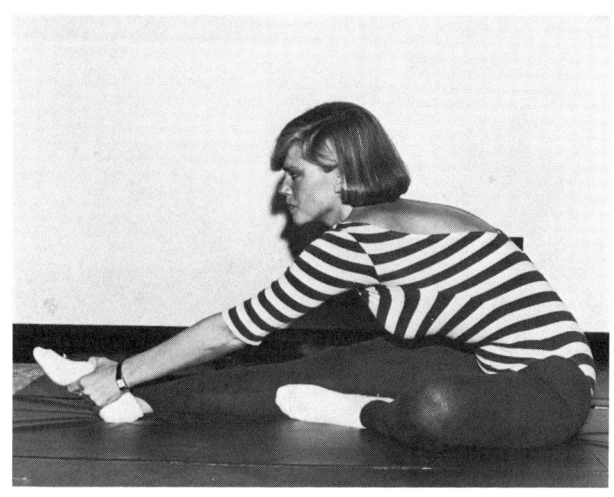

Figure 6–14. Butterfly (lotus). In a sitting position, place the soles of your feet together and pull your heels to within 10 inches of your body. Place your elbows on your knees and gently press toward the floor.

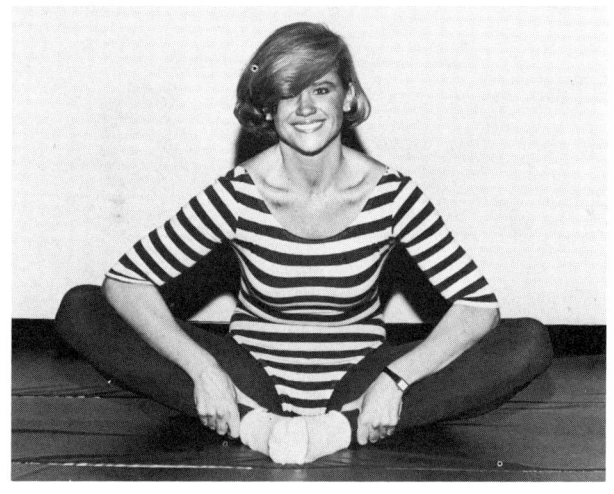

131

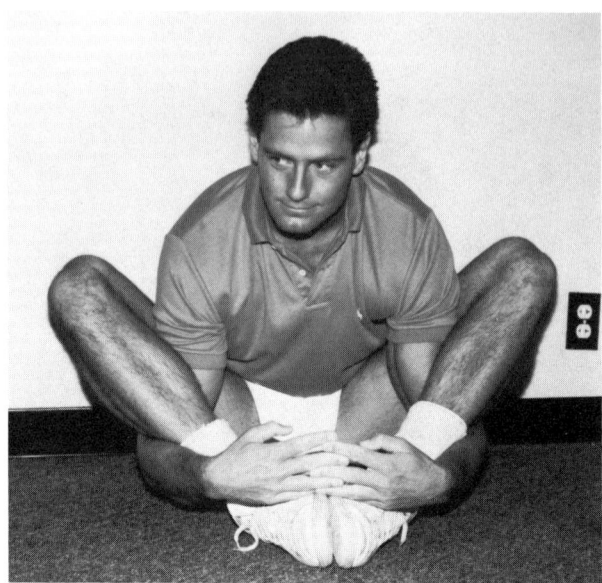

Figure 6–15. Pretzel. Assume the same position as in Figure 6–14. Place your hands through the openings in your legs and clasp them over your feet. Try this for fun!

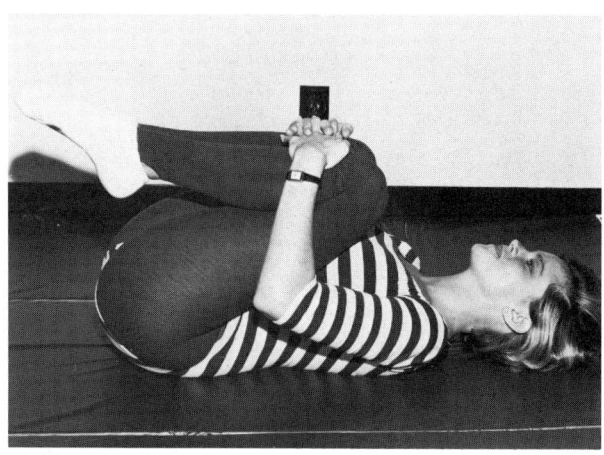

Figure 6–16. Knee tuck. In a flat lying (supine) position, pull your knees to your chest and press your lower back to the floor.

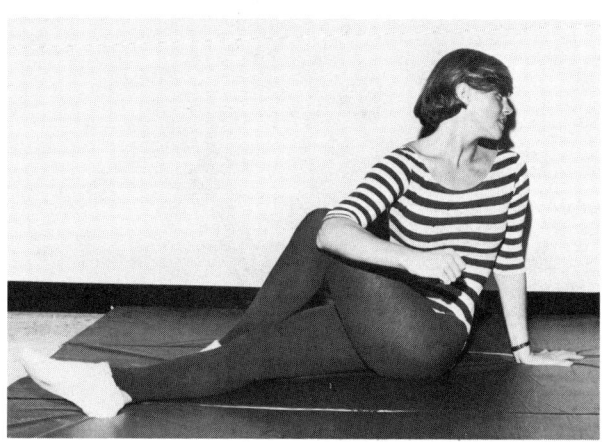

Figure 6–17. Trunk rotation. In a sitting position, cross your foot over the opposite leg and place the sole on the floor outside of the knee. Rotate your trunk in the direction toward the bent leg. Use your elbow to give a gentle push.

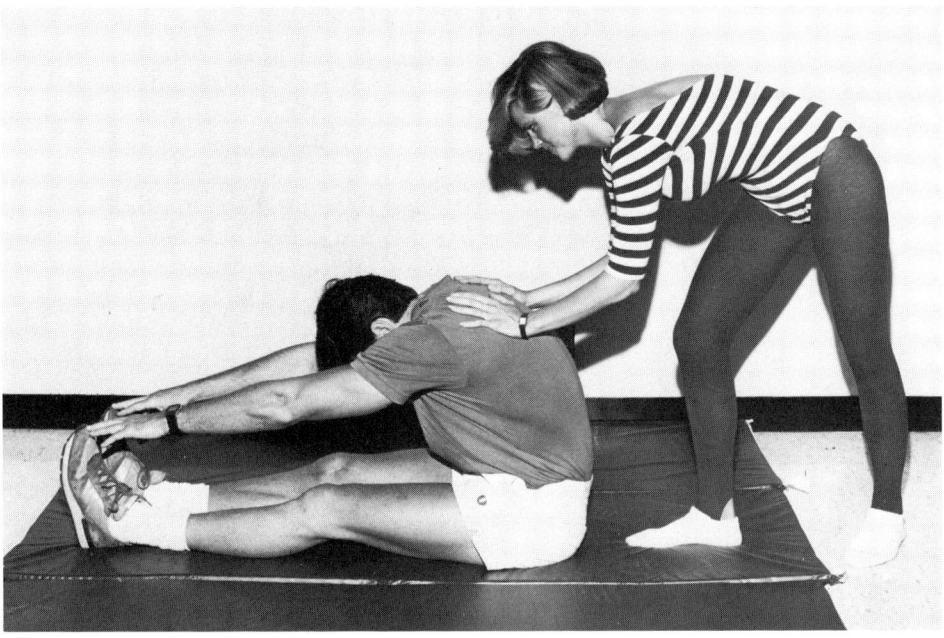

Figure 6–18. Example of using a buddy to assist in the stretching process when doing the sit and reach.

SUMMARY

◇ Although the potential for flexibility varies from person to person, each of us has an optimal range of motion that must be the subject of a regular, appropriate stretching routine if it is to be maintained.

◇ Static flexibility is the range of motion of a joint.

◇ Major limitations to flexibility include bony structures and the soft tissue associated with the joint and the muscle itself.

◇ Weight training, when done properly, will improve flexibility.

◇ Stretching exercises are important to everyone including persons with structural limitations and highly trained athletes.

◇ A good program for flexibility will include stretching exercises that challenge all major joints.

◇ Static stretching involves a gradual lengthening of the muscle group to be stretched and holding the final position for 10 to 15 seconds. This method is recommended.

◇ Ballistic stretching involves quick forceful movements. Improvement can be seen with this type stretching but drawbacks such as injury and muscle soreness make it much less desirable.

◇ The stretching routine should include each exercise done two to three times, repeated 3 to 5 days per week and preceded by a general warm-up.

◇ There is no best time to stretch but persons involved in high intensity exercise or competition would be wise to stretch before the event.

STUDY QUESTIONS

1. What is the difference between flexibility and elasticity?
2. Is it possible to overstretch a muscle? What could be the consequences of over-stretching?
3. What is likely to be the major factor that effects flexibility?
4. Why is flexibility important?
5. What are the components of the AAHPERD Health Related Fitness Test.
6. Provide an example of a stretching exercise for: (1) the shoulder; (2) the low back muscles; (3) the hamstring muscles; (4) the quadriceps muscles; and (5) the lower posterior leg muscles.
7. Describe static stretching.
8. List a series of stretching exercises that will serve as a total flexibility program.

REFERENCES AND SELECTED READINGS

Anderson, R. A.: *Stretching.* Fullerton, CA: P.O. Box 2734, 92633, 1975.

DeVries, H.: *Physiology of Exercise for Physical Education and Athletics,* 3rd edition. Dubuque, IA: W. C. Brown Co., 1980.

Dintiman, G. B.; Stone, S. E.; Pennington, J. C.; and Davis, R. G.: *Discovering Lifetime Fitness, Concepts of Exercise and Weight Control.* St. Paul, MN: West Publishing Co., 1984, pp. 115–125.

Falls, H. B.; Baylor, A. M.; and Dishman, R. K.: *Essentials of Fitness.* Philadelphia: Saunders College Publishing, 1980, pp. 166–185.

Fox, E. L.; and Mathews, D. K.: *The Physiological Basis of Physical Education and Athletics,* 3rd edition. Philadelphia: Saunders College Publishing, 1981, pp. 166–178.

Holland, G.: The physiology of flexibility: A review of the literature. *Kinesiology Review,* 49–62, 1968.

Holt, L. E.: *Scientific Stretching for Sport.* Halifax, Nova Scotia: Sport Research Ltd., 1976.

Wells, K. F.; and Luttgens, K.: *Kinesiology, Scientific Basis of Human Motion,* 6th edition. Philadelphia: W. B. Saunders Co., 1976.

Chapter 7
Nutrition
and Fitness

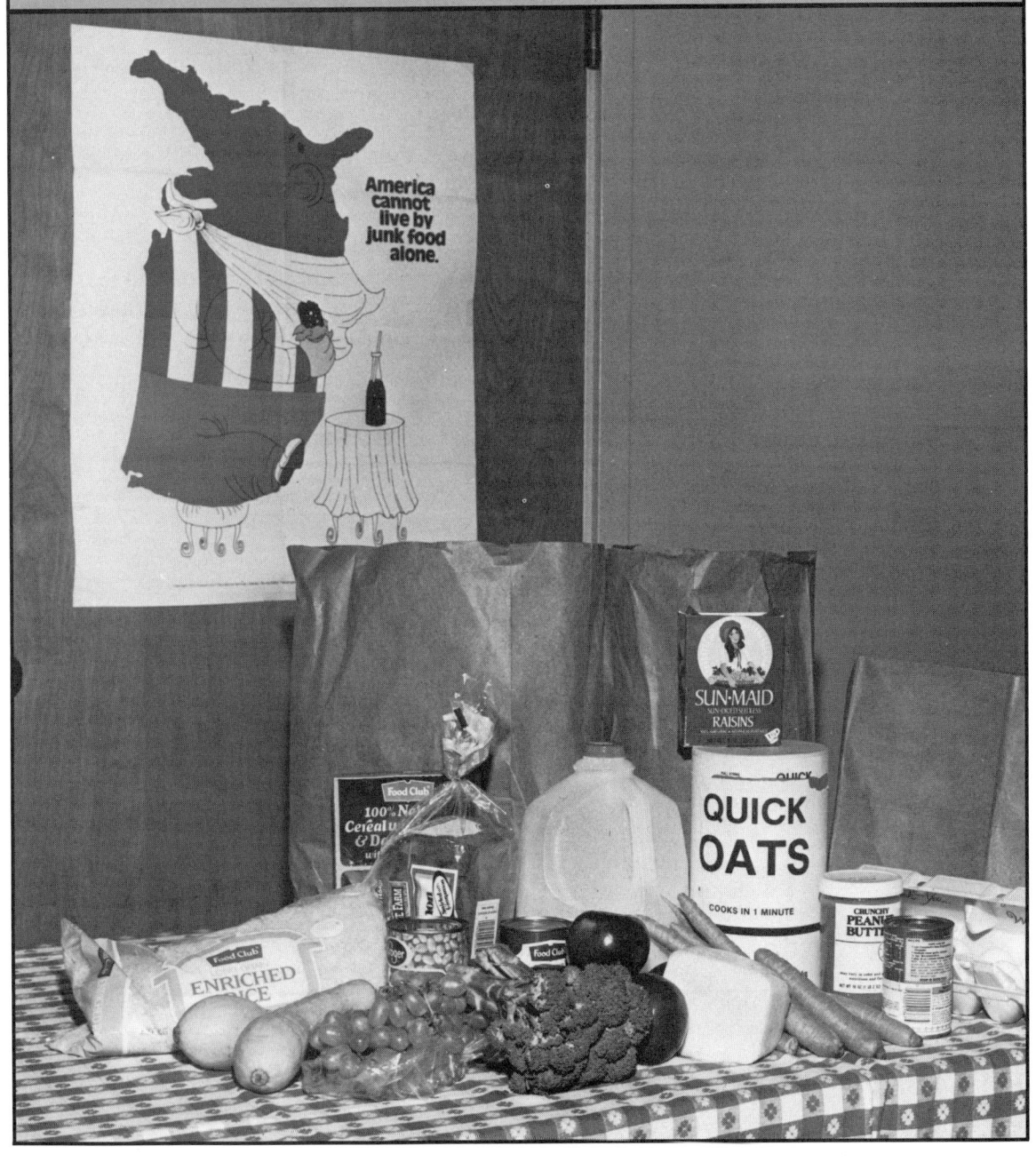

Chapter Outline

Learning Objectives

◇ To understand that nutrition is necessary for all of our body processes.

◇ To know that food nutrients have three fundamental classes: (1) energy nutrients; (2) vitamins and minerals; and (3) water.

◇ To be aware that our daily caloric intake must include all of the energy nutrients—proteins, fats, and carbohydrates.

◇ To understand that to keep body weight constant, the caloric intake must be approximately equal to the caloric expenditure.

◇ To know that a combination of a nutritionally sound diet, which reduces the daily caloric intake, along with an exercise program, which increases the daily caloric expenditure, is the best plan to follow for weight loss.

Key Words and Phrases

amino acids
blood fat levels
calorie
carbohydrate loading
carbohydrates
cholesterol
energy nutrients
fad diets
fats
fatty acids
glucose
glycogen
glycogen loading
kilocalorie
liquid pregame meals

minerals
nutrients
nutrition
nutritional fitness
nutritive snacking
pregame eating
proteins
saturated fat
spot reducing
triglyceride
unsaturated fat
vegetarian diets
vitamins
water

Introduction

"WE are what we eat" is much more than just a cliche. You will recall from Chapter 1 that **nutrition,** which is the process by which the body takes in and uses food for optimal health and performance, is necessary for all of our bodily functions. **Nutritional fitness** involves selecting foods according to their caloric and nutritive values and proper eating habits. **Nutrients** are the substances in our foods that provide nourishment and are necessary for growth, energy, reproduction, health, and the fulfillment of life. It is shocking that with the amount of research data and knowledge we have today about nutrition, 30 percent of the population of the United States has substandard diets. In other words malnutrition is definitely not limited to the underdeveloped countries of the world nor is it limited only to the economically disadvantaged of our own country. Our society places such great emphasis on being thin that many persons today are easy prey for fad diets and for downright starvation. We all know people who are more particular about the fuel that goes into their cars than the food that goes into their bodies. This chapter will teach you how to select the proper food nutrients and establish proper eating habits.

Food Nutrients

There are three fundamental classes of food nutrients: (1) energy nutrients; (2) vitamins and minerals; and (3) water.

Energy Nutrients

The only sources of food energy are carbohydrates, fats, and proteins. They are therefore called the **energy nutrients.** They supply energy for heating our bodies and for all activity. You will recall from Chapter 2 that these nutrients are the basic sources of fuel which give us the ability to do work through the breakdown of ATP.

Fats and carbohydrates (glucose and glycogen) are the primary energy nutrients. The content of the daily diet dictates to a great extent the magnitude of the stores of these nutrients within the body. The percentages of the individual nutrients required in our daily diets under normal conditions are shown in Table 7–1. Natural food sources of fats, carbohydrates, and proteins are listed in Table 7–2. Now for a few specific comments about the energy nutrients.

137

Table 7–1. Suggested Percentage
of Nutrient Contributions toward
Total Caloric Intake.

Nutrient	Percentage
Proteins	12–15
Fats	29–30
Carbohydrates	55–58

From Loviglio, L.: What's your risk: A layman's guide to cardiovascular disease. *Bostonia* 52:1, 1978, with permission.

Table 7–2. Natural Food Sources for Energy Nutrients.

Fat	Carbohydrate	Protein
Bacon	Baked beans	Cereal
Butter	Bread	Cheese
Cheese	Cakes	Eggs
Cooking fats	Cereals	Fish
Cream	Chocolate creams	Lean meat
Lard	Crackers	Liver
Margarine	Fruits (dried and fresh)	Milk
Mayonnaise	Fruit juices	Nuts
Nuts	Granulated sugar	Poultry
Peanut butter	Grean leafy vegetables	Soya beans
Pork	Honey	Yeast (brewer's)
Salad oils	Pastries	Vegetables (legumes)
Vegetable oils	Potatoes	
	Syrup	

Carbohydrates. The most efficient sources of food energy are **carbohydrates.** Plants, grains, milk, fruits, and honey all provide this nutrient. Carbohydrates are composed of the chemical compounds of simple and complex sugars. These compounds are glucose, fructose, sucrose, maltose, starch, and glycogen. All of these forms of sugar can be converted within the body according to supplies and demands. Basically, however, all sugars must be converted to **glucose** for use by the muscles and other tissues. Sugar is stored in the body in the form of **glycogen.** When the glycogen storage areas in the liver and muscles are filled, the excess amounts of glucose are converted into fats and stored in limited quantities in the fat cells throughout the body.

An average, well-nourished person must replenish carbohydrate supplies throughout the day because the readily available supply of glucose will usually be depleted by only a half-day of sedentary activities without replenishment. For an active, athletic person, the supply would last for a shorter time. Fifty-five to sixty percent of daily food intake should be in the form of carbohydrates, and, as Smith (1976) has stated, it should be well over 50 percent for active athletes.

Fats. In the United States the average per capita intake of **fats** is 40 to 45 percent of the total energy intake. According to Briggs and Calloway (1979) 30 percent would be a sufficient amount particularly where there is an incidence of cardiovascular disease. Our excessively high intake of fats undoubtedly contributes to the high incidences of obesity and cardiovascular disease in the United States. In addition, some research has suggested that there may be a correlation between fat intake and certain cancers.

Fats, however, are very necessary in our diets and are also very palatable. They are in the butter and sour cream on our potatoes, in whipped cream, in gravies, and in sauces. After they have been eaten, the slow rate at which fats are absorbed helps give us the feeling of having eaten enough. Extra fat in our daily diet—above that which we expend as energy—is stored throughout the body in the adipose tissues and is the long-term energy reserve for the body.

Some terms that apply to fats should be understood by the nutritionally knowledgeable and fitness-minded person. Fats are made up of carbon, hydrogen, and oxygen; their structural units are **fatty acids.** Fats have different chemical compositions and, therefore, are not the same. Some fat is usually solid at room temperature, particularly animal fat, eggs, and dairy products and is called **saturated fat.** Saturated fats have been related to cardiovascular diseases and atherosclerosis. **Unsaturated fat** is generally liquid at room temperature and is found in vegetable oils (such as peanut oil, corn oil, cottonseed oil, and soybean oil) and oils derived from fish. **Triglyceride** is the storage form of fats. **Cholesterol** is a fatty compound that is found in animal tissues and, in one form, is essential in our bodies. In excess, however, it is linked to atherosclerosis. Cholesterol and triglycerides are used as indexes or measures of **blood fat levels.** These are two important measurements that should be made when you have a complete physical examination. Figure 7–1 shows the relationship between cholesterol levels and coronary heart disease. Notice that the incidence of coronary heart disease of a person with a blood cholesterol level of 259 mg% is nearly five times that of a person with a blood cholesterol level under 200 mg%. Diets designed to lower cholesterol emphasize polyunsaturated fats and restrict saturated fats. Fox and Mathews (1981) noted that recent research has shown that regular exercise causes decreases in both blood cholesterol and triglyceride levels.

Proteins. Although not usually a major source of energy during exercise, **proteins** can be an energy source when carbohydrates and fats are unavailable, as in a state of starvation. **Amino acids** are the basic structural units of proteins. Proteins are the building blocks of tissue for both growth and repair. Body enzymes also are composed of proteins, as are hormones and antibodies.

Briggs and Calloway (1979) have recommended that 10 to 15 percent of

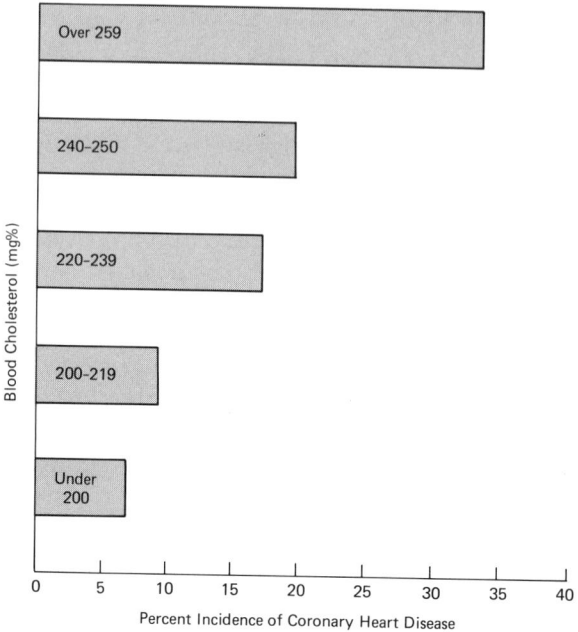

Figure 7–1. Relationships between cholesterol levels and coronary heart disease. Notice that persons with a blood cholesterol level of over 259 mg% have an incidence of coronary heart disease that is nearly five times that of persons with a blood cholesterol level under 200 mg%. (Based on data from Loviglio, L.: What's your risk: A layman's guide to cardiovascular disease. Bostonia (Boston University Alumni Magazine) *52:1, 1978.)*

the daily dietary energy intake should be in the form of protein or about 1 g/kg of body weight for a normal adult. A liberal margin over these daily recommendations can be a good way to ward off stress. Contrary to what some coaches and athletes believe, the protein requirement of the body does not significantly increase during heavy exercise. The protein requirement is based on body weight, particularly lean body weight. As muscle mass increases, greater protein intake is required. High protein diets can be harmful as they are dehydrating and can result in loss of appetite and diarrhea. Massive dosages of protein—80 to 85 percent of the total average intake—can contribute to kidney malfunction and excessive loss of calcium.

Minerals

Minerals are inorganic compounds that, along with proteins and water, are necessary for building and repairing body tissues and for proper body function. Some are needed in large amounts and some are only needed in trace amounts in our bodies. Mineral salts and vitamins act as body regulators.

Our teeth and bone structures require calcium and phosphorous from milk and green leafy vegetables. We also require iodine for the synthesis of thyroid hormones that regulate metabolism. Iodine is artificially added to salt (iodized salt is the result) to prevent goiter in areas of our country where the inhabitants do not naturally obtain it in their diets.

Iron is necessary for the red blood cells to carry oxygen. Red meats, green, leafy vegetables, dark whole grains, dates, and raisins should be parts of our diets to ensure an adequate intake of iron. A deficiency of iron reduces endurance and work performance levels. Women in particular must be sure to consume enough foods that contain iron. After heavy physical activity, the iron levels of women have been found to be significantly decreased. Some female athletes, particularly those with heavy menstrual flows, may need to supplement their diets with extra iron. Caution must always be used here, however, and the iron level should be checked medically before embarking on a supplemental iron program because iron overdoses can be toxic.

Sodium is ordinarily found in adequate if not overabundant amounts in our regular diets. Only in extreme cases is the amount of sodium lost in sweat and other body excretions great enough to require supplementation. The practice of consuming salt tablets is very ill-advised. During periods of excessive and prolonged sweating, the safest and best way to supplement salt is through the diet—adding a bit of salt to foods.

Trace amounts of potassium are essential to the functioning of muscle cells. The need is increased when there is growth or an increase in lean body mass. Potassium is lost when muscle tissue is broken down as a result of starvation, injury, or a deficiency of protein. A deficiency of potassium can cause muscular weakness, cramping, fatigue, paralysis, and even death. Disease and the use of cathartics can cause significant potassium losses since nearly all the potassium we ingest is excreted in the urine.

Vitamins

Vitamins are essential in the metabolism of fats and carbohydrates. Therefore, although they do not in themselves yield energy, they are essential to life. There are two types of vitamins: water-soluble vitamins and fat-soluble vitamins. The water-soluble vitamins are not stored in the body; rather they are eliminated in the urine. Their supply must therefore constantly be replenished. Vitamin C and B-complex vitamins are water-soluble.

The fat-soluble vitamins, A, D, E, and K, are stored in the body. These vitamins do not need to be replenished each day, and in fact, should excessive amounts accumulate, they can be toxic. Foods that are rich sources of fat-soluble and water-soluble vitamins are shown in Table 7–3. Like minerals with respect to exercise, there does not appear to be an excessive demand for vitamin supplementations if a proper diet is followed.

Water

Water makes up about 50 to 55 percent of total body weight, 72 percent of muscle weight and 80 percent of the blood. Water is probably the most

Table 7–3. Food Sources Rich in Water-soluble and Fat-soluble Vitamins.

Vitamin	Rich Food Source
Water-soluble Vitamins	
B-complex vitamins	
Vitamin B_1	Meats, whole grain cereals, milk, legumes (e.g., beans)
Vitamin B_2	Milk, fish, eggs, meats, green vegetables
Niacin	Peanut butter, whole-grain cereals, greens, meats, poultry, fish
Vitamin B_6	Whole-grain cereals, bananas, meats, spinach, cabbage, lima beans
Folic acid	Greens, mushrooms, liver
Vitamin B_{12}	Animal foods
Vitamin C (ascorbic acid)	Citrus fruits, tomatoes, strawberries, potatoes, papaya, broccoli, cabbage
Pantothenic acid	Whole grain cereals, organ meats
Biotin	Cereal, nuts, legumes, meats, egg yolk, milk
Fat-soluble Vitamins	
Vitamin A	Liver, egg yolk, milk, butter, yellow vegetables, greens
Vitamin D	Sunlight, fish, eggs, fortified dairy products
Vitamin E	Vegetable oils, greens
Vitamin K	Greens, liver

Adapted with permission from Smith, N.J.: *Food for Sport.* Palo Alto, CA: Bull Publishing Company, 1978.

essential of all nutrients for human life. A constant and uninterrupted supply of water must be a part of our daily nutritional requirements. We can survive only a matter of days without water, while we can go without food for several months. Water intake or hydration is necessary for body temperature control, for energy production in the body, and for proper elimination of wastes. During exercise, particularly under conditions of high heat or humidity, the maintenance of water levels is extremely important. To avoid dehydration drink about one-half pint of water every 20 minutes under these conditions.

Food Requirements

Two factors determine daily food requirements: (1) nutritional needs, and (2) caloric needs.

Nutritional Needs

As we discussed earlier, each of the three food nutrients—proteins, fats, and carbohydrates—must contribute to the daily calorie intake. A **calorie** is a unit of work or energy equal to the amount of heat required to raise the temperature of 1g of water 1 degree centigrade. You will also recall from Table 7–1 that the input should be approximately 15 percent protein, 30 percent fat, and 55 percent carbohydrate.

For example, if your daily caloric requirement is 3,000 kilocalories (kcal),* approximately 450 kcal should be obtained from proteins, 900 kcal from fats, and 1,650 kcal from carbohydrates. Recall once again that the fat intake should consist predominantly of unsaturated fats.

Caloric Needs

If you want to keep your body weight constant, your caloric intake must be approximately equal to your caloric expenditure for body maintenance and physical activities. Thus, if you take in 3,000 kcal per day, you must expend 3,000 kcal per day or your body weight will not remain constant. Appendix C lists the caloric costs of various activities.

Food as Fuel

We use a combination of food fuels to support our metabolism. Fats and carbohydrates provide the major contributions to our energy production, while proteins appear to contribute to a much lesser degree, with the exception of when the stores of fats and carbohydrates are depleted. Fats make the greater contribution when the body is at rest or performing low levels of exercise. Carbohydrates become a more significant source of fuel as exercise becomes more intense. This occurs because our aerobic system is more efficient when carbohydrates are the fuel source. However, since fats are stored in greater amounts in the body and carbohydrates are stored in limited amounts, we use more fats at lower levels of exercise.

Proper Eating Habits

A diet is well-balanced when proper foods are selected from the four basic food groups:

◇ Milk and milk products
◇ Meats and high protein foods
◇ Fruits and vegetables
◇ Cereal and grain foods

With a knowledge of the correct nutrient requirements for maintaining healthy bodies (Table 7–1), we must know which foods belong to each group

---

* A **kilocalorie** is a unit of work or energy equal to the amount of heat required to raise 1 kg (2.2 pounds) of water 1 degree centigrade (1.8 degrees Fahrenheit). Its abbreviation is kcal.

Table 7–4. Daily Food Guide for the Four Basic Food Groups.

Food Group	Daily Amounts	Main Contribution
I. Milk and cheese or equivalents*	Children under 9: 2 to 3 cups	Calcium
	Children 9 to 12: 3 or more cups	Protein
	Teenagers: 4 or more cups	Riboflavin
	Adults: 2 or more cups	Vitamin D
	Pregnancy: 3 or more cups	
	Lactation: 4 or more cups	
II. Meat: Beef, veal, pork, lamb, poultry, fish, eggs	Two or more servings Serving size:	
	2–3 ounces lean, boneless	Protein
	cooked meat, poultry, fish	Thiamin
Alternates: Dry	2 eggs	Iron
beans, dry peas, lentils, nuts, peanut	1 cup cooked dry beans,	Niacin
butter	dry peas or lentils	Riboflavin
	4 tablespoons peanut butter	
III. Bread and cereals (whole-grain or enriched)	Four or more servings Serving size:	
	1 slice bread	Thiamin
	½ to ¾ cup cooked cereal,	Riboflavin
	macaroni, spaghetti,	Niacin
	hominy grits, kasha,	Iron
	rice, noodles, bulgur	Protein
	1 ounce (1 cup) ready-to-eat cereal	
	5 saltines or 2 graham crackers	
IV. Vegetables and fruits	Four or more servings Serving size:	
	½ cup dark green or deep yellow every other day	Vitamin A
	½ cup or 1 medium citrus fruit (or any raw fruit or vegetable rich in ascorbic acid)	Ascorbic Acid
	Other vegetables and fruit including potato (1 medium)	Other vitamins and minerals
Water	6 to 8 glasses	

Reprinted with permission from Krause, M., and Hunscher, M.: *Food, Nutrition and Diet Therapy.* 5th ed. Philadelphia: W. B. Saunders Company, 1972.

* Milk equivalents: 1 cup whole or skimmed milk, 1 cup buttermilk, ½ cup evaporated milk, ¼ cup nonfat milk powder, 1 ounce cheddar cheese, 2 cups ice cream, 1½ cups cottage cheese. (The amount given is figured on the basis of calcium content.)

and then select from them accordingly. Table 7–4 is a daily food guide for choosing foods from the four basic food groups.

Table 7–5 gives examples of three-meal and five-meal diets. Ordinarily, three meals a day satisfy most of us, but as will be discussed later, the caloric requirements of athletes during periods of heavy activity sometimes demand that they eat five or six meals per day in order for them to ingest an adequate number of calories. Since the diets consist only of 1,200 to

Table 7–5. Examples of Basic Three- and Five-Meal Diets.

5 Meals	3 Meals
Breakfast	**Breakfast**
½ grapefruit	½ cup orange juice
⅔ cup bran flakes	1 soft-boiled or poached
1 cup skim or low-fat milk	egg
or other beverage	1 slice whole wheat toast
	1¼ teasp. margarine
Snack	1 cup skim or low-fat milk
1 small package raisins	or other beverage
½ bologna sandwich	
Lunch	**Lunch**
1 slice pizza	1½ cup Manhattan clam
carrot sticks	chowder
1 apple	2 rye wafers
1 cup skim or low-fat milk	½ cup cottage cheese
	(uncreamed)
Snack	1 medium bunch grapes *or*
2 oatmeal cookies	1 medium apple
	1 granola cookie
Dinner	**Dinner**
baked fish with	oven barbecued chicken
mushrooms (3 oz.)	(3 oz., no bone)
baked potato	½ cup green beans
2 teasp. margarine	½ cup cabbage and carrot
½ cup broccoli	salad
1 cup tomato juice or skim	⅔ cup mashed potato
or low-fat milk	½ cup applesauce
	1 cup skim or low-fat milk
	or other beverage
Total calories: about 1,400	Total calories: about 1,200

Reprinted with permission from Smith, N. J.: *Food for Sport.* Palo Alto, CA: Bull Publishing Co., 1978.

1,400 kcal, which are not enough for most of us, we will, in many cases, need to supplement calories. However, we must first be certain we eat what we need and then add what we want. Appendix B lists the caloric values of common foods.

Snacking

Although snacking is one of the primary causes of obesity, not all snacking is detrimental. **Nutritive snacking** can help maintain proper blood glucose (sugar) levels and help to fulfill the high caloric requirements of very active people. Nutritive snacks include fruits and fruit juices, sandwiches (e.g., peanut butter), yogurt, nuts, malted milk, and oatmeal cookies or other grain-enriched cookies. We should strive to eliminate foods that do not contain appropriate nutritive balances, of "junk foods" as they are called, from our diets.

Popular Fad Diets

All diets, even those designed to reduce body weight, should be nutritionally sound. There are no shortcuts to achieving the body beautiful; it requires behavioral modification and in many cases requires a lifetime commitment. Beware of **fad diets** with advertisements that claim that they will allow you to effortlessly arrive at the ideal body weight. If all of the claims were true, then there would no longer be any room for more fast-change diet programs on the market. Don't be bilked by the claims of many health spas that you can lose up to "25 inches or 14 pounds in just three days!" While it might be true that you would lose weight, this is a water loss and not a fat loss. This kind of weight loss does not last nor permanently affect your body composition. Remember that high protein diets can cause abnormally large losses of water and, in fact, can be dangerous if continued for prolonged periods of time. Other fad diets severely restrict carbohydrate intake and recommend fat intake. This can rapidly deplete carbohydrate stores, thus making physical activity or training very difficult.

Spot reducing is also a myth. People cannot selectively reduce fat stores. Falls et al. (1980), showed that regardless of which area is exercised, the fat stores are reduced all over the body, not in one selected area.

The best plan to follow for weight reduction is a nutritionally sound diet that reduces your daily caloric intake combined with an activity or exercise program that increases your daily caloric expenditure.

Vegetarian Diets

Strict **vegetarian diets** that omit all animal products make nutritional planning almost impossible. These eliminate all sources of vitamin B_{12} and many

Table 7–6. Suggestions for Dietary Supplementations for Non-Meat Eaters.

◇ Use a combination of beans; this will improve protein value. Add cooked beans to salads and soups; mash and combine with cheese for sandwich or taco filling.
◇ Also eat a variety of cereal grains, for one protein complements another, increasing the value of both.
◇ Four large mushrooms give one fourth of a day's allowance of niacin; slice them raw in salads.
◇ One cup of prune juice supplies 55 percent of an adult woman's RDA* of iron.
◇ Sesame seeds can be made into candy squares. Prepare a thick syrup of brown sugar, margarine, and water; add seeds; let cool and cut.
◇ Eat sunflower seeds as a snack; they are a good source of protein and vitamins.
◇ Brown sugar, honey, and syrup add calories and small amounts of minerals.
◇ Sprinkle brewer's yeast, a vitamin B-complex source, in soups and cereals.
◇ Add wheat germ to cooked cereal or sprinkle it over other foods. One-half ounce (2½ tablespoons) contains approximately 3 g protein plus iron and niacin.

From Smith, N.J.: *Food for Sport.* Palo Alto, CA: Bull Publishing Co., 1976.
* RDA—Recommended Daily Allowance.

sources of proteins, calcium, and iron from daily food intake. On the other hand, a modified vegetarian diet that includes eggs, milk, and other dairy products (a lacto-ovo-vegetarian diet) or a vegetarian diet that includes milk and other dairy products (a lacto-vegetarian diet) will probably not pose serious nutritional problems. You must, however, change the sources from which protein is derived. Smith (1976) has given some suggestions for dietary supplementations for non-meat eaters (Table 7–6). In addition to these suggestions, it is recommended that vegetarian dieters write The American Dietetic Association* for a complete list of food exchanges to ensure proper dietary planning.

Nutrition and Sports Performance

There are no special foods that when eaten before physical activity will lead to a superior performance. However, it is very difficult to convince some athletes of this. The eating habits they cling to are, in some cases, as irrelevant to winning performances as are their superstitions about specific pieces of apparel being their "winning hats" or "lucky shorts." Nutrition for athletes, like the daily nutrition for any person, must be wisely planned within the boundaries we have already discussed. The biggest difference between the food requirements of athletes and nonathletes is the number of calories consumed; an athlete, of course, will require more.

The eating practices of athletes before competing could fill an entire chapter or perhaps an entire volume. Most of us are familiar with the traditional steak dinners of many football teams, the bacon and eggs that soccer players prefer, the pizza or spaghetti in which runners indulge, and the dry sugared gelatin that swimmers are frequently seen eating (or accidentally dropping into the swimming pool to make a temporary colorful design) immediately before a meet. Several factors must be taken into consideration, however, for wise **pregame eating.**

First, athletes should probably avoid some foods. Generally, fats and meats are digested slowly and when eaten within a few hours before athletic competition, they may cause a feeling of fullness or sluggishness, thus impeding performance. Gas-forming foods, greasy foods, and highly seasoned foods should also be avoided. You will recall that carbohydrates help to maintain the blood sugar level and that they are easily digested. Cooked vegetables, fruits, gelatin desserts, and fish or lean meats may also be included in moderate portions. A pregame steak has a high fat content, a low carbohydrate content, and a high protein content. The consequences of this were discussed earlier.

The pregame meal should be eaten at least 2½ hours before competition and its major constituents should be carbohydrates, which are the primary source of energy during exhaustive work. Some endurance athletes (an en-

* The American Dietetic Association, 430 North Michigan Avenue, Chicago, Illinois 60611.

durance activity in this context would last 75 minutes or longer) follow such a procedure for two or three days before an event in order to increase their muscle glycogen stores. This is called **glycogen loading** or **carbohydrate loading.** Various methods are used to implement this procedure, but perhaps the most popular one is for the athlete to perform an exhaustive exercise bout, then perform no exhaustive exercise during the loading period. Bergström et al. (1967) have scientifically demonstrated in the laboratory that this is beneficial in endurance performances. Samples of diets for glycogen or carbohydrate loading are given in Table 7–7. For nonendurance athletes (e.g., sprinters) whose activities are 30 minutes or less in duration, carbohydrate loading may create a feeling of stiffness or heaviness in the muscles.

Table 7–7. Examples of Diets Designed for Muscle Glycogen Loading.

	Low-Carbohydrate Diet	High-Carbohydrate Diet
Food Groups	**Daily Amounts**	
Meats	20–25 oz	8 oz
Breads and cereals	4 servings	10–16 servings
Vegetables	3–4 servings	3–4 servings
Fruits	4 servings	10 servings
Fats	8–9 oz	4–6 oz
Desserts	1–2 servings (only fruits and un-sweetened gelatins)	2 servings (include ice cream, cookies, etc.)
Beverages	Unlimited (no sugar)	Unlimited (assuming proper calorie control)
Sample Meal Plans		
Breakfast	8 oz unsweetened orange juice 4 eggs 1 slice toast 4 tsp butter or margarine 4 strips bacon	8 oz orange juice (O.K. sweetened) 1 egg 2 slices toast 2 tsp butter or margarine 1 cup cereal
Lunch	1 meat sandwich (with butter or margarine and mayonnaise) 2–3 cheese sticks 1 tossed salad with oil dressing 1 medium apple or orange	2 sandwiches—each with 1 oz meat or cheese, ½ tsp butter or margarine 8 oz low-fat milk 2 large bananas
Dinner	10 oz meat (not ham) 1 small baked potato, with 2–3 tsp butter or margarine and 1 tbsp sour cream 1 serving vegetable (no corn), with 1–2 tsp butter or margarine 1 tossed salad 1 small apple 1 commercial "diet" dessert	4 oz meat (not ham) 1 medium baked potato, with 1 tsp butter or margarine and 1 tbsp sour cream 1 serving vegetable 2 rolls, with 1 tsp butter or margarine 2 servings fruit 2 servings commercial "diet" beverage
Snack(s)	2 meat sandwiches (with butter or margarine) 1 cheese stick 1 medium apple or banana	2 sandwiches—meat or nonmeat 1 serving fruit 8 oz low-fat milk

Reprinted with permission from Smith, N. J.: *Food for Sport.* Palo Alto, CA: Bull Publishing Co., 1978.

It is also important to consider the postgame or postperformance diet. Several days of high carbohydrate intake may be required after an endurance event, and at least several hours of such a dietary practice should be followed. Even with a high carbohydrate diet, an endurance athlete who has depleted muscle stores of glycogen will require approximately 48 hours to return those stores to normal levels.

Consumption of sugar in any amount during the hour before exercise is not recommended. Whether it is in pill form or liquid form, consuming sugar actually reduces the glucose available for use during exercise rather than making more sugar available to muscle cells. This places greater dependence upon the glycogen (sugar) stored in the muscles and the result is early fatigue.

Except for water, solid foods and certain liquids should not be consumed within the hour before physical activity. While water is the best liquid, some uncarbonated fruit-flavored drinks may also be suitable. Of course, liquids should always be available on the playing field or during competition. Remember, it is recommended that when performing heavy exercise, you should drink one-half pint of water every 20 minutes to reduce the possibility of dehydration. Electrolyte preparations can be helpful in maintaining both fluid levels and mineral concentrations. Drinks that contain sugar to enhance blood glucose may have the effect of retarding movement of water into the blood. The American College of Sports Medicine recommends a concentration of less than 2.5 g of glucose per 100 ml of water in these drinks.

Recently, some researchers have advocated the ingestion of caffeine to improve performance in endurance events. Costill et al. (1978) have shown that marathon runners can reduce their performance times by 10 to 15 minutes when they have a couple of cups of coffee about an hour before running. Some experiments with cyclists have shown similar results. Whether the practice of caffeine ingestion will, in fact, improve performance is still an open question. The stimulating effects of caffeine are apparent, but the effect on performance is yet to be satisfactorily established. Nevertheless, neither carbohydrate loading, caffeine ingestion, or other dietary manipulations will substitute in any way for appropriate training.

Commercially packaged **liquid pregame meals** are becoming increasingly popular. They are not only nutritious and palatable, but also easily digested and readily emptied from the stomach. They contribute to hydration and to energy intake since they are a liquid and a meal. They may also minimize nausea, vomiting, abdominal cramps, diarrhea, and nervous indigestion. Most of these meals (some trade names are Ensure, Ensure Plus, Nutriment, Sustagen, and Susta Cal) contain large amounts of carbohydrates plus some fats and proteins.

In summary, as long as you do not overeat or do not eat foods that cause discomfort in the gastrointestinal tract, your performance will not be affected by the foods you consume on the day you exercise. There are no absolute "dos" or "don'ts." Basically, however, your diet on the day of competition or exercise should not differ significantly from your normal diet. You should

Table 7–8. Guidelines for Eating before Exercising.

How much?

Food consumption should provide sufficient caloric intake to prevent weakness or famished feelings during the entire activity period. Foods ingested immediately prior to activity or sport participation do not contribute significantly to short-term energy needs; however, they do contribute to the maintenance of adequate blood sugar levels. Pre-game consumption of foods and liquids should also help ensure proper hydration during the activity period.

What?

The pre-exercise diet should include foods that will not cause gastrointestinal distress.

When?

Timing of food and liquid consumption should ensure that the stomach feels empty during sport or activity participation.

Why?

The pre-activity diet should appeal to your appetite and contribute positively to your performance aspirations while achieving the other guidelines set forth.

not miss meals but you should regularly eat food in modest proportions.

During times of exercise or competition, you will also learn to eliminate from your diet foods that can be eaten under normal circumstances but that cause distress in nervous or tense situations. Guidelines in planning what to eat before exercising are given in Table 7–8.

SUMMARY

◇ Nutrition is necessary for all of our body functions.

◇ Nutrition is the process by which the body takes in and uses food for optimal health and performance.

◇ Nutritional fitness is concerned with the selection of foods according to their caloric and nutritive values and with proper eating habits.

◇ Nutrients are the substances in our foods that provide our nourishment and are necessary for growth, energy, reproduction, health, and the fulfillment of our lives.

◇ Food nutrients have three fundamental classes: (1) energy nutrients; (2) vitamins and minerals; and (3) water.

◇ The most efficient sources of food energy are carbohydrates.

◇ Exercise, as well as dietary restrictions, causes decreases in blood cholesterol and triglyceride levels.

◇ The protein requirement does not significantly increase during heavy exercise.

◇ After heavy exercise, the iron levels of women have been found to be significantly decreased.

◇ Water is probably the most essential nutrient for human life.

◇ Our daily caloric intake should include 15 percent protein, 30 percent fat, and 55 percent carbohydrate.

◇ A well-balanced diet is ensured by selecting proper foods from the four basic foods groups: milk or milk products; meat and high protein foods; fruit and vegetables; and cereal and grain foods.

◇ To keep your body weight constant, your caloric intake must be approximately equal to your caloric expenditure.

◇ The best plan to follow for weight reduction is a nutritionally sound diet that reduces daily caloric intake along with an exercise program that increases the daily caloric expenditure.

◇ There are no foods that when eaten before physical activity will lead to a superior performance.

◇ Basically, the diet on the day of competition or exercise should not differ from the normal diet.

STUDY QUESTIONS

1. What are the food nutrients and how does each individually contribute to our daily diets?

2. Discuss how different forms of fat affect one's health.

3. Plan a well-balanced, nutritionally sound 2,500 kcal diet for one day.

4. Why is "spot" reducing a myth?

5. What factors must be considered for wise pregame or pre-physical activity eating?

REFERENCES AND SELECTED READINGS

Bergström, J.; Hermansen, L.; Hultman, E.; and Saltin, B.: Diet, muscle glycogen and physical performance. *Acta Physiologica Scandinavica* 71:140–150, 1967.

Briggs, G. M.; and Calloway, D. H.: *Bogart's Nutrition and Physical Fitness*, 10th ed. Philadelphia: W. B. Saunders, 1979.

Costill, D. L.; Dalsky, G.; and Fink, W.: Effects of caffeine ingestion on metabolism and exercise performance. *Medicine and Science in Sports* 10:155–158, 1978.

Falls, H. B.; Baylor, A. M.; and Dishman, R. K.: *Essentials of Fitness.* Philadelphia: Saunders College Publishing, 1980.

Fox, E. L.: *Lifetime Fitness.* Philadelphia: Saunders College Publishing, 1983.

Fox, E. L.: *Sports Physiology*, 2nd ed. Philadelphia: Saunders College Publishing, 1984.

Fox, E. L.; and Mathews, D. K.: *The Physiological Basis of Physical Education and Athletics*, 3rd ed. Philadelphia: Saunders College Publishing, 1981.

Krause, M.; and Hunscher, M.: *Food, Nutrition, and Diet Therapy*, 5th ed. Philadelphia: W. B. Saunders, 1972.

Loviglio, L.: What's your risk: A layman's guide to cardiovascular disease. *Bostonia* (Boston University Alumni Magazine) 52:1, 1978.

Smith, N. J.: *Food for Sport.* Palo Alto, CA: Bull Publishing Co., 1976.

Young, E. A.; Brennan, E. H.; and Irving, G. L. (guest eds.): Perspectives on fast foods. *Public Health Currents* 19:1970.

Chapter 8
Exercise, Body Composition, and Body Weight Control

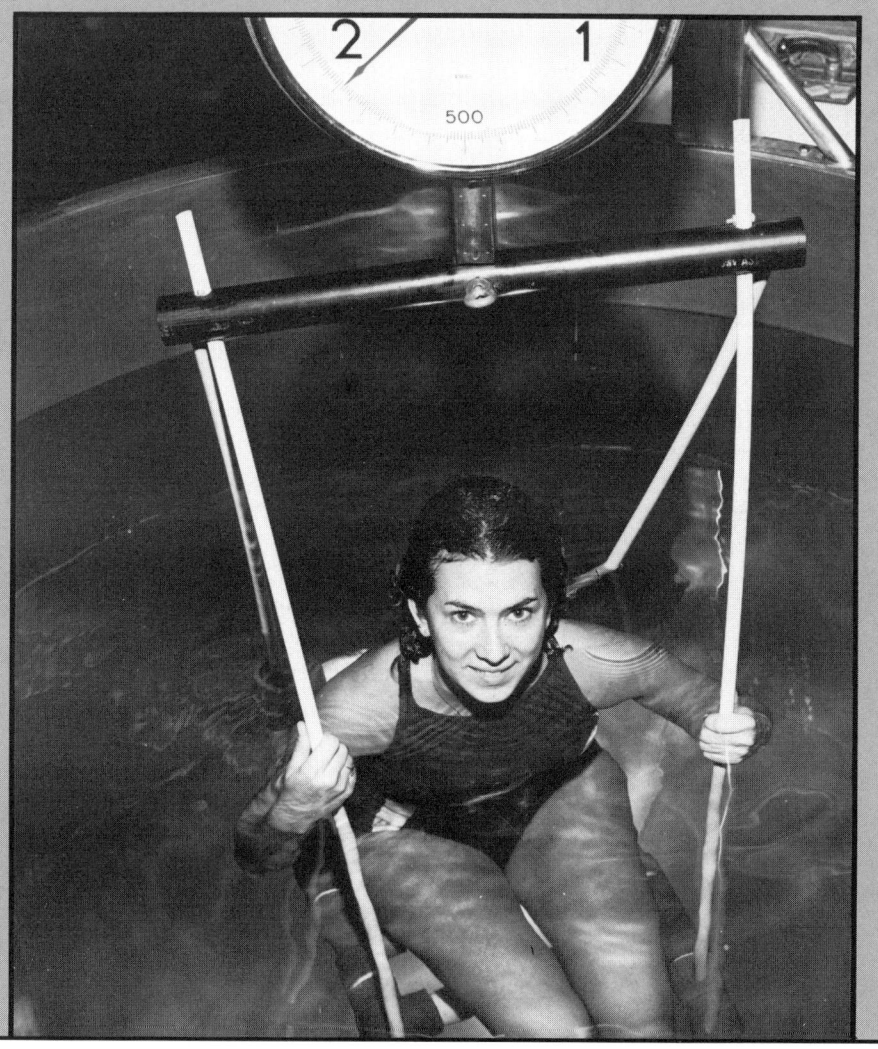

Chapter Outline

Learning Objectives

◇ To understand that weight change is usually a gradual process.
◇ To learn what body composition is and how diet and exercise can change it.
◇ To know that obesity is primarily caused by inactivity, NOT by overeating.
◇ To understand how body fat is lost or lean body weight is gained.
◇ To know how to calculate caloric intake and caloric expenditure.
◇ To understand that to maintain present weight, caloric intake and caloric expenditure must be equal.
◇ To know that to lose weight, caloric expenditure must be greater than caloric intake.
◇ To understand that to gain lean body weight, caloric intake must be greater than caloric expenditure.
◇ To understand that exercise is as important as dietary considerations in programs to lose weight or gain lean body weight.

Key Words and Phrases

adipocytes
anorexia nervosa
body composition
body fat weight
bulimia
caloric deficit
caloric expenditure
caloric intake
daily activity level
ectomorph
endomorph
fat-free weight
lean body weight

mesomorph
muscle weight
negative energy balance
obesity
overfatness
overweight
physical activity rate
positive energy balance
resting or basal rate
secondary amenorrhea
skinfold measurement
somatotyping
underwater weighing

Introduction

W HEN many of us consider why we should control our body weights, we think in terms of aesthetics—we all enjoy looking trim and svelte. The reasons for weight control, of course, cover a much broader spectrum. Many diseases are associated with overweight, or rather overfatness: heart disease, bone and joint diseases, atherosclerosis, and diabetes to name a few. Also motor performance is impeded by fatness. At the other end of the scale are anorexia and bulimia. Both weight problems can cause psychological and behavioral changes as well as physiological changes in our bodies.

Weight change for many of us is often very gradual but still significant. An increase of one pound in a year seems of little consequence, but after 25 years of this seemingly harmless increase we may find that losing 25 pounds requires substantial effort. In fact, this insidious overfatness affects the average man and woman considerably and is the main cause of our overweight and overfat society.

In Chapter 7 we discussed the importance of good nutritional fitness; in Chapters 3 and 4 we covered cardiorespiratory fitness; and in Chapter 5 muscular strength and endurance fitness. In this chapter, we shall learn the importance of nutrition and exercise in controlling body weight. Since we are, fortunately, not a cloned society, we have different starting points and aspirations. Although many of us must be concerned with avoiding the addition of extra pounds or even with shedding a few pounds, there are also a few who must strive to gain. Our starting point therefore is learning what body composition is and how diet and exercise can change it.

Body Composition

Body composition refers to the component parts of the body. Although the parts are many, for our purposes in this chapter we shall regard the body basically as having two components: (1) **body fat weight;** and (2) **fat-free weight** (also referred to as **lean body weight** or **muscle weight).** We should mention at this time some sexual differences regarding these two components. When compared with the average adult male, the average adult female (1) is 3 to 4 inches shorter; (2) is 25 to 30 pounds lighter in total body weight; (3) has 10 to 15 pounds more fat (adipose) tissue; and (4) has 40 to 45 pounds less fat-free weight (mainly located in muscle, bone, and organs).

Generally, these differences are true for nonathletic as well as athletic men and women. With these points in mind, we shall now learn more about the two components.

Body Fat

Two factors determine the amounts of body fat that our bodies store: (1) the number of fat-storing cells, which are called **adipocytes;** and (2) the capacity or size of the adipocytes. Once we reach adulthood, the number of adipocytes cannot be reduced by dietary restrictions or by exercise. Only the size of the adipocytes can be changed at that point. The factors that determine the number of adipocytes are controversial but include genetic influences and early childhood diet and nutritional habits.

The old saying that "a fat baby is a healthy baby" is far from true. The control of fat cells must begin early in childhood. Research has shown that exercise and diet programs introduced at that point can lead to a reduction in both the number and size of fat cells during adulthood. This is true even if we don't continue exercising as adults. It is obvious from this that it is imperative that good eating habits be established in early childhood.

Body Fat Percentages. Body fat accounts for approximately 22 to 25 percent of the total body weight of the average college-aged woman; for the average college-aged man, body fat represents approximately 12 to 15 percent of total body weight. These values are statistical averages and are not presented as optimal levels of body fat. In our illustration in Chapter 1, we said that if the college-aged man has a total body weight of 160 pounds, 19 to 24 pounds* would be fat and the rest (136–141 pounds) would be lean body weight.

The percentage of body fat of athletes, regardless of sports preference, is usually lower than that of the average nonathlete and, as mentioned earlier, it differs on the basis of sex. For example, the body fat of male marathon runners ranges between 1 and 9 percent of total body weight and averages under 5 percent. Female long-distance runners are also extremely lean but the lowest individual values for them are about 6 percent body fat. Figure 8–1 gives the percentages of body fat for various male and female athletes.

It should be mentioned that menstrual irregularities are being noted in women whose body fat stores are reduced significantly enough to cause excessive weight loss. Since many athletes have low body fat values (particularly long distance runners and gymnasts), it is a possible cause of the **secondary amenorrhea** experienced by these athletes. Amenorrhea in such situations is ordinarily a temporary condition and can be precipitated by other factors in addition to low body fat values. Although more research is required in this area, you should be aware of this possibility.

Performance and Body Fat. Fat cells and adipose tissue are not biochemically active in generating ATP energy, at least not in the same sense that muscle cells generate ATP energy (see Chapter 2). For this reason, exces-

---

* $160 \times 0.12 = 19$ pounds and $160 \times 0.15 = 24$ pounds

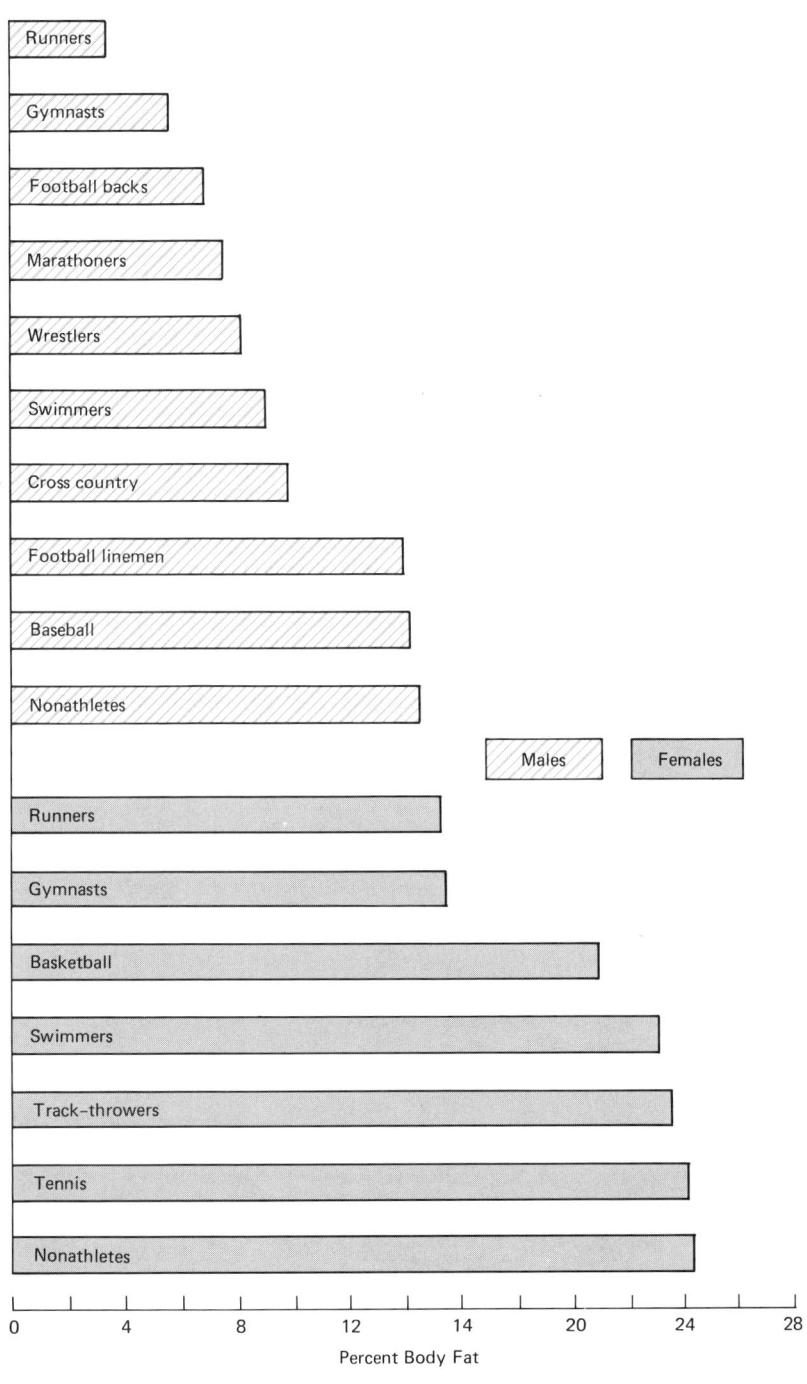

Figure 8–1. Percentages of body fat for male and female athletes of various sports. The body fat percentages are usually lower among athletes than among nonathletes. (Based on Boileau, R. A. and Lohman, T. G.: The measurement of human physique and its effects on physical performance. Orthop. Clin. North Am. 8(3):563–581, 1977.)

157

sive fat contributes weight to the body but does not contribute to its movement. Excessive fat therefore is a hindrance in activities that require weight-bearing skills such as walking, running, and gymnastics. Women are at a greater disadvantage here than men because, as we have discussed, their fat-to-muscle ratio is greater than that of men (even those of the same body weight). The workload of a woman is thus increased by her extra fat-to-muscle ratio and is analogous to performing against her male counterpart in a weight-bearing activity with weights strapped on her back. In swimming, however, women have the advantage over men because the greater fat content in a woman's body leads to less body drag (due to greater buoyancy) in the water, and hence to less energy expenditure per distance swum. The body fat percentages for athletes in various sports are shown in Figure 8–1.

Obesity or Overfatness. As stated in Chapter 1, **obesity** can be defined as a body weight greater than 20 percent above the ideal weight for one's height. Using this definition yet recognizing the difficulty in establishing ideal weight, there are probably between 50 and 80 million obese persons in the United States today. It is obvious that obesity or overfatness refers to an above-average amount of fat contained in the body. This is, of course, dependent upon the fat content of each fat cell and the total number of fat cells in the body.

Obesity is primarily caused by inactivity *not* by overeating. Some athletes eat 6,000 to 10,000 kcal per day during their competitive seasons and do not gain a single pound; in fact, some even lose weight. *Exercise is the key!*

Notice that we use the term **overfatness.** We must point out that the use of height-weight charts for assessing body size can be very misleading. A person can be **overweight** according to these charts and yet not be overfat. As we said previously, athletes (football players, for example) can be over-

Table 8–1. Suggested Body Weights for Various Heights.

Height (inches)	Body Weight in Pounds			
	Men		Women	
	Suggested	Obese	Suggested	Obese
60			109	>130
62			115	>138
64	133	>160	122	>146
66	142	>170	129	>155
68	151	>181	136	>163
70	159	>190	144	>173
72	167	>200	152	>182
74	175	>210		
76	182	>218		

From Fox, E. L.: *Lifetime Fitness.* Copyright © 1983 by CBS Publishing. Reprinted by permission of CBS College Publishing.

weight according to these charts and yet a very small percentage of their weights is body fat. For this reason, height-weight charts must be used carefully.

Table 8–1 can be used as a guide to suggest whether you may be overfat and by approximately how much. (For more specific determinations of appropriate body weight based on body composition, see Chapter 9.) Remember from our above discussion to use this table wisely, particularly if you are an athlete. The body weights in the table are those of college-aged men and women who are generally not obese. In fact a guideline that is frequently suggested for determining a suggested weight later in life is whether or not the person weighs the same as when in college (20 to 25 years old). By this standard a person whose weight exceeds his or her college weight by 20 percent is considered to be obese or overfat (Table 8–1). If we are realistic about our body concepts, most of us should know when the couple of extra pounds we have added repeatedly spill over into obesity.

Fat-Free Weight (Lean Body Weight or Lean Body Mass)

Fat-free weight or **lean body mass** is the weight remaining when the weight of body fat is subtracted from total body weight.

Total Body Weight − Body Fat Weight = Lean Body Weight

Skeletal muscle weight is the main component of fat-free weight (FFW), which also includes the weight of other organs and tissues such as skin and bones. Forty to 50 percent of the fat-free weight is composed of muscle weight or mass. The average fat-free weight of a college-aged woman is about 75 percent of her total body weight, while that of a college-aged man is 85 percent of his total body weight.

Changing Body Weight

How do you lose body fat or gain lean body weight? As discussed in Chapter 7, the basic principle involved in changing the amount of body fat is the balance between energy taken in as food and energy expended through physical activity and the support of the body processes. Body fat therefore can be lost by reducing the number of calories taken in or by increasing the number of calories expended through exercise or by both. Therefore, in order to change your amount of body fat, you need to know how many calories you expend in activities each day and your daily consumption of calories through food intake. Lean weight can be lost through lack of use

Table 8–2. *Estimated Energy Expenditures in Kilocalories Per Day for Different Body Weights and Activity Levels for Men.*

Activity Level	Body Weight											
	110 lb (50 kg)	120 lb (54 kg)	130 lb (59 kg)	140 lb (64 kg)	150 lb (68 kg)	160 lb (73 kg)	170 lb (77 kg)	180 lb (82 kg)	190 lb (86 kg)	200 lb (91 kg)	210 lb (95 kg)	220 lb (100 kg)
Sedentary Activity limited to routine sitting and walking	1680	1830	1985	2135	2288	2440	2595	2745	2900	3050	3205	3355
Semisedentary Activities involve standing and walking only	1800	1960	2125	2290	2450	2615	2780	2940	3105	3270	3430	3595
Semiactive Physically active but limited	1920	2090	2265	2440	2615	2790	2965	3140	3310	3485	3660	3835
Active Regular participation in sports activities or physical fitness programs	2040	2220	2410	2595	2780	2965	3150	3335	3520	3705	3890	4075
Very active Engaged in competitive sports or in vigorous daily fitness programs	2160	2355	2550	2745	2940	3140	3335	3530	3725	3920	4120	4315

From, Fox, E. L.: *Lifetime Fitness.* Copyright © 1983 by CBS College Publishing. Reprinted by permission of Saunders College Publishing, CBS College Publishing.

Table 8–3. *Estimated Energy Expenditures in Kilocalories Per Day for Different Body Weights and Activity Levels in Women.*

Activity Level	Body Weight									
	90 lb (41 kg)	100 lb (45 kg)	110 lb (50 kg)	120 lb (54 kg)	130 lb (59 kg)	140 lb (64 kg)	150 lb (68 kg)	160 lb (73 kg)	170 lb (77 kg)	180 lb (82 kg)
Sedentary Activity limited to routine sitting and walking	1235	1375	1510	1650	1790	1920	2060	2195	2335	2470
Semisedentary Activities involve standing and walking only	1325	1470	1620	1764	1915	2061	2205	2355	2500	2645
Semiactive Physically active but limited	1410	1570	1730	1880	2039	2195	2355	2510	2670	2825
Active Regular participation in sports activities or physical fitness programs	1500	1665	1835	2000	2170	2335	2500	2670	2835	3000
Very active Engaged in competitive sports or in vigorous daily fitness programs	1590	1765	1945	2120	2295	2470	2645	2825	3000	3175

From Fox, E. L.: *Lifetime Fitness*. Copyright © 1983 by CBS College Publishing. Reprinted by permission of Saunders College Publishing, CBS College Publishing.

of skeletal muscle, which results in atrophy. Conversely, weight can also be gained through activity that increases muscle size. In fact it is possible to lose fat weight and gain lean weight through exercise with a net increase in weight and an improvement in body composition.

Estimating Caloric Expenditure

Your **daily activity level** determines your **caloric expenditure** each day. There are two parts of the daily activity level: (1) a **resting** or **basal rate,** which is the minimal activity level required by the body in order to live; and (2) the **physical activity rate,** or your activities above the basal level. Both of these factors are rather difficult to assess accurately. However, reasonable estimates based on body weights and physical activity levels are given in Table 8–2 for men and Table 8–3 for women. Both parts of your daily activity are combined in these tables. For example, let's say that you are a man who weighs 170 pounds (77 kg) and that you are semiactive; in other words, the amount of your daily physical exercise is limited. From looking at the table, your estimated energy expenditure over a 24-hour period would be approximately 2,965 kcal. To lose weight your daily intake of kilocalories would have to be less than 2,965.

Estimating Caloric Intake

Appendix B lists the caloric values of common foods, including many "fast" foods. Counting the number of calories you consume takes time because you must record every food you eat as well as how many servings of it you have eaten. By referring to the caloric values of foods, you can estimate your 24-hour **caloric intake.** For example, let's say your breakfast included:

  ◇ ¾ cup orange juice
  ◇ ½ cup granola cereal
  ◇ 2 slices whole wheat bread or toast
  ◇ 1 tsp margarine on the toast
  ◇ 2 cups regular instant coffee (black)

Using Appendix C, you can estimate the number of kilocalories to be 85 for orange juice; 215 for the granola cereal; 130 (65 per slice) for the bread or toast; 35 for the margarine and 6 for the two cups of coffee for a total of 471 kcal. After doing this for each meal plus all snacks eaten during a 24-hour period, you will have an estimate of your daily caloric intake.

Another less accurate way of calculating your caloric intake is based on your energy expenditure as estimated in the caloric costs of various activities in Appendix C. To calculate this, your body weight must be fairly constant.

(Weigh yourself at the same time of day for several days to determine this.) After recording all of your daily activities, you can check Appendix C to get a total energy expenditure.

Using this technique, once you have determined the number of calories that you expend daily (basal rate + activities rate), you can estimate the number of calories you consume. Now you are ready to adjust your caloric intake so you can lose body fat.

As an illustration, let's assume that Willy Walkalot is a 180-pound man who wishes to sensibly lose 1 pound a week—that's 3,500 kcal. If this is done by diet alone, it means a reduction in caloric intake of 700 kcal per day. This can be done, of course, but it would be much nicer for Willy to add a brisk 30-minute, 2-mile walk to his daily routine. If we check in Appendix C, we find that for a 180-pound man walking on an asphalt road a deficit of 6.6 kcal/minute or 198 kcal per 30 minutes is created. Let's round that number off to 200 kcal for our illustration. Now, we see that by taking the 2-mile walk, Willy only has to reduce his caloric intake by 500 calories. If he increases his walking to 4 miles, thus creating a loss of 400 kcal, then his caloric intake reduction is down to 300 kcal per day.

In Appendix D there is a chart with which you can calculate your present caloric intake, caloric expenditure, and the deficit required to lose appropriate amounts of fat weight.

Assessing Body Composition

As we have said, height-weight charts are very superficial and sometimes misleading means of assessing whether we need to lose fat or gain lean muscle weight. There are, however, other means by which we can more accurately evaluate our body composition.

Somatotyping

Although exact assessment of body composition cannot be made by **somatotyping** (the physical classification of the human body), it would be remiss not to briefly mention this procedure. Many coaches use this means of predicting in which athletic events or positions an athlete will best perform. Also, somatotyping is sometimes used to predict which body type is most susceptible to various diseases.

In somatotyping, three body types are distinguished: **endomorph, mesomorph,** and **ectomorph** (Figure 8–2). An endomorph's body is round and soft; this body has extra adipose tissue. A mesomorph has a square body with a rugged, hard musculature; the bones are large and covered with thick muscle. Finally, an ectomorph's body possesses linearity, fragility, and deli-

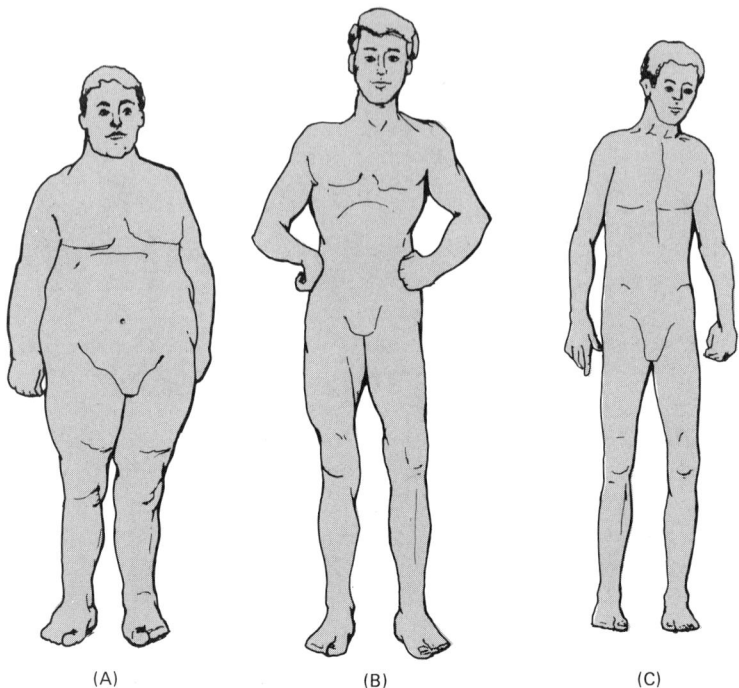

Figure 8–2. Three body types used in somatotyping. (A) Endomorph; (B) mesomorph; (C) ectomorph. Most of us are combinations of body types.

cacy. The bones are small, the muscles are thin and frequently an ectomorph has drooping shoulders. Of course, many of us are combinations of body types. To "type" a person's body according to these definitions, measurements or photographs or both are taken of the body. These are then compared with standards, some of which have been established by Sheldon (1954) and by Heath and Carter (1967).

Skinfold Measurements

Body composition and hence body fat may be reasonably estimated by taking measurements of the subcutaneous fat at various skinfolds of the body. These **skinfold measurements,** which are relatively easy to do, can be made by physicians, trainers, coaches, or physical educators to assess body composition with respect to acceptable values of body fat. For details including illustrations of the techniques and standards of evaluation for these measurements, see Chapter 9.

Underwater Weighing

The most precise method of assessing body composition in humans is **underwater weighing** along with the measurement of residual lung volume. Because of the equipment required for making these determinations, these measurements are not always easily obtained (see Figure 9–8 on p. 188).

What is actually measured in this procedure is body density. Density (D) is defined as mass (M) per unit volume (V) or:

$$D = M/V$$

Since in healthy young adults the body is 45 to 60 percent water (Briggs and Calloway, 1979), its density is very close to that of water (1 g/cc of volume). The density of pure fat tissue is, however, only about 0.9 g/cc, whereas fat-free tissue has a density of about 1.10 g/cc. Therefore, when the density of the body is known, the percentage of body fat can be calculated.

Body Fat Loss

Water Loss Versus Fat Loss

Once again, we need to stress that to lose body fat, you must expend more kilocalories than you consume. In fact, to lose 1 pound of pure fat, you must expend 3,500 calories more than you consume. This reinforces our earlier recommendation that the most effective way to lose weight is to combine an exercise or activity program with a diet program. Increasing your caloric expenditure and decreasing your caloric intake to produce a **caloric deficit** with the activity–diet combination will ensure that fat is lost and that lean body weight or muscle weight is preserved or possibly increased. Greater amounts of muscle are lost when dieting alone is instituted.

Also remember that there are no easy roads to weight (fat) loss. We referred to the health spa claims of losing many inches and pounds in a few days. This, of course, is sheer water loss, which is reclaimed as rapidly as it is sloughed. Also recall that fat is lost all over the body, not just in one spot; hence claims for spot reduction are myths.

Making Weight

Not a myth, however, is the reality in some sports of "making weight." Smith (1976) has noted that to effectively compete in athletic events body weight should be at a level that includes effective hydration, lack of excessive body fat, and an optimal quantity of muscle mass. "Making weight" frequently does not incorporate these criteria. In some cases, competitors will lose up to 5 percent of their body weight through water loss within two or three days of competition. Not only can this be damaging to the person involved, but it is damaging to the sport and is leading to the exclusion of certain sports from some school curricula. It is strongly recommended that all competitors adhere to the examples of good nutrition, including hydration, as presented in this chapter and in Chapter 7.

Correctly Losing Weight

Ideally, the weight loss for adults should be between 2 and 3 pounds per week; an absolute maximum loss would be 4 pounds per week for someone who is obese. The caloric deficit for adults should not exceed 2,000 to 2,500 kcal per day. This should represent an increased caloric expenditure through exercise as well as a reduced caloric intake of food. For boys and girls, a well-selected daily caloric intake of 1,400 kcal can provide all necessary nutrients needed in order not to compromise growth; however, an intake of 2,000 kcal permits a little more latitude for some preferred selections to be added to the basics. In any weight loss plan it is important to maintain an adequate caloric intake and appropriate nutrient intake. This will often require the supervision of your physician or a trained professional to meet individual needs.

Always keep in mind during your dieting procedure that "Rome was not built in a day." Your weight likewise did not accumulate in a day or a week; therefore, you should not expect your weight loss to occur over night. It will take you several months or longer to lose 25 pounds, but persevere!

Anorexia and Bulimia

We are beginning to see a greater incidence of diseases that stem from improper means of weight control. Two diseases with the most devastating outcomes are **anorexia nervosa** and **bulimia.**

Anorexia nervosa means a nervous loss of appetite. It is a disease that primarily affects young women (it is estimated that only 10 percent of all anorexics are male) from the middle and upper social classes—affluent enough to be able to refuse food. Typically the anorexic has a history of being a model child who is a high achiever and a perfectionist. Sufferers of this disease are so obsessed with excessive thinness that it becomes the focal point of their lives. Even when the anorexic becomes thin, fears of being obese do not diminish; the feeling of being fat still exists.

Usually anorexia is preceded by a stressful life situation; change of any kind is particularly stressful. Table 8–4 compiled by Neuman and Halvorson (1983) lists some identifying signals to help in identifying anorexia.

As anorexia progresses, fluid and electrolyte imbalances can occur, which can lead to dehydration, potassium deficiencies, and even death. Recovery

Table 8–4. Identifying Signals for Anorexia.

1. Loss of menstrual period
2. Dieting with relish when not overweight
3. Claiming to "feel fat" when an overweight condition does not exist
4. Preoccupation with food, calories, nutrition, or cooking
5. Denial of hunger
6. Excessive exercising; being overly active
7. Frequent checking of weight on scales
8. Use of laxatives or vomiting or both to control weight
9. Leaving for the bathroom after meals (secretive vomiting)
10. Strange food-related behaviors
11. Complaints of feeling bloated or nauseated when eating normal amounts of food
12. Intermittent episodes of "binge-eating"

From Neuman, P. A.; and Halvorson, P. A.: *Anorexia Nervosa and Bulimia, A Handbook for Counselors and Therapists.* Copyright © 1983 by Van Nostrand Reinhold Co. by permission of the publisher.

from anorexia nervosa is possible but diagnosis and treatment by trained medical personnel are imperative.

Bulimia victims may share the anorexic's fear of becoming fat but may or may not be obsessed with excessive thinness. They are trying to escape negative feelings and stressful situations.

Bulimia is characterized by binge-eating and then by purging one's self to control weight through vomiting or the use of laxatives or diuretics. Unlike the anorexic, for the bulimic eating is an obsession. The bulimic usually maintains near normal body weight. This disease tends to be chronic—it comes and goes—unlike anorexia, which is more constant. Like anorexia, the victims of bulimia are usually female (5 to 10 percent are male) in their late adolescence or early twenties. Table 8–5, again formulated by Neuman and Halvorson (1983), lists early identifying signals of bulimia. Anorexia nervosa and bulimia are compared in Table 8–6.

Table 8–5. Identifying Signals for Bulimia.

1. Excessive concern about weight
2. Strict dieting followed by eating binges
3. Frequent overeating, especially when distressed
4. Binging on high calorie, sweet food (some bulimics may binge on salads or other foods)
5. Expressing guilt or shame about eating
6. Being secretive about binges and vomiting
7. Planning binges or opportunities to binge
8. Feeling out of control
9. Disappearing after a meal
10. Depressive moods

From Neuman, P. A.; and Halvorson, P. A.: *Anorexia Nervosa and Bulimia, A Handbook for Counselors and Therapists.* Copyright © 1983 by Van Nostrand Reinhold Co. by permission of the publisher.

Table 8–6. Comparison of Bulimia and Anorexia.

Anorexics	*Bulimics*
1. Refusal to maintain recommended minimal weight	1. Normal or near-normal weight—may be overweight
2. Afflicts younger age group	2. Afflicts older age group
3. Loss of menstrual period	3. Menstrual period may or may not be lost; irregularities common
4. Distorted body image common	4. Usually do not have a distorted body image
5. The existence of a food-related problem is generally denied	5. Eating is recognized as being abnormal
6. More self control	6. More impulsivity—alcohol and drug abuse common
7. Anemia and vitamin deficiencies rare	7. Anemia and vitamin deficiencies are uncommon but not as rare
8. Vomiting less pervasive	8. Greater incidence of vomiting and other purging behavior
9. Eating rituals	9. Generally appear to eat in a normal manner when not binging and when eating in public
10. 4–25 percent mortality rate	10. Mortality rate undetermined

From Neuman, P. A.; and Halvorson, P. A.: *Anorexia Nervosa and Bulimia, A Handbook for Counselors and Therapists.* Copyright © 1983 by Van Nostrand Reinhold, Co. by permission of the publisher.

Lean Body Weight Gain (Muscle Weight)

Gaining weight is easy for most of us; unfortunately, in most cases it is a body fat gain rather than an increase in lean muscle weight. When a person consumes more calories than he or she expends, a **positive energy balance** is said to exist and weight will be gained. A **negative energy balance** exists when more calories are expended than consumed and, consequently, weight is lost. If, for example, a young, adult, nonathletic man were to consume 3,500 kcal in a day yet expend only 3,000 kcal, then he would be in a positive energy balance and gain body weight. The crucial point is would this weight be fat weight or fat-free weight? It could be fat-free weight if he were involved in an exercise program during this positive energy balance. In other words, he could be gaining muscle weight, not fat weight. It requires about 2,500 kcal of excessive calorie intake to gain 1 pound of fat-free weight or muscle mass. With the 500 kcal excess in our illustration it would therefore take five days (500 × 5 = 2,500) to gain 1 pound of lean body mass. The exercise programs given in Chapter 4, particularly the weight training program, as well as the caloric values of food listed in Appendix B will help you in establishing a regimen for gaining lean body weight. Just like the loss of excessive fat, the gain of lean body weight or muscle tissue is also a slow process.

When starting this process, it is wise for one to keep caloric intake at a level that does not exceed caloric expenditure by more than 1,000 to 1,500 kcal or about 2 to 3 pounds per week. The most practical approach would be the example stated of a daily excess of 500 kcal combined with the weight training program suggested in Chapter 4. This would result in a weekly weight increase of approximately 1 pound. Once again, exercise and persevere!

SUMMARY

◇ Many diseases are associated with overfatness—heart disease, bone and joint diseases, atherosclerosis, and diabetes to name a few.

◇ Insidious overfatness affects the average man and woman considerably and is the main cause of our overweight and overfat society.

◇ Body composition has two components: (1) body fat weight; and (2) fat-free weight (lean body weight or muscle weight).

◇ Two factors determine the amount of body fat that our bodies store: (1) the number of fat-storing cells (adipocytes); and (2) the capacity or size of the adipocytes.

◇ When we reach adulthood, the size but not the number of our adipocytes can be changed by dietary restrictions.

◇ The control of fat cells must begin early in childhood.

◇ Body fat accounts for approximately 22 to 25 percent of the total body weight of the average college-aged woman and 12 to 15 percent of the average college-aged man.

◇ The percentage of body fat of athletes is usually lower than that of their nonathletic counterparts.

◇ Menstrual irregularities can occur in women with very low body fat values.

◇ Obesity is primarily caused by inactivity, *not* by overeating.

◇ Height-weight charts must be carefully used.

◇ Anorexia nervosa and bulimia are two diet-related diseases that have devastating effects and may even cause death.

◇ Body composition can be assessed by somatotyping, skinfold measurements, or underwater weighing.

◇ Spot reducing is a myth.

◇ Two to three pounds per week is an ideal amount of weight for an adult to lose on a weight-loss program.

◇ Exercise is as important as dietary considerations when trying to lose fat weight or gain lean muscle weight.

STUDY QUESTIONS

1. Discuss the validity of the saying that "a fat baby is a healthy baby."
2. How does body fat affect physical performance?
3. What is obesity and how can it be avoided or overcome?
4. Why must height-weight charts be carefully used?
5. What is anorexia nervosa? What are signs of this disease?

6. What is bulimia? What are its symptoms?
7. How do you lose body fat?
8. How do you gain lean body weight?
9. Why is "making weight" for an athletic event hazardous and undesirable?
10. Using Appendix C, calculate your caloric expenditure for one day, and for the same day, using Appendix B, calculate your caloric intake.
11. Why is exercise as important as dietary restrictions in a weight-loss program?

REFERENCES AND SUGGESTED READINGS

Briggs, G. M.; and Calloway, D. H.: *Bogert's Nutrition and Physical Fitness*, 10th ed. Philadelphia: W. B. Saunders Co., 1979.

Fox, E. L.: *Lifetime Fitness*. Philadelphia: Saunders College Publishing, 1983.

Fox, E. L.: *Sports Physiology*, 2nd ed. Philadelphia: Saunders College Publishing, 1984.

Fox, E. L.; and Mathews, D. K.: *The Physiological Basis of Physical Education and Athletics*, 3rd ed. Philadelphia: Saunders College Publishing, 1981.

Heath, B.; and Carter, J.: A modified somatotype method. *American Journal of Physical Anthropology* 27:57–74, 1967.

Neuman, P. A.; and Halvorson, P. A.: *Anorexia Nervosa and Bulimia, A Handbook for Counselors and Therapists*. New York: Van Nostrand Reinhold Co. Inc., 1983.

Sheldon, W.: *Atlas of Men*. New York: Harper and Brothers, 1954.

Smith, N. J.: *Food for Sport*. Palo Alto, CA: Bull Publishing Co., 1976.

Chapter 9
Evaluation of Fitness

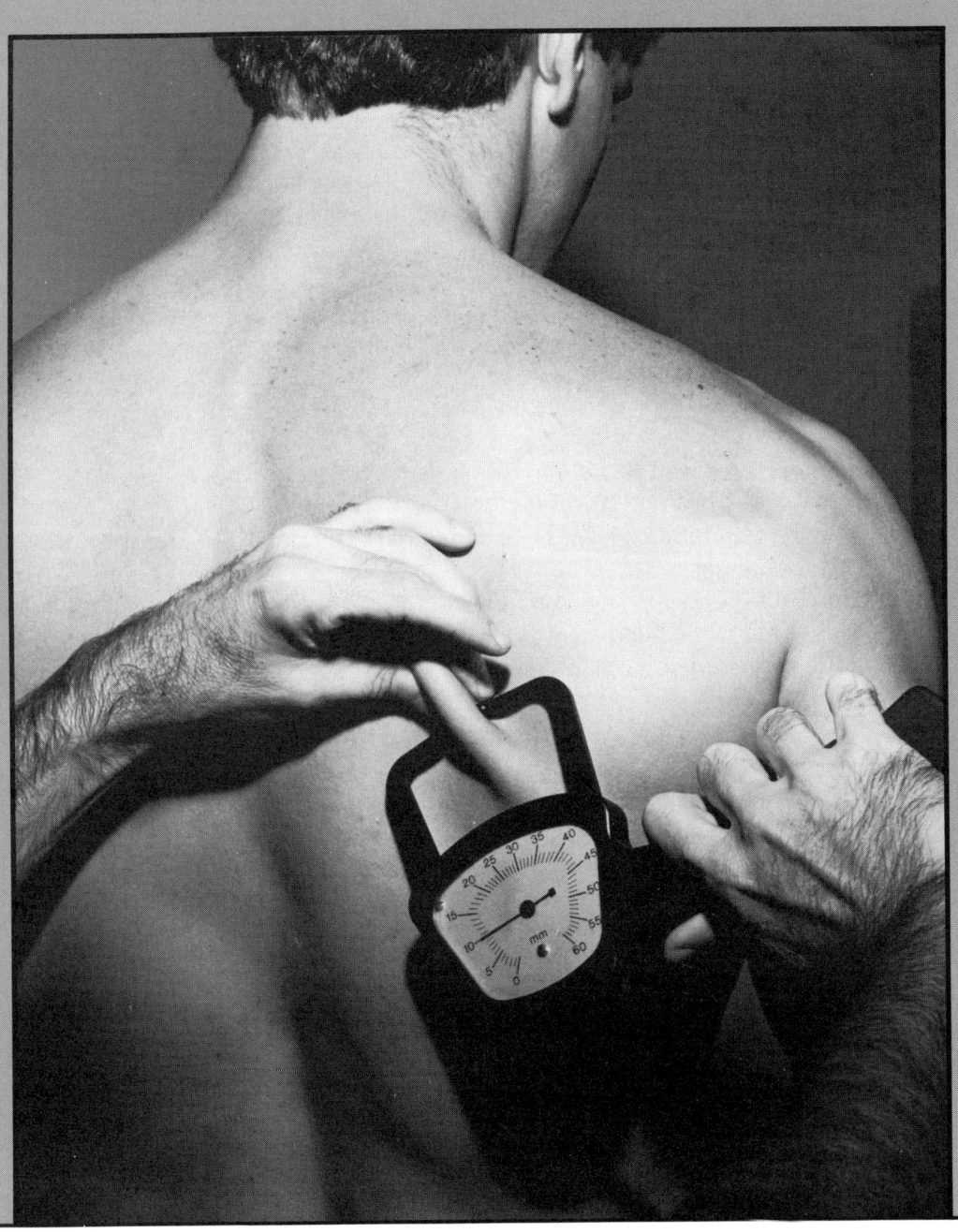

Chapter Outline

Learning Objectives

◇ To know what factors should be evaluated to determine a person's fitness level.

◇ To know the changes that occur with a fitness program.

◇ To be able to identify the specific changes that occur after cardiorespiratory training in the following variables: (1) heart rate; (2) maximal oxygen consumption; (3) cardiac output; and (4) stroke volume.

◇ To be able to identify the specific change that occurs after strength training.

◇ To understand the effects that detraining have on cardiorespiratory fitness and muscle strength and endurance.

◇ To understand and be able to implement evaluation of cardiorespiratory fitness with: (1) submaximal tests using a bicycle ergometer and a step test; and (2) a field test.

◇ To understand and be able to implement an evaluation of muscular strength.

◇ To understand and be able to implement flexibility evaluations using the sit-and-reach test and a test of shoulder flexibility.

◇ To understand the concept of body composition determination by underwater weighing.

◇ To be able to evaluate body composition using skinfold measurements.

◇ To be able to evaluate scores of fitness measurements, and to identify the recommended levels of each.

Key Words and Phrases

aerobic power
Åstrand-Rhyming bicycle
  ergometer test
contractility
Cooper's 12-minute run test
detraining
graded exercise test (GXT)
Ohio State University step test

PWC_{170} test
sit-and-reach test
skinfold caliper
skinfold measurement
Sloan-Weir method
three-site method of Pollock,
  Schmidt, and Jackson
underwater weighing

Introduction

T O properly evaluate fitness the term must be clearly defined. In Chapter 1 we answered the question "What is fitness?" In subsequent chapters further insight was provided into an interpretation of that definition. Fitness was earlier defined as a physiological or functional capacity that permits an improved quality of life. The question to be answered in this chapter is "How can we assess physiological or functional capacity?" Also, there are other factors we cannot assess that may affect the quality of life.

Evaluation

Evaluating the factors that indicate your fitness level can be a significant aid in developing and maintaining an appropriate fitness program. An evaluation of your fitness level before beginning a program will provide a benchmark against which you can compare future evaluations. Be it good, bad, or in-between, an unbiased evaluation usually serves as an excellent motivator. Little else will have the impact that a comparison of fitness values, before and after training, will have on our motivation levels to continue an exercise training program.

Frequency of Evaluation

How often should we evaluate our progress? Changes in each factor will occur at different rates for each person and according to the specific factor being measured. Change is unlikely to occur after 3 to 4 weeks of appropriate exercises unless there are changes in the intensity, frequency, or duration of a cardiovascular program. With gradual increases in one or more of the criteria, a large percentage of the benefits to be gained, from a health-related standpoint, is likely to occur in 3 to 4 months. An evaluation should be made at the start of your program, then after 3 months and every 6 to 12 months thereafter.

Factors Included in Evaluation

The factors that should be included in your evaluation are: (1) cardiorespiratory fitness; (2) body composition; (3) flexibility; and (4) muscular strength and endurance. Each of these factors is discussed in detail below. Before your evaluation or before starting an exercise program, remember that a medical examination and clearance from your physician are important prerequisites.

Some factors associated with the changes that occur as a result of an exercise training program do not lend themselves to an evaluation or are very difficult to evaluate with acceptable precision. We often hear testimony from people who have been involved in a regular exercise program about how much better they feel. There is little doubt that most people do feel better when they exercise regularly but this is difficult to measure accurately. Other similar changes associated with an exercise training program are an increased productivity on the job or in school, less chronic fatigue, an improvement in self-concept and other psychological variables, and an increased ability to deal with stressful situations. Each of these factors has been and continues to be an area of investigation and the results that have been produced often support the concept that regular exercise does improve the quality of life. In a fitness program it is likely that you will experience improvement in at least one or perhaps all of these areas but they are nevertheless very difficult to quantify.

Changes in Fitness Variables

If we are going to evaluate change, it is useful not only to have absolute values with which we can compare new values but also to have a knowledge of the changes that can be expected.

Cardiovascular Changes. A basic change that occurs after a cardiovascular conditioning program can be seen in Figure 9–1. The line representing the heart rate response has shifted up and to the left, indicating a decreased heart rate at any given level of work. This decreased heart rate also can be seen at rest or at work at the same level of oxygen consumption. This is mainly because of the increase in stroke volume and improvement in efficiency that occur as a result of training. Figure 9–2 provides an indication of the changes that occur in some physiological and functional variables when measuring fitness.

The increase in maximal oxygen consumption or **aerobic power** ($\dot{V}O_2max$) that can be anticipated for college-aged men or women following 3 months of appropriate training will range between 5 and 20 percent. As you know from Chapter 4, maximal oxygen consumption is a measure of the functional capacity of your aerobic system. It is generally considered by most exercise physiologists to be the best single measure of cardiorespiratory endurance fitness.

The increased maximal cardiac output (Figure 9–2) is a factor largely responsible for an increased $\dot{V}O_2max$. The cardiac output, as described earlier

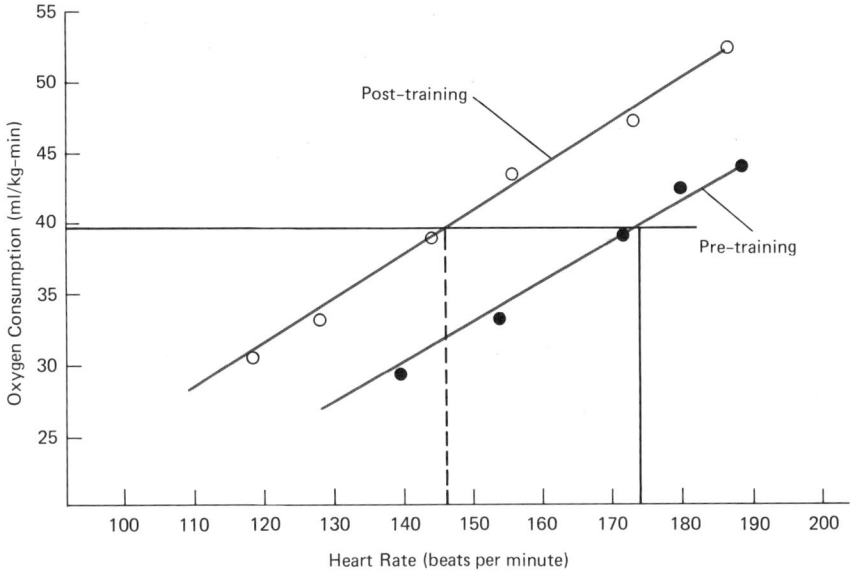

Figure 9–1. The change in heart rate at any given level of work after training. In this example when the subject was working at 40 ml/kg-min the pretraining heart rate was 172 and the post-training heart rate is 147.

in Chapter 2, is the product of stroke volume and heart rate. After training maximal heart rate remains unchanged or perhaps decreases slightly and so the change in cardiac output is the result of increases in stroke volume.

The stroke volume changes (Figure 9–2) that are a result of training are related to an increase in the size of the left ventricle (hypertrophy) and its ability to hold more blood, and to an increased efficiency of the ventricle to pump blood **(contractility).**

Strength Changes. Changes in muscle strength when measuring the large leg muscles (leg press) are approximately the same in men and women. After 3 months of training, there is an increase of approximately 25 percent in men and 28 percent in women. Women, however, show greater gains than men in the bench press. This is probably because women have not previously challenged the muscle groups responsible for doing the bench press. After training, women show about a 30 percent increase in 1 RM bench press while men have about a 15 percent increase (Wilmore, 1974).

Flexibility Changes. Flexibility as measured by the sit-and-reach test is less likely to improve equally in men and women. The degree of improvement is not well established. The after-training value in Figure 9–2 is based on the 75th percentile achieved by college-aged students at the Ohio State University and may not be an accurate representation of the effects of a regular stretching program.

Body Fat Changes. The decrease in the percentage of fat that occurs with training and is represented in Figure 9–2 is for the average college-

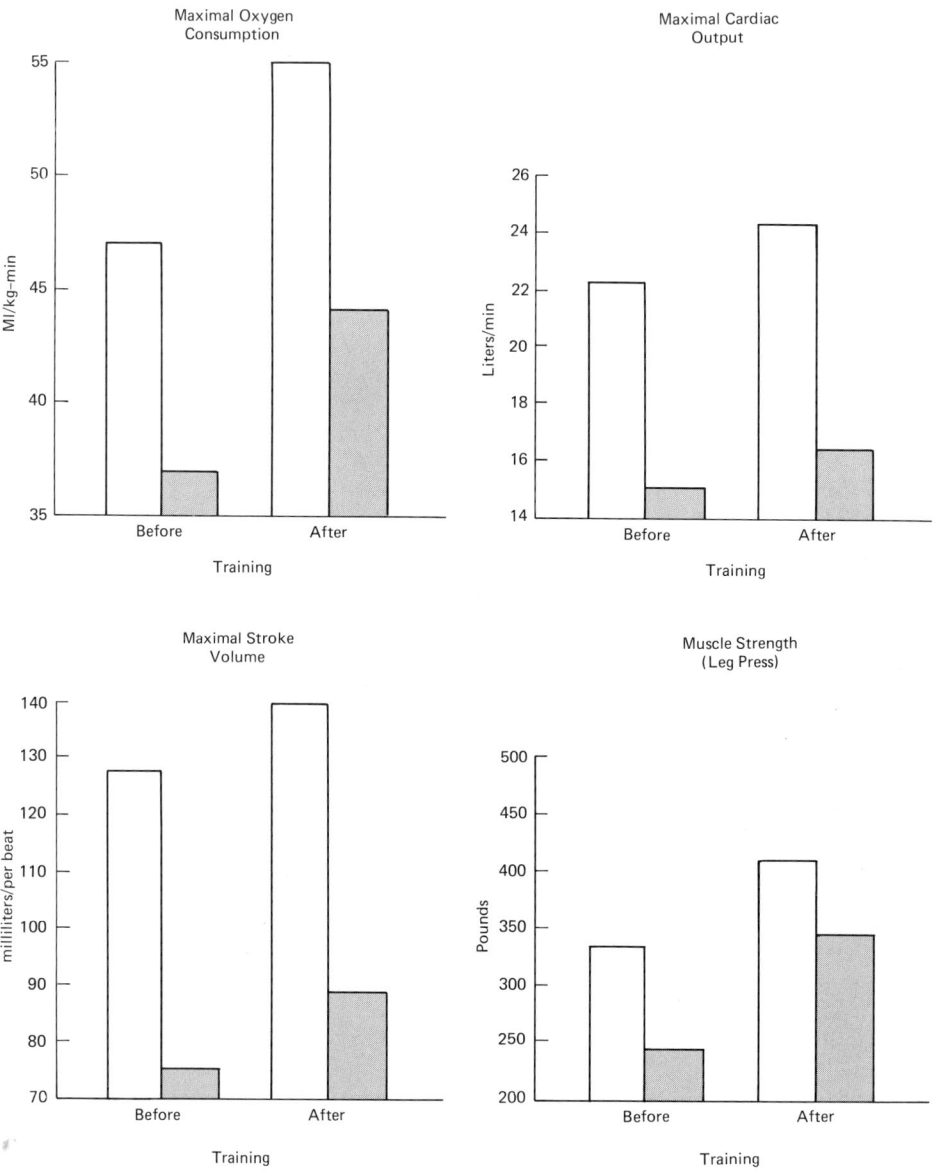

Figure 9–2. Expected changes that are likely to occur in the average 20-year-old (160 lb. male, 120 lb. female) after an appropriate training program of 3 months. Open bars represent males, shaded bars females.

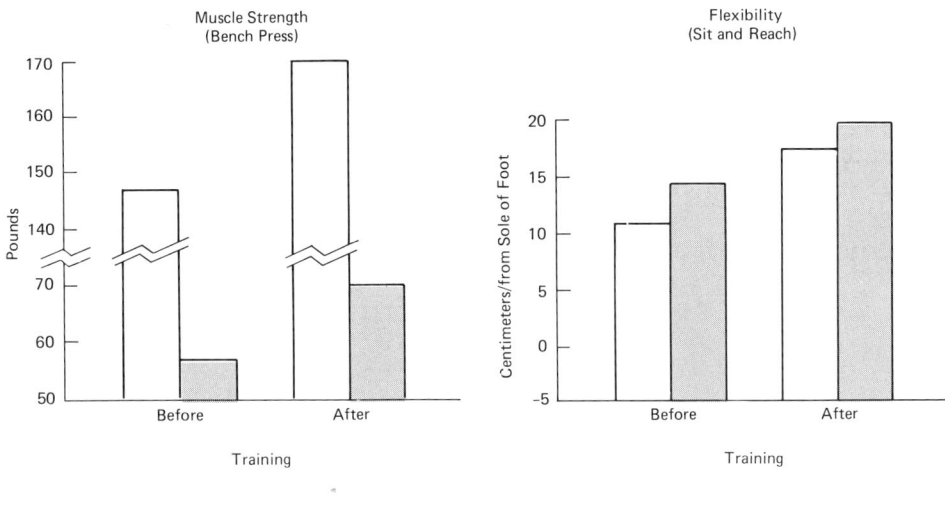

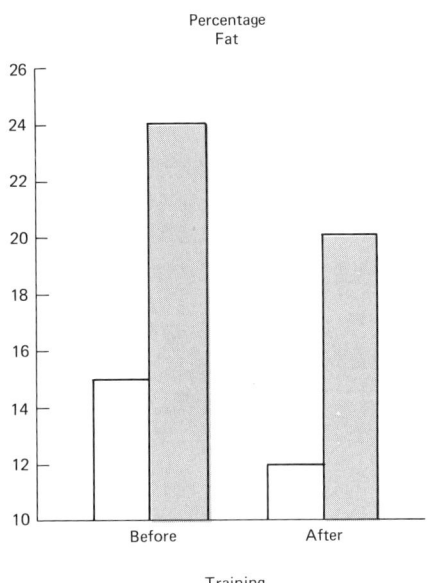

Figure 9–2 (Continued)

aged male and female. A change such as this may not result in a significant weight change because of the increase that can occur in lean body weight. If no weight resistance exercise were included in your program, the changes in the percentage of fat are likely to be accompanied by a total weight loss.

Losses in Training Effects. The effects of training on the cardiorespiratory system are lost within a relatively short period of time. When the training criteria in Chapter 4 arc no longer met, between 15 and 20 percent of the increase in $\dot{V}O_2$max will be lost per week. This means that after 4 to 8 weeks of **detraining** you will have reached the point at which you began. The loss of the effect of a weight training program, however, is much slower.

Although there is limited information on the effects of detraining after a weight resistance program is stopped, it appears that 75 percent or more of the strength and muscular endurance gained in the program are retained after 12 weeks of detraining and perhaps 40 to 50 percent of the original increase remains after one year (Fox and Mathews, 1981).

Cardiorespiratory Fitness Evaluation

As was mentioned previously, measurement of maximal oxygen consumption is the most valid means of determining cardiorespiratory fitness or maximal aerobic power. Both direct and indirect measurements of oxygen consumption are available. A direct measurement involves the subject working on a stationary bicycle ergometer or treadmill. Most direct measures use a **graded exercise test (GXT)** protocol, which allows for gradual increases in the work accomplished; each stage is 2 to 3 minutes in length. The protocols used should be designed so that the subject will reach his or her maximum ability to do work in approximately 10 minutes. The subject's maximum ability to do work at $\dot{V}O_2$max is attained when the measured values for $\dot{V}O_2$ do not increase with an increasing level of work. The expensive, sophisticated laboratory equipment and expertise needed to conduct maximal tests with a direct measure of oxygen consumption make such tests undesirable in many situations and therefore go beyond the scope of most programs. For this reason, a number of submaximal tests and field tests have been developed and provide more feasible methods with which to evaluate cardiorespiratory fitness. Four of these tests are the Astrand-Rhyming ergometer test, the PWC_{170} test, the Ohio State University step test, and Cooper's 12-minute run.

Åstrand-Rhyming Bicycle Ergometer Test. The **Åstrand-Rhyming bicycle ergometer test** (Åstrand, 1960) is a submaximal test based on the linear relationship that exists between workload ($\dot{V}O_2$) and heart rate. This linear relationship is most reliable with heart rates ranging between approximately 120 and 170 beats per minute. The originators of this evaluation have established an estimated $\dot{V}O_2$max for a heart rate response to a given workload on the bicycle ergometer with corrections made for the subject's age.

The procedure is as follows:

1. Set the bicycle ergometer seat height so that the subject's knee is nearly completely extended when the pedal is at bottom for greatest efficiency.
2. Have the subject pedal at 50 rpm (18 km/hr)—set the workload for the first trial at 300 kpm/min for women or 600 kpm/min for men.

Figure 9–3. Adjusted nomogram for calculating estimated $\dot{V}O_2$ max from submaximal heart rate and the associated workload in kpm/min on a bicycle ergometer. Estimate the $\dot{V}O_2$ cost of the submaximal work by reading horizontally from the "work load" scale to the "O_2 uptake" scale. This point should be connected to the corresponding point for heart rate on the "pulse scale," and the predicted $\dot{V}O_2$ can be read on the middle scale. For example a male subject reaches a heart rate of 166 at a workload of 1200 kpm/min. The drawn line indicates that his maximal oxygen consumption is 3.6 L/min. (From Astrand, I. Aerobic work capacity in men and women with special reference to age. Acta. Physiol. Scand. 49(suppl 169), 1–92, 1960.)

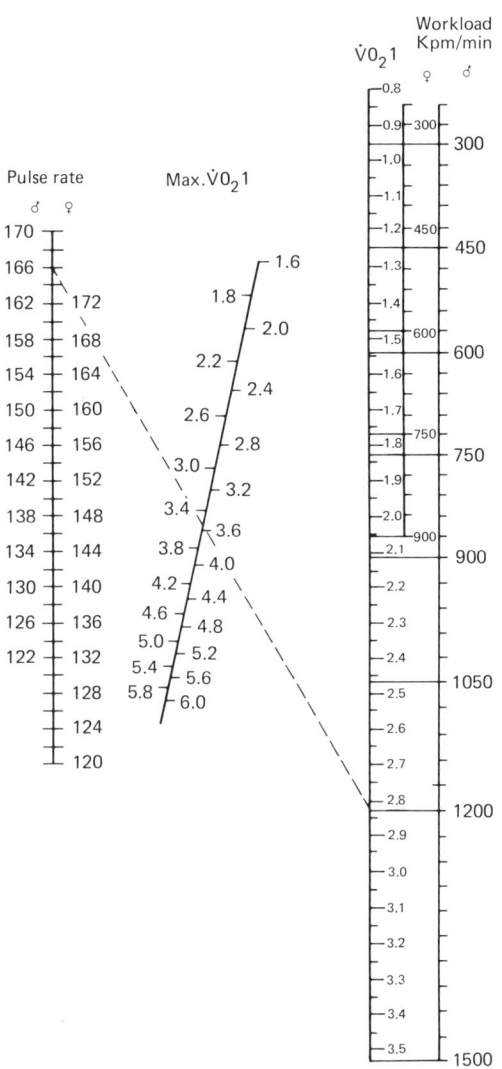

3. Adjust the workload during fourth minute of exercise if the heart rate is not between 120 and 170.

4. The average HR for minutes 5 and 6 is entered in the nomogram (Figure 9–3). The HR for minutes 5 and 6 (A) must be within the 120–170 range and (B) must be within 5 beats per minute of each other or the subject should continue to minute 7.

5. Apply the age correction factor (Table 9–1) [i.e., age factor × est. $\dot{V}O_2$ (liters per minute)].

6. Determine the $\dot{V}O_2$max estimate of the subject in milliliters per kilogram-minute.

Table 9–1. Age Correction Factors for Estimating the Maximal Oxygen Intake.

Age	Factor	Maximum Heart Rate	Factor
15	1.10	210	1.12
25	1.00	200	1.00
35	0.87	190	0.93
40	0.83	180	0.83
45	0.78	170	0.75
50	0.75	160	0.69
55	0.71	150	0.64
60	0.68		
65	0.65		

Reprinted with permission from Astrand, I.: Aerobic work capacity in men and women with special reference to age. *Acta Physiologica Scandinavica* 49(Suppl. 169):55, 1960.

Table 9–2. Maximal Oxygen Consumption ($\dot{V}O_2max$) Evaluation Chart.*

$\dot{V}O_2max$ Classification	Age				
	20–29	*30–39*	*40–49*	*50–59*	*60+*
Men					
Superior	>53	>50	>48	>45	>44
Excellent	46–53	45–50	44–48	41–45	36–44
Good	42–46	41–45	39–44	36–41	32–35
Fair	36–42	35–41	33–39	31–36	26–32
Poor	<36	<35	<33	<31	<26
Women					
Superior	>43	>42	>39	>37	>33
Excellent	38–43	37–42	35–39	33–37	29–33
Good	34–38	33–37	31–35	29–33	25–29
Fair	30–34	29–33	27–31	25–29	21–25
Poor	<30	<29	<27	<25	<21

* Values are expressed in milliliters per kilogram-minute (ml/kg-min).

7. Evaluate your $\dot{V}O_2max$ (ml/kg-min) by using Table 9–2.

$$\dot{V}O_2(\text{ml/kg-min}) = \frac{\dot{V}O_2(\text{liters/min}) \times 1{,}000}{\text{Weight (kg)}}$$

For example, a 25-year-old, 160-pound man was found to have a heart rate of 165 at the end of minute 5 and a rate of 167 at the end of minute 6 when the workload was 1,200 kpm/min. Using Figure 9–3 we see his predicted $\dot{V}O_2max$ is 3.6 liters/min. Following steps 5–7 we find:

5. Age correction from Table 9–1 is 1.0

$$1.0 \times 3.6 = 3.6 \text{ liters/min}$$

6. $\dot{V}O_2\text{(ml/kg-min)} = \dfrac{\dot{V}O_2\text{(liters/min)} \times 1{,}000}{\text{Weight (kg)}}$

$$= \dfrac{3.6 \times 1{,}000}{72.7}$$

$$\dot{V}O_2\text{(ml/kg-min)} = 49.5$$

7. Based on Table 9–2 we find our subject has an excellent maximal oxygen consumption.

The PWC$_{170}$ Test. The **PWC$_{170}$ test** or physical working capacity at a heart rate of 170 (Sinning, 1975) requires the subject to work at approximately 85 percent of his or her maximal heart rate and thus determines the level of work attainable at that heart rate. Since this evaluation was developed for a college-aged population and 170 beats per minute is 85 percent of the predicted maximum heart rate for a 20-year-old, the test was named the PWC$_{170}$ test. As a basis for evaluation to assess the change resulting from a training program, you would compare the amount of work attainable before training and after training at this given submaximal heart rate. The work could involve any mode (speed of walking, running, swimming, etc.); however, the original test used the bicycle ergometer, which provided for precise measurement.

The Ohio State University Step Test. The **Ohio State University Step Test** (Mathews, 1968) is a submaximal cardiovascular test devised to estimate the fitness of college-aged men. The test is certainly appropriate for women, but as yet no norms for women have been reported. Men and women follow the procedures outlined below. The test is based on the findings that the time required for the heart rate to increase to 150 beats per minute is a valid indicator of a subject's cardiovascular capacity for exhaustive work.

The activity requires minimum skill and lends itself well to large groups. The procedure for taking heart rate measurements in recovery is simple and can be taught very easily.

The test requires one specialized piece of equipment, which is a split-level bench, 15 inches high at one level and 20 inches high at the other, with an adjustable hand bar (Figure 9–4). It is helpful to record the test on a tape recorder, which can be timed periodically to ensure accurate replication.

The test is composed of 18 innings of 50 seconds duration (total time, 15 minutes). Each inning is divided into a 30-second work period and a 20-second rest period, during which a pulse count is taken for 10 seconds beginning with second 5 and stopping at second 15. The test is terminated when the pulse rate reaches 25 beats (150 beats per minute) or when the

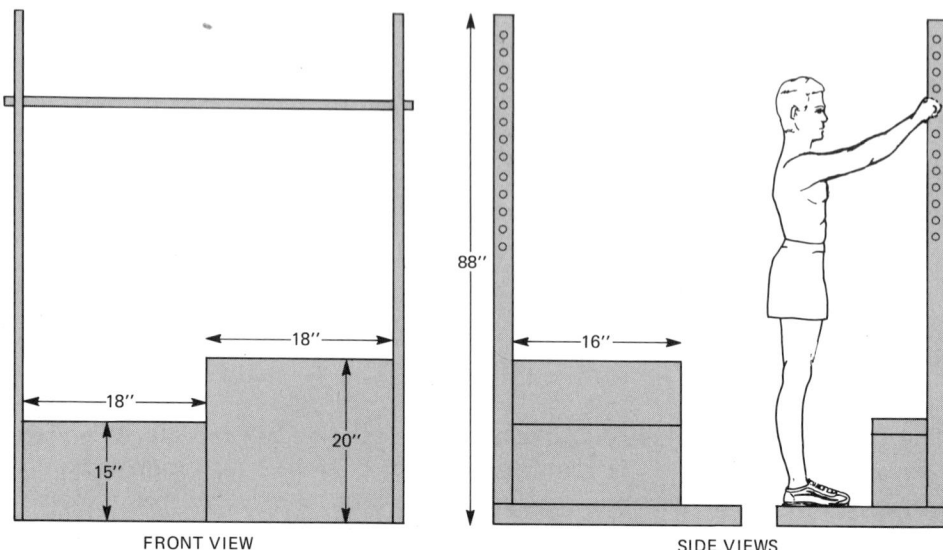

FRONT VIEW   SIDE VIEWS

Figure 9–4. Apparatus used in conducting The Ohio State University Step Test.

subject completes the entire 18 innings. Scoring is by the number of innings completed. There are three different work loads:

1. Phase I consists of 6 innings at a cadence of 24 steps per minute on the 15-inch bench.
2. Phase II consists of 6 innings at a cadence of 30 steps per minute on the 15-inch bench.
3. Phase III consists of 6 innings at a cadence of 30 steps per minute on the 20-inch bench. Phases I, II, and III are consecutive.

To take the test, the subject stands in front of the 15-inch platform and grasps the bar with both hands. When the commands "ready" and "up" are given by the examiner, the subject places one foot and then the other on the platform, straightens his legs and back, and immediately steps down again, one foot at a time. The pace "up, up, down, down," can be recorded on the tape and given every 2½ seconds. At the end of 30 seconds, the commands "stop" and "find your pulse" are given.

At exactly 5 seconds into the rest period the examiner commands "count," and at 15 seconds into the rest period the examiner commands "stop" and "prepare to exercise." He records the number of beats counted during the 10-second period and continues this procedure for 6 innings (or until a pulse rate of 150 is reached).

After the 10-second pulse count and before the seventh inning, the examiner informs the subject that the cadence will be increased and continues the same procedure. The 30-step-per-minute cadence during the seventh through twelfth innings requires that the commands "up, up, down, down" be given every 2 seconds.

Table 9–3. Interpretation of Results of the Ohio State University Step Test.

Level of Fitness		Result
Poor	−	Phase I; inning 1–2
	0	Phase I; inning 3–4
	+	Phase I; inning 5–6
Fair	−	Phase II; inning 1–2
	0	Phase II; inning 3–4
	+	Phase II; inning 5–6
Good	−	Phase III; inning 1
	0	Phase III; inning 2
	+	Phase III; inning 3
Excellent	−	Phase III; inning 4
	0	Phase III; inning 5
	+	Phase III; inning 6

Reprinted with permission from Mathews, D. K.: *Measurement in Physical Education.* Copyright © 1968 by W. B. Saunders Co. Reprinted with permission of Saunders College Publishing, CBS College Publishing.

After the 10-second pulse count and before the thirteenth inning, the subject is told to move over to the 20-inch platform, where the cadence of 30 steps per minute is continued for the thirteenth through eighteenth innings.

The end point of the test is the eighteenth inning or when the subject's heart rate reaches 25 beats in the 10-second pulse count (150 beats per minute), whichever occurs first. Only those with superior aerobic capabilities will reach the eighteenth inning. The minimum and maximum times for the test are 50 seconds and 15 minutes, respectively. Usually it is easier for the subject to step up with the same foot each time rather than to alternate the feet. However, alternating is permissible if one leg becomes tired. The examiner must be sure that the subject steps completely onto the platform during the test. No crouching should be permitted.

The subject's score is the inning during which his or her heart rate reaches 150 beats per minute (25 beats during the 10-second pulse count). Table 9–3 provides a basis for comparison and an interpretation of the results.

Cooper's 12-Minute Run Test. **Cooper's 12-minute run** (Cooper, 1977) requires a near maximal effort and is highly dependent upon the motivation of the subject. To complete this evaluation the subject should run for 12 minutes on a measured track and note the distance covered to the nearest hundredth of a mile. Cooper found that this distance was highly correlated with direct measures of oxygen consumption made in the laboratory. Figure 9–5 provides a classification of distances and the associated $\dot{V}O_2$max for men and women ages 20 to 29 years. Information for other age groups can be found in Cooper's text.

Other field tests commonly used are the 9-minute run and the 1- or 1.5-mile run for time. Regardless of the method used to directly measure or

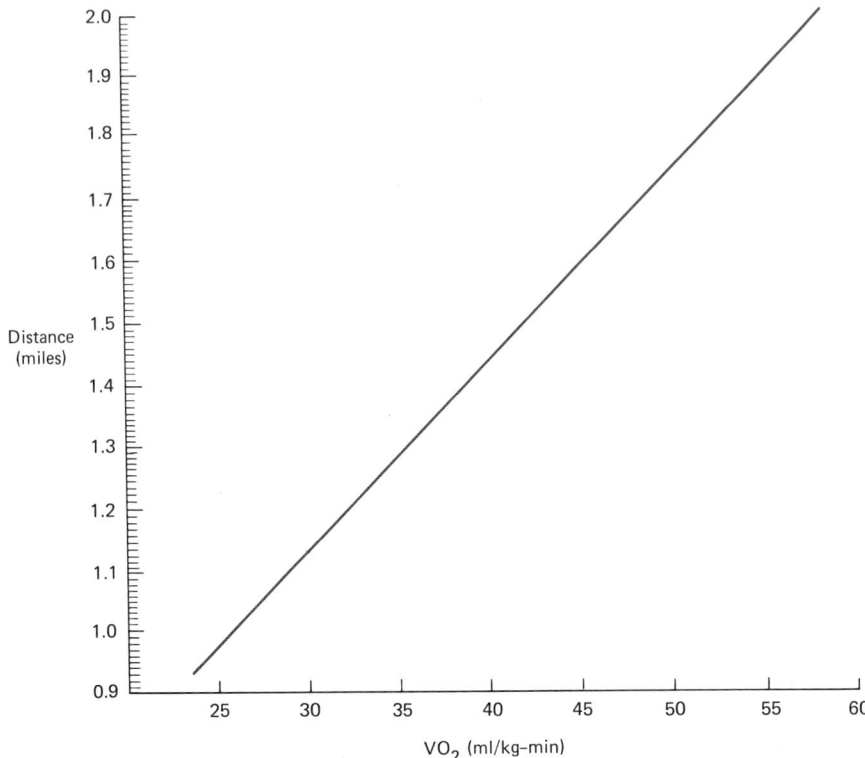

Figure 9–5. The relationship between oxygen consumption and total distance covered during a 12-minute run.

estimate $\dot{V}O_2$max, the chart in Table 9–2 provides a comparison to normal standards and an indication of your present level of cardiorespiratory fitness. The categories presented here coincide with Table 4–4 in Chapter 4, which determined your starting stage for a walk/run program based on $\dot{V}O_2$max.

Evaluation of Muscle Strength and Endurance

You will recall that strength has been defined as the amount of force produced (resistance overcome) during a single repetition maximum (1 RM). For any given muscle group an appropriate determination of strength would be a determination of the amount of weight that can be lifted one time for the particular exercise that uses that muscle group. Repeated attempts, with appropriate rest periods in between, should be conducted until the subject reaches a weight that cannot be moved through the range of motion of the exercise. Those involved in weight training have recognized the lack of reliability of this type of measure. Motivation, day-to-day changes, nonavaila-

Table 9–4. An Evaluation of Strength Based on a Single Repetition Maximum Load Capability.*

Strength	Bench Press	Standing Press	Arm Curl	Leg Press
		Male		
Excellent	>105	>85	<60	<240
Very Good	90–105	70–85	50–60	210–240
Good	75–89	60–69	40–49	180–209
Fair	60–74	45–59	30–39	150–179
Poor	<60	<45	<30	<150
		Female		
Excellent	>90	>65	<45	<205
Very Good	75–90	50–65	35–45	175–205
Good	60–74	40–49	25–34	145–174
Fair	45–59	25–39	15–24	115–144
Poor	<45	<25	<15	<115

Adapted from Wilmore, J. H.: Alterations in strength, body composition, and anthropometric measurements consequent to a 10-week training program. *Medicine and Science in Sports* 6:133–138, 1974; and Pollock, M. L.; Wilmore, J. H.; and Fox, S. M.: *Health and Fitness Through Physical Activity.* New York: John Wiley & Sons, 1978.

* Values indicate percentages of subject total body weight.

bility of precise loads, and other factors all contribute to the difficulty of obtaining highly reliable results. To implement this strength evaluation, use the lowest charted weight (i.e., poor) from Table 9–4 for the initial trial. Add or subtract weight as appropriate to find the maximum weight.

Isokinetic testing devices are another means by which to evaluate strength. These devices are thought by many to be more precise because of their ability to measure maximal force production at each angle of pull within the range of motion (see Chapter 5). The problem of subject reliability still exists with these devices but the variability may be less. Such testing devices, however, are very expensive and are not available to most persons who would like to evaluate strength. When this equipment is available, some question exists about its usefulness as a testing device when training has been isotonic.

A single RM can be determined for each of the weight training exercises discussed in Chapter 5. Listed in Table 9–4 is an evaluation based on body weight for selected exercises.

Flexibility Evaluation

It is difficult to specifically and reliably measure the range of motion of a given joint. Some widely used testing devices are available but they usually lack joint specificity. The most widely used test is the **sit-and-reach test.** There are other more specific measurement devices, for example, the goniometer and the Leighton flexometer, but these have their limitations as well. The goniometer is used to measure the angle through which a subject is able to move. It is easily used and readily available but requires a subjective determination concerning the axis of the bones constituting the joint.

The sit-and-reach test has excellent reliability and is objective, but it includes a combined measure of the flexibility of the hip and the lower and upper back. As discussed in Chapter 6, our major interest in flexibility from a health-related standpoint is hip flexibility and its relation to low back pain. The sit-and-reach test is outlined below because it provides the best available evaluation with standards to judge performance. You should keep in mind, however, that this measure falls short of the ideal measure of hip flexibility and ignores other joints of particular importance such as the shoulders.

Figure 9–6 shows an example of the sit-and-reach test being administered. The testing apparatus is a box $16 \times 16 \times 16$ inches with the top board extending approximately 10 inches toward the subject. The top of the apparatus should be marked in centimeters (cm), with the 23-cm mark at the bottom of the foot and used as a measuring scale.

The subject should remove his or her shoes, sit down with the knees fully extended and feet flat against the front board as shown and about shoulder-width apart. The arms are extended forward with the right hand placed evenly on top of the left. The subject reaches as far forward as possible, palms down, four times slowly, holding the fourth trial for 1 second; the reading then is taken. The tester should read the score to the nearest centimeter ensuring that the subject has not bent his or her knees. A warm-up should be allowed and encouraged. In Table 9–5 are the standards for a college-

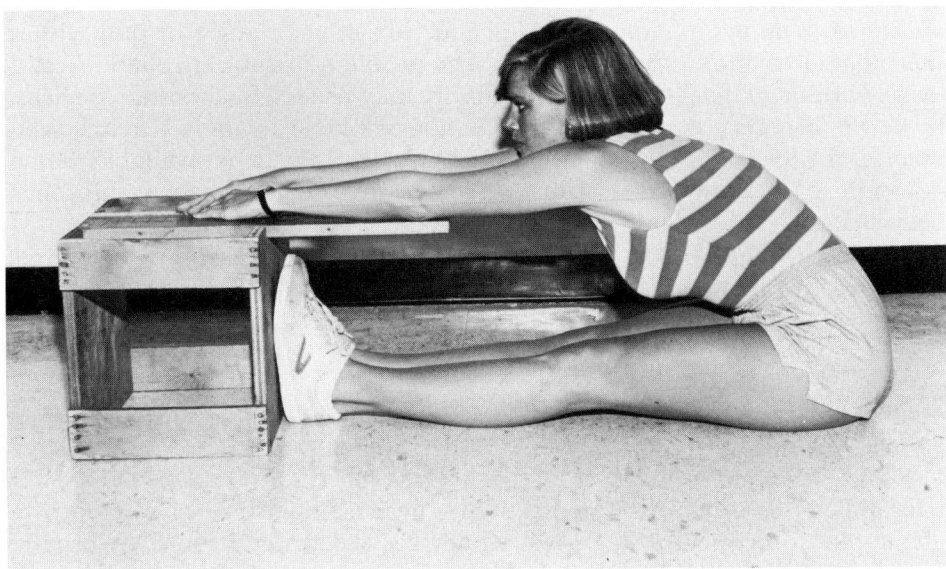

Figure 9–6. The sit-and-reach test is used to evaluate flexibility of the hips and lower back region.

Table 9–5. Evaluation of Flexibility
Using the Sit-and-Reach Test.*

Result	Men	Women
Excellent	>40	>43
Very Good	37–40	39–43
Good	33–36	37–38
Fair	28–32	32–36
Poor	<27	<32

* Values are in centimeters, with 23 cm being even with the bottom of the foot.

aged population developed while using this testing procedure on 200 students at The Ohio State University.

A simple test used by the authors to assess shoulder flexibility is demonstrated in Figure 9–7. The subject is asked to reach behind his or her back with each hand and slide the hand up his or her back as far as possible, keeping the wrist straight.

Body Composition Evaluation

The discussion of body composition provided in Chapter 8 (pp. 155–159) indicated many of the ways people evaluate their body compositions and ideal weights. Some of these were noted as appropriate, others somewhat lacking in capabilities to evaluate body composition appropriately.

Figure 9–7. Test of shoulder flexibility. Scored as follows: 5 = excellent; 4 = very good; 3 = good; 2 = fair; 1 = poor.

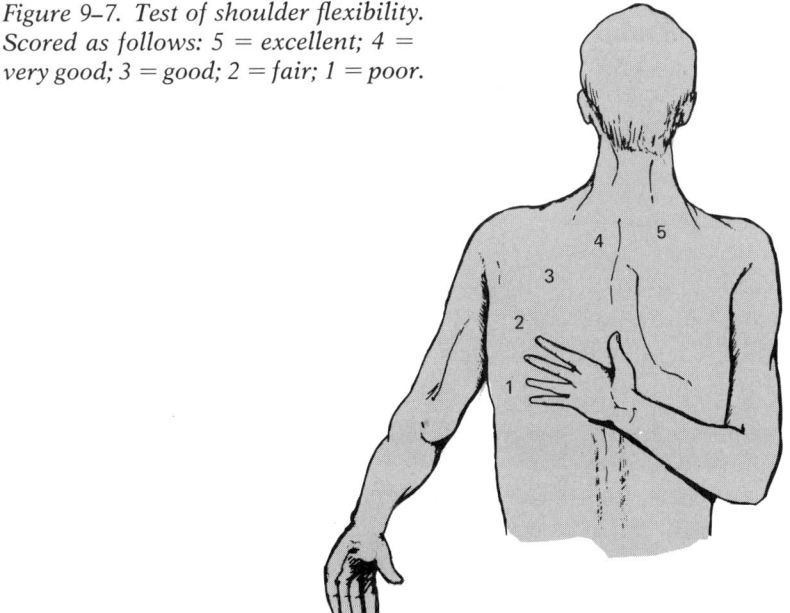

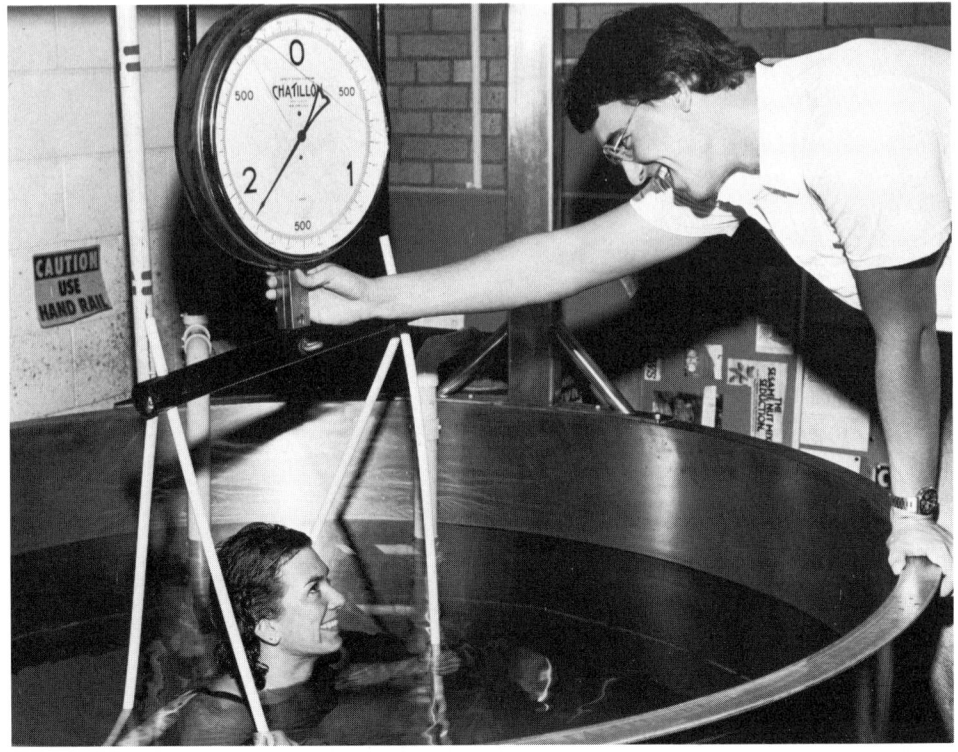

Figure 9–8. Determining body composition using underwater weighing method.

Underwater Weighing. The determination of body density (Db) using **underwater weighing** has been a widely used method for determining fat percentage. This method is based on Archimedes' Principle and requires a tank such as that shown in Figure 9–8. The formulas for determining Db and percentage of fat are:

$$Db = \frac{Wa}{\dfrac{Wa - Ww}{Dw} - RV}$$

where Db is body density in grams per cubic centimeter; Wa is the weight of the subject in air in grams; Ww is the weight of the subject in water in grams; Dw is the density of the water; and RV is the residual volume in cubic centimeters.

$$\% \, Fat = \left(\frac{4.95}{Db} - 4.50\right) \times 100*$$

This method requires that the subject be completely submerged and the lungs deflated as much as possible so that only the residual volume remains. Residual volume can be estimated as 28 percent of the vital capacity for

* SIRI formula from Fox and Mathews (1981).

women and 24 percent for men, or approximately 1,300 ml for men and 1,000 ml for women.

Skinfold Measurements. In the hands of an experienced evaluator, a more practical, reliable, and accurate method is the determination of body fat by **skinfold measurement.** Numerous equations using many skinfold sites have been developed for different populations. The two methods provided below have been developed for college-aged students, although the second covers a wider age range.

The **Sloan-Weir method** predicts fat percentage from two skinfold measurements (Sloan and Weir, 1970). In men, a vertical skinfold on the anterior midline of the thigh, halfway between the inguinal ligament and top of the patella (Fig. 9–9A) and a subscapular skinfold running downward and laterally in the natural fold of the skin along the inferior border of the scapula (Fig. 9–9B) are measured. In women, a vertical skinfold over the iliac crest in the midaxillary line (Fig. 9–9C) and a vertical skinfold over the triceps muscle halfway between the acromial process and olecranon process of the ulna (Fig. 9–9D) is used. All skinfold measurements should be taken on the right side of the body. Figure 9–10 contains the nomograms used to find body density from the two skinfold measures.

A second method is the **three-site method of Pollack, Schmidt, and Jackson** (1980). This method uses the sum of three skinfolds and directly provides a fat percentage based on the subject's age (Tables 9–6 and 9–7). The three sites used for men are the thigh, described above; the abdomen, which is a vertical skinfold 1 to 2 inches to the right of the navel; and the chest, which is a diagonal skinfold taken midway between the acromial process and the nipple. The sites used for women are the triceps, the suprailiac, and the thigh—all described above.

When using the skinfold method the recommended procedure is as follows:

1. Firmly grasp the skin between thumb and forefinger, with a finger pointed down, and lift it away from underlying muscle.
2. Place the contact surfaces of the caliper 1 cm below the finger.
3. Slowly release open calipers enabling them to exert pressure (10 g/mm²) on the skinfold for 1 to 2 seconds and take reading.
4. Two successive readings within 1 mm of each other constitute a successful trial.

Figure 9–11 shows some of the **skinfold calipers** presently available. Those on the left are expensive and reliable; those on the right are low in cost. The inexpensive calipers have demonstrated excellent accuracy; however, their reliability over the long-term to produce consistent pressure is unproved.*

* Available from Ross Laboratories, 625 Cleveland Avenue, Columbus, Ohio 43215.

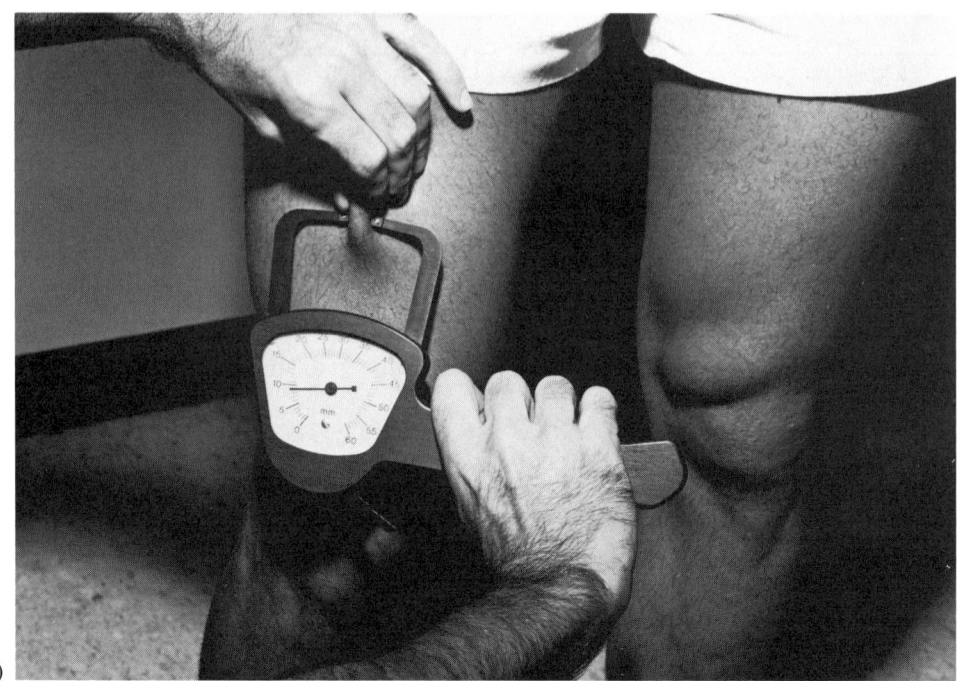

(A)

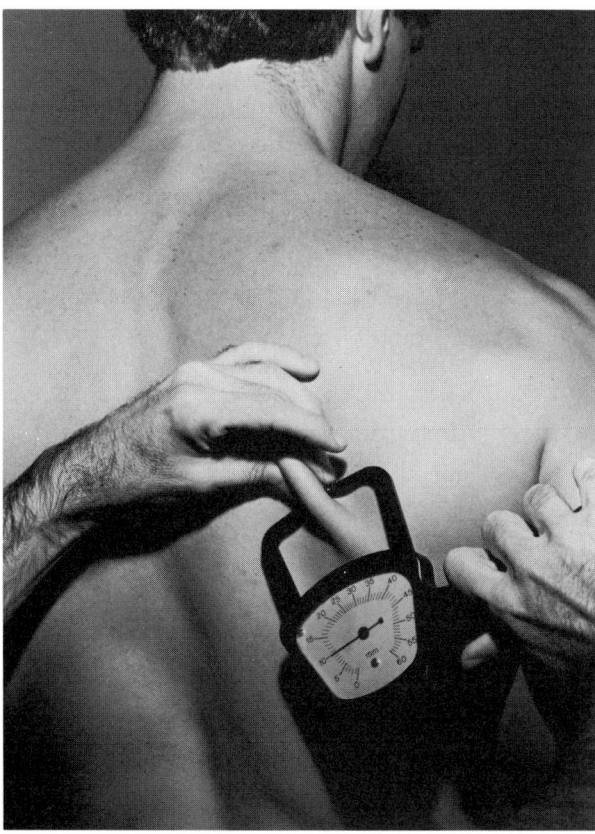

(B)

Figure 9–9. Locations and technique to be used with a Sloan Weir nomogram for (A) male thigh, (B) subscapular skinfold, (C) female tricep, and (D) iliac crest skinfold measures.

190

Figure 9–9. (Continued)

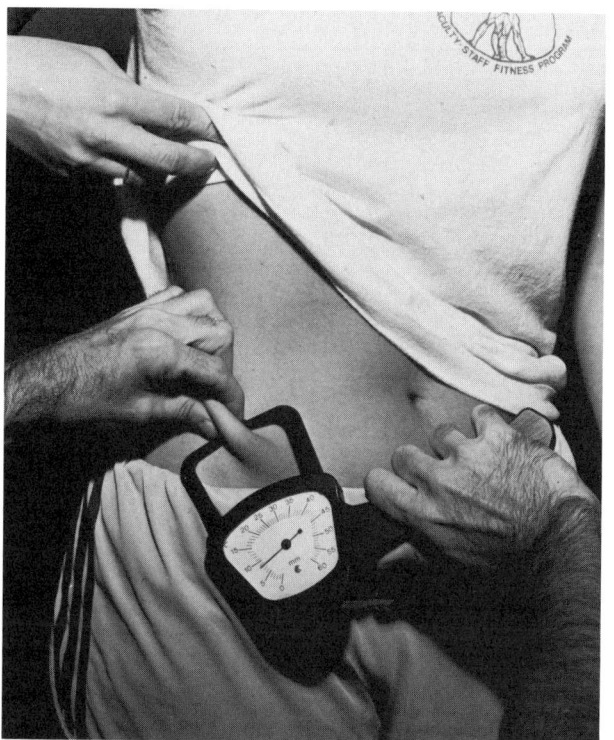

(C)

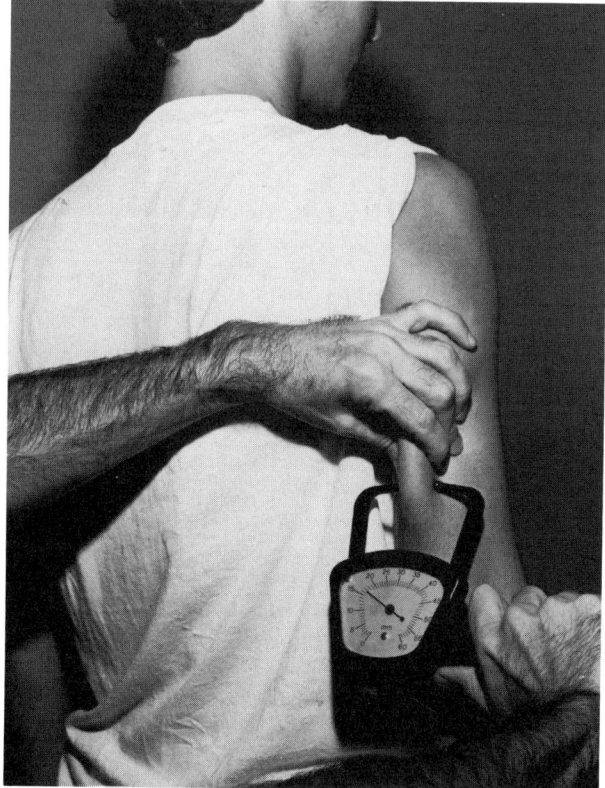

(D)

191

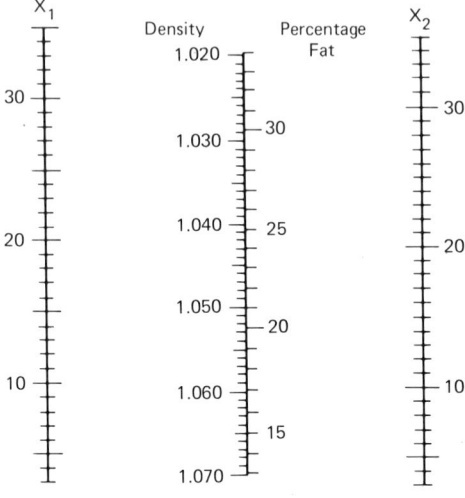

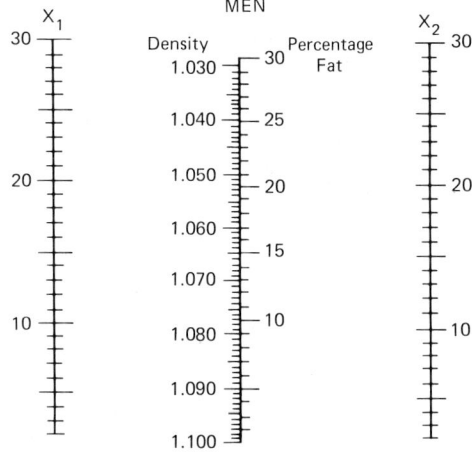

Figure 9–10. Sloan-Weir nomograms for men and women for the prediction of body density and percentage fat. (From Sloan, A. and Weir, J.: Nomograms for prediction of body density and total body fat from skinfold measurements. J. Appl. Physiol. *28(2):221–222, 1970.)*

Table 9–6. Estimating the Percentage of Body Fat in Males.

Sum of Skin Folds (mm)*	Age to the Last Year								
	Under 22	23–27	28–32	33–37	38–42	43–47	48–52	53–57	Over 58
8–10	1.3	1.8	2.3	2.9	3.4	3.9	4.5	5.0	5.5
11–13	2.2	2.8	3.3	3.9	4.4	4.9	5.5	6.0	6.5
14–16	3.2	3.8	4.3	4.8	5.4	5.9	6.4	7.0	7.5
17–19	4.2	4.7	5.3	5.8	6.3	6.9	7.4	8.0	8.5
20–22	5.1	5.7	6.2	6.8	7.3	7.9	8.4	8.9	9.5
23–25	6.1	6.6	7.2	7.7	8.3	8.8	9.4	9.9	10.5
26–28	7.0	7.6	8.1	8.7	9.2	9.8	10.3	10.9	11.4
29–31	8.0	8.5	9.1	9.6	10.2	10.7	11.3	11.8	12.4
32–34	8.9	9.4	10.0	10.5	11.1	11.6	12.2	12.8	13.3
35–37	9.8	10.4	10.9	11.5	12.0	12.6	13.1	13.7	14.3
38–40	10.7	11.3	11.8	12.4	12.9	13.5	14.1	14.6	15.2
41–43	11.6	12.2	12.7	13.3	13.8	14.4	15.0	15.5	16.1
44–46	12.5	13.1	13.6	14.2	14.7	15.3	15.9	16.4	17.0
47–49	13.4	13.9	14.5	15.1	15.6	16.2	16.8	17.3	17.9
50–52	14.3	14.8	15.4	15.9	16.5	17.1	17.6	18.2	18.8
53–55	15.1	15.7	16.2	16.8	17.4	17.9	18.5	19.1	19.7
56–58	16.0	16.5	17.1	17.7	18.2	18.8	19.4	20.0	20.5
59–61	16.9	17.4	17.9	18.5	19.1	19.7	20.2	20.8	21.4
62–64	17.6	18.2	18.8	19.4	19.9	20.5	21.1	21.7	22.2
65–67	18.5	19.0	19.6	20.2	20.8	21.3	21.9	22.5	23.1
68–70	19.3	19.9	20.4	21.0	21.6	22.2	22.7	23.3	23.9
71–73	20.1	20.7	21.2	21.8	22.4	23.0	23.6	24.1	24.7
74–76	20.9	21.5	22.0	22.6	23.2	23.8	24.4	25.0	25.5
77–79	21.7	22.2	22.8	23.4	24.0	24.6	25.2	25.8	26.3
80–82	22.4	23.0	23.6	24.2	24.8	25.4	25.9	26.5	27.1
83–85	23.2	23.8	24.4	25.0	25.5	26.1	26.7	27.3	27.9
86–88	24.0	24.5	25.1	25.7	26.3	26.9	27.5	28.1	28.7
89–91	24.7	25.3	25.9	26.5	27.1	27.6	28.2	28.8	29.4
92–94	25.4	26.0	26.6	27.2	27.8	28.4	29.0	29.6	30.2
92–97	26.1	26.7	27.3	27.9	28.5	29.1	29.7	30.3	30.9
98–100	26.9	27.4	28.0	28.6	29.2	29.8	30.4	31.0	31.6
101–103	27.5	28.1	28.7	29.3	29.9	30.5	31.1	31.7	32.3
104–106	28.2	28.8	29.4	30.0	30.6	31.2	31.8	32.4	33.0
107–109	28.9	29.5	30.1	30.7	31.3	31.9	32.5	33.1	33.7
110–112	29.6	30.2	30.8	31.4	32.0	32.6	33.2	33.8	34.4
113–115	30.2	30.8	31.4	32.0	32.6	33.2	33.8	34.5	35.1
116–118	30.9	31.5	32.1	32.7	33.3	33.9	34.5	35.1	35.7
119–121	31.5	32.1	32.7	33.3	33.9	34.5	35.1	35.7	36.4
122–124	32.1	32.7	33.3	33.9	34.5	35.1	35.8	36.4	37.0
125–127	32.7	33.3	33.9	34.5	35.1	35.8	36.4	37.0	37.6

From Pollock, M. L.; Schmidt, D. H.; and Jackson, A. S.: Measurement of cardiorespiratory fitness and body composition in the clinical setting. *Comprehensive Therapy* 6(9), pp. 12–27, 1980. Published with permission of the Laux Company, Inc., Harvard, Mass.

* Sum of chest, abdominal, and thigh skinfolds.

Table 9–7. Estimating Percent Body Fat in Females.

Sum of Skinfolds (mm)*	Age to the Last Year								
	Under 22	23–27	28–32	33–37	38–42	43–47	48–52	53–57	Over 58
23–25	9.7	9.9	10.2	10.4	10.7	10.9	11.2	11.4	11.7
26–28	11.0	11.2	11.5	11.7	12.0	12.3	12.5	12.7	13.0
29–31	12.3	12.5	12.8	13.0	13.3	13.5	13.8	14.0	14.3
32–34	13.6	13.8	14.0	14.3	14.5	14.8	15.0	15.3	15.5
35–37	14.8	15.0	15.3	15.5	15.8	16.0	16.3	16.5	16.8
38–40	16.0	16.3	16.5	16.7	17.0	17.2	17.5	17.7	18.0
41–43	17.2	17.4	17.7	17.9	18.2	18.4	18.7	18.9	19.2
44–46	18.3	18.6	18.8	19.1	19.3	19.6	19.8	20.1	20.3
47–49	19.5	19.7	20.0	20.2	20.5	20.7	21.0	21.2	21.5
50–52	20.6	20.8	21.1	21.3	21.6	21.8	22.1	22.3	22.6
53–55	21.7	21.9	22.1	22.4	22.6	22.9	23.1	23.4	23.6
56–58	22.7	23.0	23.2	23.4	23.7	23.9	24.2	24.4	24.7
59–61	23.7	24.0	24.2	24.5	24.7	25.0	25.2	25.5	25.7
62–64	24.7	25.0	25.2	25.5	25.7	26.0	26.7	26.4	26.7
65–67	25.7	25.9	26.2	26.4	26.7	26.9	27.2	27.4	27.7
68–70	26.6	26.9	27.1	27.4	27.6	27.9	28.1	28.4	28.6
71–73	27.5	27.8	28.0	28.3	28.5	28.8	29.0	29.3	29.5
74–76	28.4	28.7	28.9	29.2	29.4	29.7	29.9	30.2	30.4
77–79	29.3	29.5	29.8	30.0	30.3	30.5	30.8	31.0	31.3
80–82	30.1	30.4	30.6	30.9	31.1	31.4	31.6	31.9	32.1
83–85	30.9	31.2	31.4	31.7	31.9	32.2	32.4	32.7	32.9
86–88	31.7	32.0	32.2	32.5	32.7	32.9	33.2	33.4	33.7
89–91	32.5	32.7	33.0	33.2	33.5	33.7	33.9	34.2	34.4
92–94	33.2	33.4	33.7	33.9	34.2	34.4	34.7	34.9	35.2
95–97	33.9	34.1	34.4	34.6	34.9	35.1	35.4	35.6	35.9
98–100	34.6	34.8	35.1	35.3	35.5	35.8	36.0	36.3	36.5
101–103	35.3	35.4	35.7	35.9	36.2	36.4	36.7	36.9	37.2
104–106	35.8	36.1	36.3	36.6	36.8	37.1	37.3	37.5	37.8
107–109	36.4	36.7	36.9	37.1	37.4	37.6	37.9	38.1	38.4
110–112	37.0	37.2	37.5	37.7	38.0	38.2	38.5	38.7	38.9
113–115	37.5	37.8	38.0	38.2	38.5	38.7	39.0	39.2	39.5
116–118	38.0	38.3	38.5	38.8	39.0	39.3	39.5	39.7	40.0
119–121	38.5	38.7	39.0	39.2	39.5	39.7	40.0	40.2	40.5
122–124	39.0	39.2	39.4	39.7	39.9	40.2	40.4	40.7	40.9
125–127	39.4	39.6	39.9	40.1	40.4	40.6	40.9	41.1	41.4
128–130	39.8	40.0	40.3	40.5	40.8	41.0	41.3	41.5	41.8

From Pollack, M. L.; Schmidt, D. H.; and Jackson, A. S.: Measurement of cardiorespiratory fitness and body composition in the clinical setting. *Comprehensive Therapy* 6(9), pp. 12–27, 1980. Published with permission of the Laux Company, Inc., Harvard, Mass.

* Sum of triceps, suprailiac, and thigh skinfolds.

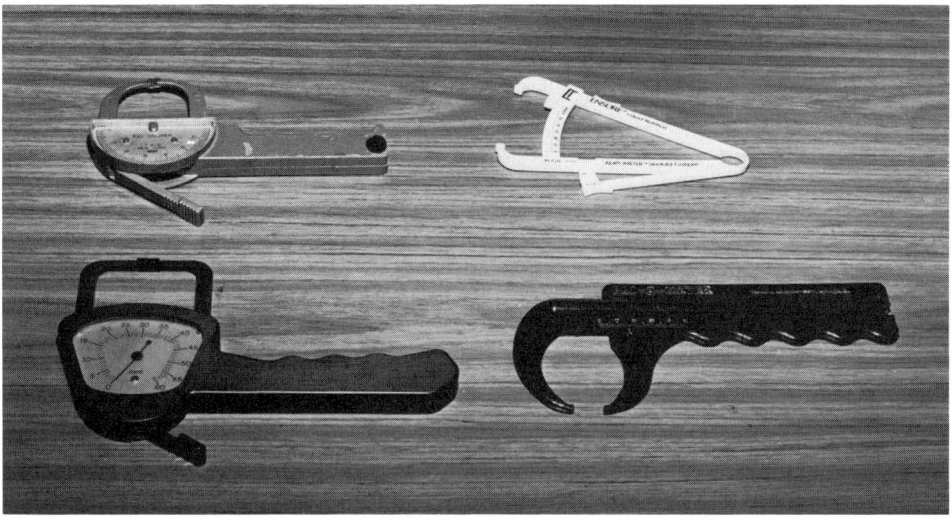

Figure 9–11. Calipers used to measure skinfold thickness. Upper left: Lange; lower left: Lafayette; upper right: Ross Labs; lower right: Fat-O-Meter.

SUMMARY

◊ Evaluation of fitness variables serves as a basis for exercise prescription and as an excellent motivational tool.

◊ In order to place sufficient demand upon the cardiovascular system early in an exercise program one component of the exercise prescription should be increased every 3 to 4 weeks, with most of the change occurring in a 3 to 4 month period.

◊ Changes to be expected with a cardiovascular training program are (1) decreased submaximal exercise and resting heart rate; (2) increased oxygen consumption; and (3) increased stroke volume and cardiac output.

◊ The change in muscle strength with weight training is approximately the same for men and women for the. leg muscles but greater in women for upper body exercises.

◊ Detraining will result in a 15 to 20 percent loss per week of the increased oxygen uptake gained. Strength gains are less dramatically affected, showing a 25 percent loss in increase after 12 weeks with approximately 50 percent loss in 1 year.

◊ Maximal oxygen consumption, the best measure of cardiorespiratory fitness, can be estimated using either the Åstrand-Rhyming bicycle ergometer test, or the 12-minute run for distance. Other measures that estimate cardiorespiratory fitness levels include the PWC_{170} test and The Ohio State University step test.

◊ The most commonly used measure for evaluating muscle strength is the single repetition maximum (1 RM). The more sophisticated determination of force production using isokinetic dynamometers is very expensive and usually not available to most people.

◇ Flexibility evaluation is difficult and usually subjective. The sit-and-reach test is objective but not as specific as one would desire.

◇ Underwater weighing to determine body density and fat percentage is the most accurate means of assessing body composition but requires special facilities. Skinfold determinations are simple and accurate, in the hands of a practiced technician. Two methods of skinfold measurement are the Sloan-Weir method for college-aged students and the three-site method of Pollack, Schmidt, and Jackson.

STUDY QUESTIONS

1. How often should fitness levels be evaluated?

2. What measurements should be included in a fitness evaluation?

3. Why does the resting heart rate decrease after a training program?

4. What is the single best measure of cardiorespiratory fitness?

5. What factors are responsible for increased oxygen consumption?

6. What magnitude of change in strength can be expected with a weight training program in men and women?

7. What is the most widely used practical measure of strength?

8. How does detraining affect an increase in (1) cardiorespiratory fitness; (2) muscular strength?

9. Name two tests to estimate maximal oxygen consumption and two others that evaluate cardiorespiratory fitness.

10. Describe the relationship between workload and heart rate.

11. Identify a test of flexibility.

12. Compare the use of underwater weighing, skinfold measures, and height-weight tables as measures of ideal weight.

REFERENCES AND SELECTED READINGS

Åstrand, I.: Aerobic work capacity in men and women with special reference to age. *Acta Physiologica Scandinavica* 49(Suppl. 169):45–60, 1960.

Cooper, K. H.: *The Aerobics Way.* New York: Bantam Books, 1977.

Falls, H. B.; Baylor, A. M.; and Dishman, R. K.: *Essentials of Fitness.* Philadelphia: Saunders College Publishing, 1980.

Fox, E. L., and Mathews, D. K.: *Physiological Basis of Physical Education and Athletics.* Philadelphia: Saunders College Publishing, 1981.

Mathews, D. K.: *Measurement in Physical Education.* Philadelphia: W. B. Saunders Co., 1968, pp. 223–226.

Pollack, M. L.; Schmidt, D. H.; and Jackson, A. S.: Measurement of cardiorespiratory fitness and body composition in the clinical setting. *Comprehensive Therapy* 6:12–27, 1980.

Pollack, M. L.; Wilmore, J. H.; and Fox, S. M. III: *Health and Fitness Through Physical Activity.* New York: John Wiley & Sons, 1978.

Sinning, W. E.: *Experiments and Demonstrations in Exercise Physiology.* Philadelphia: W. B. Saunders Co., 1975.

Sloan, A.; and Weir, J.: Nomograms for prediction of body density and total body fat from skinfold measurements. *Journal of Applied Physiology* 28:221–222, 1970.

Wilmore, J.: Alterations in strength, body composition and anthropometric measurements consequent to a 10-week training program. *Medicine and Science in Sports* 6:133–138, 1974.

Chapter 10
Lifetime Sports and Fitness

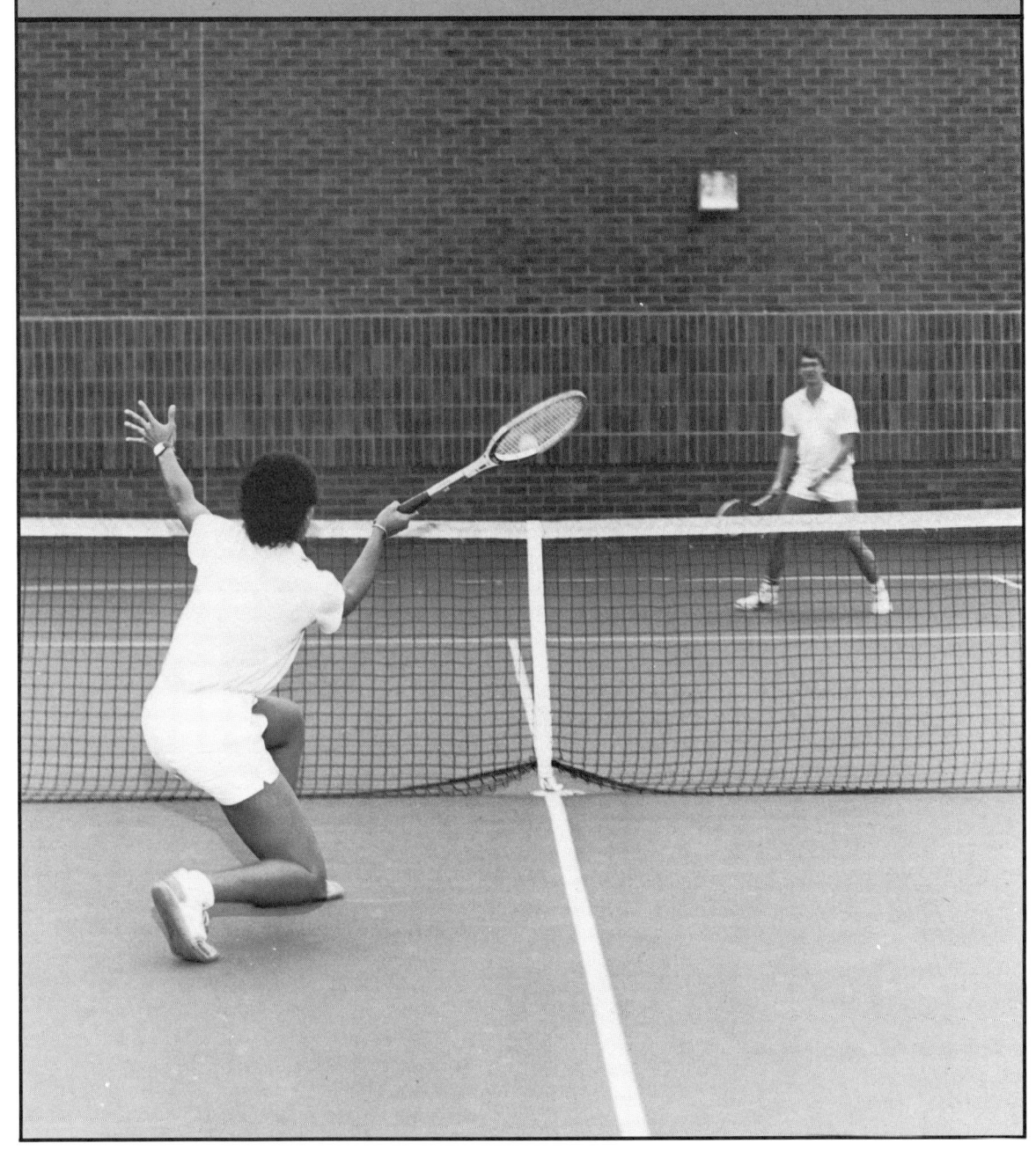

Chapter Outline

Learning Objectives

◇ To be able to identify the potential contributions of lifetime sports activities to various aspects of fitness.

◇ To appreciate the role of various lifetime sports activities in motivating people to continue participation and in enhancement of the quality of life.

◇ To recognize the limited values of occasional participation in any sports activity.

Key Words and Phrases

aerobic base
caloric expenditure
cardiorespiratory fitness
flexibility

lifetime sports
muscular endurance
muscular strength
quality of life

Introduction

W E have reached the point in developing the bases of fitness at which we must consider the potential benefits of sports activities as lifetime pursuits. Not all sports activities will help you to achieve or maintain fitness, but there are many sports activities suitable as "lifetime" endeavors that meet the criteria necessary to improve **cardiorespiratory fitness.** Most of these were discussed in Chapter 4. Many other sports activities improve **muscular strength and endurance** and **flexibility.** Some of us choose an activity based on its potential for physiological improvement. Most of us, however, need more than a potential physiological change to motivate us to become involved in a regular exercise program. We are most apt to remain involved in a program of regular exercise that we enjoy. The task then is to become involved in a program of exercise that is enjoyable enough to maintain your interest and that has the potential for physiological improvement.

Benefits of Lifetime Sports Activities

The purpose of this chapter is to identify the benefits that can be gained from and the positive aspects of common **lifetime sports.**

Physiological Benefits

When developing a habit of exercise that will become a part of your lifestyle, emphasis must be placed on cardiovascular benefit. Exercise activities that improve cardiovascular fitness have significant health-related implications that are important to us all. The American Heart Association believes that a very large percentage of the premature deaths resulting from cardiovascular disease are preventable. Regular exercise that meets the criteria for improving cardiovascular fitness can have a significant influence on the risk of cardiovascular disease.

If the activity you enjoy does not have the potential to improve cardiorespiratory conditioning, you would be wise to supplement this activity by participating at least 3 days per week in a sports activity that does improve cardiorespiratory conditioning. In addition to the health-related benefits of such a program, most coaches will tell you that a well-developed and well-maintained **aerobic base** will enhance your enjoyment of other sports activities. This gives you the chance to use the skills you have worked hard to develop. A strong aerobic base is particularly important when playing against someone with equal or greater skills. Those sports activities in Table 10–1 rated as excellent for developing cardiorespiratory fitness would serve to support those not rated as excellent. Keep in mind that this table only refers to the potential of the activity. Simply because you go for a walk five times per week does not necessarily mean that you are deriving an excellent cardiorespiratory benefit. You must meet all the criteria noted in Chapter 4.

Today more of us are remaining active in team sports for enjoyment and fitness. Table 10–2 evaluates some popular team activities as they are ordinarily played for their potential in improving cardiorespiratory fitness, muscular strength and endurance, and flexibility. Many "summertime athletes" feel they can "play" themselves into shape each year or maintain a good level of fitness by playing a sport two or three times per week. This is not the case. They may adjust to the rigors of the activity and notice a reduction in delayed muscle soreness but this is not a measure of fitness.

Many of the individual and team sports activities listed in Tables 10–1

Table 10–1. A Rating of the Potentials for Various Sports Activities to Develop and Maintain Cardiorespiratory Fitness, Muscular Strength and Endurance, and Flexibility.

	Cardiovascular Fitness	Muscular Strength/ Endurance	Flexibility
Archery	3*	3	3
Backpacking	2	2	3
Badminton	2	2	2
Bicycling	1	2	3
Bowling	3	3	3
Calisthenics	3	2	1
Canoeing	2	2	3
Dance			
Aerobic	1	2	1
Modern	2	2	1
Social	3	3	3
Fencing	3	2	2
Golf	3	3	3
Gymnastics	3	1	1
Handball	2	2	2
Ice Skating	2	2	3
Jogging/Running	1	2	3
Judo	3	2	1
Karate	3	2	1
Sailing	3	3	3
Scuba Diving	2	2	3
Skiing			
Downhill	2	2	3
Cross Country	1	2	2
Squash	2	2	2
Swimming	1	1	2
Tennis	2	2	2
Walking	1	2	3
Weight Training	3	1	2

* 1 = excellent; 2 = fair; 3 = poor.

Table 10–2. The Potential for Various Team Sports to Develop and Maintain Cardiorespiratory Fitness, Muscular Strength and Endurance, and Flexibility.

	Cardiovascular Fitness	Muscular Strength/ Endurance	Flexibility
Baseball/Softball	3*	3	3
Basketball	2	2	2
Football	3	2	2
Soccer	2	2	2
Volleyball	3	2	2

* 1 = excellent; 2 = fair; 3 = poor.

and 10–2 that are not highly rated for their potential contributions to cardio-respiratory fitness are nevertheless activities that require high levels of work output or intensity. Table 10–3 provides the requirements for many lifetime sports. The fact that the work is of very high intensity for short periods of time make many sports unsuitable as appropriate activities for improving

Table 10–3. MET Values for Selected Lifetime Sports Activities.

Activity	Range of METs*
Archery	3–4
Backpacking	5–11
Badminton	4–9+
Basketball	7–12+
Bowling	2–4
Canoeing	3–8
Calisthenics	3–8+
Cycling	3–8+
Dancing (aerobic)	6–9
Fencing	6–10+
Football (touch)	6–10
Golf	2–7
Handball	8–12+
Ice Skating	5–8
Running	9–16+
Sailing	2–5
Scuba Diving	5–10
Skiing	
Downhill	5–8
Cross Country	6–12+
Soccer	5–12+
Swimming	4–8+
Tennis	4–9+
Volleyball	3–6

Adapted with permission from American College of Sports Medicine: *Guidelines for Graded Exercise Testing and Exercise Prescription*, 2nd ed. Copyright © 1980. Lea & Febinger, Philadelphia.

* 1 MET — 3.5 ml/kg·min (resting metabolic cost); 1 MET = 1 cal/kg-hour.

cardiovascular fitness. Since such a large variation exists from person to person, with respect to the intensity with which any given activity is done, it is impossible to precisely identify the requirements of most sports activities. A sports activity's potential for enhancing fitness, however, can be generally applied.

Lifetime Activity Requirements

Each of the sports activities listed in Tables 10–1 and 10–3 has specific energy demands and as such has an optimum training program that will enhance your ability to perform it. As noted, a good foundation in aerobic fitness or an aerobic base is appropriate for every activity, but the potential for performance in a specific sport can be improved with training designed for that sports activity.

A knowledge of the requirements of each activity is essential to the development of the energy system(s), the strength, and the flexibility involved. Brief descriptions of the training requirements (not including skill development) follow for each of the activities listed in the Tables 10–1 and 10–3.

Archery.   Use of the bow and arrow is older than recorded history. While the activity itself produces little in the way of physiological benefits, archers should possess a good kinesthetic sense, hand–eye coordination, patience, and control. Arm and shoulder strength and flexibility may be important to a regular participant.

Backpacking.   Carrying moderate to heavy loads over miles of often rugged terrain certainly requires that the participant have a well-conditioned cardiovascular system as well as muscle strength and endurance. This is an activity that requires a base of both aerobic and anaerobic training for the serious participant. The muscular strength and endurance program should be a well-rounded program such as that described in Chapter 5.

Badminton.   The serious indoor game, not the backyard version, places great demands on anaerobic capacity and flexibility. Since badminton is fairly continuous it also requires input from the aerobic system as well. A good badminton player usually possesses a high degree of flexibility, which improves his or her ability to move quickly to return the difficult placements. Most of the emphasis in training should be placed on the anaerobic energy systems and improving flexibility.

Bicycling.   See Chapter 4.

Bowling.   Certainly skill and coordination are necessary for success in bowling. There are no apparent physiological benefits to be gained and the activity is done at a low intensity level. No physiological preparation therefore seems necessary.

Canoeing. Paddling at high intensity can require considerable muscular endurance as well as cardiovascular endurance. We were tempted to rate this activity as excellent in Table 10–1 but since the activity is done only with the relatively smaller muscle mass of the upper body with no contribution from the legs we refrained. It may well have an excellent potential for developing cardiorespiratory fitness. It does require training using the arms for improving both aerobic and anaerobic capabilities.

Dance. The demands of dance are variable depending on the type of dancing to be done. All vigorous forms of dance require excellent flexibility and muscular endurance. Aerobic dance and its correlates are well recognized as excellent forms of cardiovascular conditioning. Particular attention should be given to the different levels of intensity that would be appropriate for different participants, which is an important fact that is not always taken into consideration.

Fencing. Fencing is a more vigorous activity than many people realize. Its requirement for energy expenditure, however, is limited to the anaerobic systems because power movements are the essence of this activity. The fencer reaches full velocity as rapidly as possible from a nearly motionless start. Movements such as this place great demand on the neuromuscular system and require good flexibility.

Golf. Golf is an activity that is demanding in its requirement for skill, concentration, and coordination. The better golfers are usually aerobically fit but this is not a requirement for success. Anaerobic power and flexibility will enhance the golfer's swing and add distance to the long game. Walking the 18 holes of a golf course may require the player to cover over 4 miles. This aspect of the game indicates the need for prior aerobic conditioning and provides a potential for improving cardiorespiratory endurance. Unfortunately many golfers ride in carts or spend too much time between shots or holes to produce any training effect.

Gymnastics. Even the casual observer of this activity recognizes the demands of various gymnastic events. While there is a minimal requirement for cardiorespiratory endurance, few if any sports require the high degree of muscular strength, endurance, and flexibility that characterize the successful gymnast.

Handball/Squash/Tennis. While the specific skills required for court games such as these are different, the physiological demands nevertheless are similar. A well-developed aerobic base is helpful, particularly in the later stages of a match, and the anaerobic requirements of these activities are most important. For this reason a well-rounded weight training program combined with high-intensity work of short duration will benefit those who play these sports. Certainly flexibility is essential to the player who wishes to perform at optimal levels.

Ice Skating. Ice skating is another activity done at various intensities. The requirements for ice hockey, speed skating, and figure skating are very different. Cardiorespiratory endurance is essential to most forms of ice skating. Because skating can be rhythmical, continuous, and uses the large muscles of the legs, it has great potential for cardiovascular fitness.

Jogging/Walking/Running. See Chapter 4.

Judo/Karate. The martial arts require precision, concentration, a high degree of neuromuscular coordination, and well-developed flexibility. Most derive a minimal contribution from the aerobic system but require strength and power. Those participating in these activities could prepare through an overall weight training program and an aggressive flexibility development routine.

Sailing. In its advanced form, upper body strength is required of the sailor to meet the demands of quick responses under rapidly changing conditions. Most sailing is done for enjoyment and requires little physiological capability.

Skiing. Cross country skiing is rapidly becoming a major activity in those areas of the United States in which sufficient amounts of snowfall make it possible. Indoor trainers are now becoming popular as well. The elite cross country skier is able to generate the largest measured oxygen consumption values of any athlete. The requirement for this activity as well as its potential influence is largely aerobic. Downhill skiing requires more strength and equal muscular endurance but does not have the cardiorespiratory requirements.

Swimming. See Chapter 4.

Weight Training. See Chapter 5.

Enhancement of the Quality of Life

There are other benefits from participation in many lifetime sports activities that should be considered. The potentials of many of these activities to enhance the **quality of life** for each of us as individuals account for the increased participation we see today. Regardless of the intensity with which we exercise, there is a **caloric expenditure** associated with the work accomplished. The rate at which calories are burned is noted in Table 10–3. For a more extensive list of the caloric expenditure of various sports activities see Appendix C. Any sports activity carries with it a potential for increasing caloric expenditure as long as it does not include the potential for increasing caloric intake during participation (for example, eating potato chips and drinking beer while bowling).

We have stressed the concept of regularly including exercises that improve cardiovascular fitness in your fitness program. To ensure a health-related benefit, however, it should be noted that studies designed to assess the influence of activity on the risk of developing coronary diseases have found that a generally active lifestyle decreases the risk of death from heart attack. We cannot say with absolute certainty that optimum fitness and participation in sports activities will increase the quantity of your life, but they surely will enhance the quality!

SUMMARY

◇ Lifetime sports activities have a wide range of potential values for improving cardiorespiratory fitness, muscular strength and endurance, and flexibility.
◇ Activities that have good potentials for enhancing the quality of life but lack the potentials to improve cardiorespiratory fitness should be supplemented with conditioning exercises that meet the criteria for cardiorespiratory improvement.

STUDY QUESTIONS

1. What considerations would you make when deciding upon a sports activity in which to participate on a regular basis?
2. List three lifetime sports activities that have the potential to improve cardiorespiratory fitness.
3. List three individual lifetime sports activities and three team sports that would enhance the quality of life but not improve cardiovascular fitness.
4. Discuss the reason why there is such a wide range of energy expenditures for any given sports activity.

REFERENCES AND SELECTED READINGS

American College of Sports Medicine: *Guidelines for Graded Exercise Testing and Exercise Prescription.* Philadelphia: Lea & Febiger, 1980.
Cooper, K. H.: *The Aerobics Way.* New York: Bantam Books, 1977.
Getchell, B.: *Physical Fitness: A Way of Life.* New York: John Wiley & Sons, 1976.
Paffenberger, R. S. Jr.; and Hale, W. E.: Work activity and coronary heart mortality. *New England Journal of Medicine* 292:545–550, 1975.

Appendix A

Commonly Asked Questions and Answers About Fitness

Question: If I do aerobic exercise regularly and meet the criteria that should be met will I be immune from death from heart attack?

Answer: Some have supported the concept that large amounts of aerobic exercise are a guarantee against heart attack. Don't believe such a theory. There are *NO* guarantees. We should reduce our risk as best we can and can expect training to assist in that regard, but training does not serve as absolute protection. (See Chapter 3.)

Question: How often should I increase my aerobic work and what should I change?

Answer: Increase your working level at least every 3 to 4 weeks or no further improvement will occur. The most effective way to increase your work comfortably is to increase the workload to maintain the same relative intensity and gradually increase duration until you find a suitable time frame in which to work. (See Chapter 4.)

Question: Is there any time of day that is particularly good for exercise?

Answer: The best time of day to exercise is when you feel most comfortable and are the most likely to stay on your exercise routine. It is wise to find a certain time of the day and stick to it. (See Chapter 4.)

Question: Will weight training make me a better runner?

Answer: Increased strength is an asset in any endeavor. However, without an appropriate challenge to the aerobic system through cardiovascular training, weight training will in fact inhibit your ability to do aerobic exercise. (See Chapter 4.)

Question: How useful is breathing pure oxygen to enhance performance?

Answer: For the person who is limited to his or her ability to exchange or transfer oxygen, pure oxygen can be a lifesaver. For a normal healthy person, breathing oxygen during the rest periods between activity is of virtually no value. (See Chapter 3.)

Question: Is golf beneficial from a fitness standpoint or is it just fun?

Answer: Golf can be useful in burning calories if you walk the course. The average golfer will walk at least 3 miles in a round of golf, which results in about 300 to 400 calories being lost. That can be useful in helping to maintain your weight. Flexibility could be enhanced as well if the game is played properly. (See Chapter 10.)

Question: I would like to make sure I'm training at the activities I can do best. How can I tell if I have a larger ratio of fast-twitch or slow-twitch muscle fibers.

Answer: The most accurate assessment is a muscle biopsy, which requires that a small piece of muscle be removed. The procedure is not casually done for interest's sake, so it is not feasible. Your innate ability to run fast over short distances can give you a good relative indication. Try a variety of activities and you will soon find those for which you are genetically predisposed. Stay with each activity long enough to give yourself the best opportunity for success. (See Chapter 2.)

Question: What coronary artery disease risk factors are affected by exercise?

Answer: It appears that most controllable risk factors are influenced to some degree by a regular training program. There is evidence to support the positive role played by exercise in all three of the major risk factors (high cholesterol, hypertension, and cigarette smoking). The specific role of exercise is not clearly established but its general effect to reduce risk is undeniable. (See Chapter 3.)

Question: How should I breathe when I exercise?

Answer: Breathe through both your mouth and nose. Restricting air intake by keeping your mouth closed increases the oxygen cost of respiration and reduces tidal volume, both of which can be detrimental to performance. The rhythm with which you breathe should be left to what comes naturally. If you can relax, your pattern of breathing will be fine.

Question: Is "athlete's heart" something to be careful of?

Answer: Don't worry, the change in heart size associated with training is beneficial. In the somewhat distant past some people believed that since an enlarged heart occurred in those with heart disease any enlarged heart was detrimental. Exercise training can only improve upon the capabilities of a normal healthy heart. (See Chapter 4.)

Question: Is it too late to start an exercise program at 60 years of age?

Answer: No, absolutely not. Each of us should consult our physician before starting to exercise but age is not a hindrance. Follow the recommendations in Chapter 4 and in a few months you may feel like you are 30! In fact the older we get the more important it is to be engaged in a regular exercise program. (See Chapter 4.)

Question: Should women have some special weight program if they want to avoid bulging muscles?

Answer: No, it's not necessary. By virtue of their gender women have less testosterone, which is a hormone responsible in a large measure for the increase in muscle bulk. Because of this, women need not be concerned about bulging muscles. (See Chapter 5.)

Question: If I am a well-trained swimmer will I do well running since they are both aerobic activities?

Answer: Training is very specific and the transfer from one activity to another is limited. In response to training, physiological changes are both central and peripheral (see Chapter 4). The central changes will be helpful when crossing over but the peripheral specificity must be gained by actually doing that activity. (See Chapter 2.)

Question: With inactivity will muscle turn to fat?

Answer: Muscle tissue will gradually atrophy if not overloaded. The rate and extent of atrophy (diminished size) depends on the level of activity. Muscle does not become fat, nor does fat become muscle. Fat gain and muscle loss are independent of each other, although a sedentary life-style promotes both. (See Chapter 5.)

Question: How will I know if my exercise program is working?

Answer: You can evaluate yourself using the appropriate evaluation presented in Chapter 9. Good indicators are that you feel better; you can exercise longer and harder and feel no worse; and you begin to look forward to the exercise session. (See Chapter 9.)

Question: What is obesity?

Answer: Obesity is a body weight greater than 20 percent above the "ideal" weight for one's height. Using this definition, yet recognizing the difficulty in establishing ideal weight, there are probably between 50 to 80 million obese people in the United States today. It is obvious that obesity or overfatness refers to an above-average amount of fat contained in the body. This is, of course, dependent upon the fat content of each fat cell and the total number of fat cells in the body. Obesity is primarily caused by inactivity, *not* by overeating. (See Chapter 3.)

Question: How do you lose body fat or gain lean body weight?

Answer: The basic principle involved is the balance between energy taken in as food and energy expended through physical activity and the support of normal body processes. Body fat therefore can be lost by reducing the number of calories taken in or by increasing the number of calories expended through exercise or both. Therefore, in order to change your body fat weight, you need to know how many calories you expend in activities each day and your daily consumption of calories through food intake. (See Chapter 8.)

Question: What are nutrition and nutritional fitness?

Answer: Nutrition is necessary for all of our bodily functions. It is defined as the process by which the body takes in and uses food for optimal health and performance. Nutritional fitness is concerned with the selection of proper foods according to their caloric and nutritive values and with proper eating habits. (See Chapter 7.)

Question: Are the nutritional needs of athletes different from nonathletes?

Answer: From a nutritional view, athletes are no different from anybody else. However, their caloric needs are generally much greater (5,000 to 7,000 kcal per day during heavy training). (See Chapter 7.)

Question: Of what should a preexercise, preactivity, or pregame meal consist?

Answer: First, it should be emphasized that no foods when eaten several hours before activity or competition will lead to a spectacular performance. Carbohydrates should be the major foodstuff of pregame meals and may be consumed up to 2½ hours before the activity or competition. Consumption of sugar in large amounts in a liquid or pill form is not recommended within less than an hour before exercise. Fats, which are digested slowly, should be consumed 3 to 4 hours before the event. Basically, a pregame meal should not differ drastically from the normal diet. (See Chapter 7.)

Question: What are the major components of the body? How do they relate to sports participation?

Answer: Fat and fat-free weight are the body's two major components. The amount of stored body fat is determined by both the number and size of the fat-storing cells. Once adulthood is reached, the number of fat cells is fixed and cannot be changed. Fat-free weight is mainly skeletal muscle and the weight of other tissues and organs as well. Athletes generally have a lower body fat weight and a higher fat-free weight than nonathletes. Fat-free weight is positively related to athletic performance. Since women generally have a greater relative body fat weight and a lesser absolute fat-free weight component, they are at a disadvantage in most sports activities except for water activities. (See Chapter 8.)

Question: Is it wise to follow a vegetarian diet?

Answer: Strict vegetarian diets that eliminate all animal products from the diet make nutritional planning almost impossible. Absent from daily intake are vitamin B_{12} and many sources of proteins, calcium, and iron. A modified vegetarian diet that includes eggs and dairy products is much wiser nutritionally. Additional supplements help to ensure proper nutrient intake. (See Chapter 7.)

Question: What are the most important considerations in gaining weight?

Answer: First of all, you should gain fat-free weight rather than fat. Second, in order to gain weight, caloric intake must be greater than caloric expenditure. In order to gain 1 pound of fat-free weight (mainly muscle), an extra 2,500 kcal must be consumed. It is recommended that not more than 2 or 3 pounds per week be gained. To ensure that the excess calories will be laid down primarily as muscle, a vigorous training program, mainly weight training, should be undertaken during the high-caloric diet period. (See Chapter 8.)

Question: What is anorexia nervosa and what are its warning signs?

Answer: Anorexia nervosa literally means a nervous loss of appetite. This illness mainly strikes young women of the middle and upper classes who are high achievers and who have recently undergone a stressful life situation. The victim becomes completely obsessed with thinness and starves and dehydrates her body to achieve her goal. Dehydration and potassium deficiency are frequently some of the results, with death ensuing in some cases. Amenorrhea, love of dieting in the absence of overfatness, frequently weighing oneself, a preoccupation with food, and the use of laxatives are some of the symptoms. (See Chapter 8.)

Question: What is bulimia? How does it differ from anorexia nervosa?

Answer: Bulimia is characterized by binge eating and then purging the stomach to control weight. Bulimics may share with anorexics the fear of becoming fat, but they may or may not desire to be excessively thin. Usually, sufferers of this illness maintain near normal weight and even occasionally appear to eat normally. They love sweet foods and frequently disappear after a meal. Generally, their eating habits are not normal. (See Chapter 8.)

Question: Are there some helpful tips that particularly apply to the beginning exerciser?

Answer: We use a concise list of "Dos and Don'ts." Perhaps this list can be helpful. This list is certainly not all-inclusive but it will help remind you of some important factors.

Dos

◊ Do exercise regularly. Regularity is the key to improvement. Three times a week is the minimum.

◊ Do warm up with moderate stretching exercises before moving on to more vigorous exercise.

◇ Do taper off after exercise by decreased activity and walking. It is dangerous to stop suddenly because blood tends to pool in the legs resulting in a decrease in return to the heart.

◇ Do take your heart rate by feeling the pulse at the wrist or neck. Make sure you are obtaining your desired training heart rate.

◇ Do get a good pair of shoes for use during exercise. Use shoes that are designed for the activity.

◇ Do adjust your exercise intensity and duration to the climatic conditions. Be careful of hot and humid conditions.

◇ Do keep your knees bent at 90° when doing sit ups. This helps to isolate abdominal muscles.

◇ Do start slowly and progress gradually.

◇ Do drink frequently, every 15 to 20 minutes, in hot or humid weather. Water is the drink of choice for most activities.

◇ Do obtain the clearance of your physician before beginning an exercise training program.

◇ Do find a good time of day to exercise and stick with it!

◇ Do dress properly in cold weather. Layer your clothing, cover your hands and face when necessary, and be careful not to overdress.

◇ Do on cold days when walking, running, or cycling go into the wind first and with it on your return.

Don'ts

◇ Don't exercise when you are ill, or have a fever or serious infections.

◇ Don't exercise within two hours after a full meal or longer if digestion is delayed.

◇ Don't smoke before exercising. Smoke that you inhale from your cigarette, cigar, or pipe contains small amounts of carbon monoxide, a very selective poison. It displaces oxygen from the hemoglobin molecule in your red cells, thus immediately reducing the effectiveness of your oxygen transport system.

◇ Don't start exercising with arm work (push-ups, pull-ups, weight lifting, or isometrics).

◇ Don't hold your breath and strain during exercise. Breathe regularly and through the mouth. Holding your breath can cause an increase in the blood pressure in the arteries along with a marked increase in the pressures within the chambers of the heart.

◇ Don't take a hot shower, sauna, steam bath, or whirlpool bath after exercise. The excessive heat released into the blood is not able to dissipate if the skin temperature is high.

◇ Don't wear plastic or rubber suits when exercising. These can cause a retention of body heat resulting in an increased core temperature.

Appendix B

Caloric and Other Values for Selected Common Foods, Including "Fast" Foods

Table B–1. Selected Common Foods.*

DAIRY PRODUCTS (CHEESE, CREAM, IMITATION CREAM, MILK; RELATED PRODUCTS)

Butter. See Fats, oils; related products

Foods, approximate measures, units and weight (edible part unless footnotes indicate otherwise)	Amount	Weight (grams)	Water (per cent)	Food Energy (calories)	Protein (grams)	Fat (grams)	Carbohydrate (grams)	Calcium (milligrams)	Phosphorus (milligrams)	Iron (milligrams)	Potassium (milligrams)	Vitamin A Value (I.U.)	Thiamin (milligrams)	Riboflavin (milligrams)	Niacin (milligrams)	Ascorbic Acid (milligrams)
Cheese:																
Natural:																
Blue	1 oz	28	42	100	6	8	1	150	110	0.1	73	200	0.01	0.11	0.3	0
Camembert (3 wedges per 4-oz container)	1 wedge	38	52	115	8	9	Trace	147	132	0.1	71	350	0.01	0.19	0.2	0
Cheddar:																
Cut pieces	1 oz	28	37	115	7	9	Trace	204	145	0.2	28	300	0.01	0.11	Trace	0
	1 cu in	17.2	37	70	4	6	Trace	124	88	0.1	17	180	Trace	0.06	Trace	0
Shredded	1 cup	113	37	455	28	37	1	815	579	0.8	111	1,200	0.03	0.42	0.1	0
Cottage (curd not pressed down):																
Creamed (cottage cheese, 4% fat):																
Large curd	1 cup	225	79	235	28	10	6	135	297	0.3	190	370	0.05	0.37	0.3	Trace
Small curd	1 cup	210	79	220	26	9	6	126	277	0.3	177	340	0.04	0.34	0.3	Trace
Low fat (2%)	1 cup	226	79	205	31	4	8	155	340	0.4	217	160	0.05	0.42	0.3	Trace
Low fat (1%)	1 cup	226	82	165	28	2	6	138	302	0.3	193	80	0.05	0.37	0.3	Trace
Uncreamed (cottage cheese dry curd, less than ½% fat).	1 cup	145	80	125	25	1	3	46	151	0.3	47	40	0.04	0.21	0.2	0
Cream	1 oz	28	54	100	2	10	1	23	30	0.3	34	400	Trace	0.06	Trace	0
Mozzarella:																
Whole milk	1 oz	28	48	90	6	7	1	163	117	0.1	21	260	Trace	0.08	Trace	0
Part skim milk	1 oz	28	49	80	8	5	1	207	149	0.1	27	180	0.01	0.10	Trace	0
Parmesan, grated:																
Cup, not pressed down	1 cup	100	18	455	42	30	4	1,376	807	1.0	107	700	0.05	0.39	0.3	0
Tablespoon	1 tbsp	5	18	25	2	2	Trace	69	40	Trace	5	40	Trace	0.02	Trace	0
Ounce	1 oz	28	18	130	12	9	1	390	229	0.3	30	200	0.01	0.11	0.1	0
Provolone	1 oz	28	41	100	7	8	1	214	141	0.1	39	230	0.01	0.09	Trace	0
Ricotta:																
Whole milk	1 cup	246	72	428	28	32	7	509	389	0.9	257	1,210	0.03	0.48	0.3	0
Park skim milk	1 cup	246	74	340	28	19	13	669	449	1.1	308	1,060	0.05	0.46	0.2	0
Romano	1 oz	28	31	110	9	8	1	302	215	—		160	—	0.11	Trace	0
Swiss	1 oz	28	37	105	8	8	1	272	171	Trace	31	240	0.01	0.10	Trace	0
Pasteurized process cheese:																
American	1 oz	28	39	105	6	9	Trace	174	211	0.1	46	340	0.01	0.10	Trace	0
Swiss	1 oz	28	42	95	7	7	1	219	216	0.2	61	230	Trace	0.08	Trace	0
Pasteurized process cheese food, American.	1 oz	28	43	95	6	7	2	163	130	0.2	79	260	0.01	0.13	Trace	0
Pasteurized process cheese spread, American.	1 oz	28	48	82	5	6	2	159	202	0.1	69	220	0.01	0.12	Trace	0
Cream, sweet:																
Half-and-half (cream and milk)	1 cup	242	81	315	7	28	10	254	230	0.2	314	260	0.08	0.36	0.2	2
	1 tbsp	15	81	20	Trace	2	1	16	14	Trace	19	20	0.01	0.02	Trace	Trace

Food and measure															
Light, coffee, or table	1 cup	240	74	470	6	46	9	231	192	0.1	292	1,730	0.08	0.36	0.1	2
	1 tbsp	15	74	30	Trace	3	1	14	12	Trace	18	110	Trace	0.02	Trace	Trace
Whipping, unwhipped (volume about double when whipped):																
Light	1 cup	239	64	700	5	74	7	166	146	0.1	231	2,690	0.06	0.30	0.1	1
	1 tbsp	15	64	45	Trace	5	Trace	10	9	Trace	15	170	Trace	0.02	Trace	Trace
Heavy	1 cup	238	58	820	5	88	7	154	149	0.1	179	3,500	0.05	0.26	0.1	1
	1 tbsp	15	58	80	Trace	6	Trace	10	9	Trace	11	220	Trace	0.02	Trace	Trace
Whipped topping, (pressurized)	1 cup	60	61	155	2	13	7	61	54	Trace	88	550	0.02	0.04	Trace	0
	1 tbsp	3	61	10	Trace	1	Trace	3	3	Trace	4	30	Trace	Trace	Trace	0
Cream, sour	1 cup	230	71	495	7	48	10	268	195	0.1	331	1,820	0.08	0.34	0.2	2
	1 tbsp	12	71	25	Trace	3	1	14	10	Trace	17	90	Trace	0.02	Trace	Trace
Cream products, imitation (made with vegetable fat):																
Sweet:																
Creamers:																
Liquid (frozen)	1 cup	245	77	335	2	24	28	23	157	0.1	467	220[1]	0	0	0	0
	1 tbsp	15	77	20	Trace	1	2	1	10	Trace	29	10[1]	0	0	0	0
Powdered	1 cup	94	2	515	5	33	52	21	397	0.1	763	190[1]	0	0.16[1]	0	0
	1 tsp	2	2	10	Trace	1	1	Trace	8	Trace	16	Trace[1]	0	Trace[1]	0	0
Whipped topping:																
Frozen	1 cup	75	50	240	1	19	17	5	6	0.1	14	650[1]	0	0	0	0
	1 tbsp	4	50	15	Trace	1	1	Trace	Trace	Trace	1	30[1]	0	0	0	0
Powdered, made with whole milk.	1 cup	80	67	150	3	10	13	72	69	Trace	121	290[1]	0.02	0.09	Trace	1
	1 tbsp	4	67	10	Trace	Trace	1	4	3	Trace	6	10[1]	Trace	Trace	Trace	Trace
Pressurized	1 cup	70	60	185	1	16	11	4	13	Trace	13	330[1]	0	0	0	0
	1 tbsp	4	60	10	Trace	1	1	Trace	1	Trace	1	20[1]	0	0	0	0
Sour dressing (imitation sour cream) made with nonfat dry milk.	1 cup	235	75	415	8	39	11	266	205	0.1	380	20[1]	0.09	0.38	0.2	2
	1 tbsp	12	75	20	Trace	2	1	14	10	Trace	19	Trace[1]	0.01	0.02	Trace	Trace
Ice cream. See Milk desserts, frozen																
Ice milk. See Milk desserts, frozen																
Milk:																
Fluid:																
Whole (3.3% fat)	1 cup	244	88	150	8	8	11	291	228	0.1	370	310[2]	0.09	0.40	0.2	2
Lowfat (2%):																
No milk solids added	1 cup	244	89	120	8	5	12	297	232	0.1	377	500	0.10	0.40	0.2	2
Milk solids added:																
Label claim less than 10 g of protein per cup.	1 cup	245	89	125	9	5	12	313	245	0.1	397	500	0.10	0.42	0.2	2
Label claim 10 or more grams of protein per cup (protein fortified).	1 cup	246	88	135	10	5	14	352	276	0.1	447	500	0.11	0.48	0.2	2

Note: Dashes (—) denote lack of reliable data for a constituent believed to be present in measurable amount.

* Adams, C. F., and Richardson, M.: Nutritive Value of Foods. Homes and Garden Bulletin 72, Agricultural Research Service, U.S. Department of Agriculture, Washington, D.C., revised 1977. Adapted from Robinson C. H. and Lawler, M. R.: Normal and Therapeutic Nutrition, 16th ed. New York: Macmillan, 1982, pp. 736–764.

[1] Vitamin A value is largely from beta carotene used for coloring. Riboflavin values for powdered creamer apply to product with added riboflavin.

[2] Applied to product without added vitamin A. With added vitamin A, value is 500 International Units (I.U.).

Table B-1. (Continued)

Foods, approximate measures, units and weight (edible part unless footnotes indicate otherwise)	Amount	Weight (grams)	Water (per-cent)	Food Energy (calories)	Protein (grams)	Fat (grams)	Carbohydrate (grams)	Calcium (milligrams)	Phosphorus (milligrams)	Iron (milligrams)	Potassium (milligrams)	Vitamin A Value (I.U.)	Thiamin (milligrams)	Riboflavin (milligrams)	Niacin (milligrams)	Ascorbic Acid (milligrams)
DAIRY PRODUCTS (CHEESE, CREAM, IMITATION CREAM, MILK; RELATED PRODUCTS)																
Lowfat (1%):																
No milk solids added	1 cup	244	90	100	8	3	12	300	235	0.1	381	500	0.10	0.41	0.2	2
Milk solids added:																
Label claim less than 10 g of protein per cup.	1 cup	245	90	105	9	2	12	313	245	0.1	397	500	0.10	0.42	0.2	2
Label claim 10 or more grams of protein per cup (protein fortified).	1 cup	246	89	120	10	3	14	349	273	0.1	444	500	0.11	0.47	0.2	2
Nonfat (skim):																
No milk solids added	1 cup	245	91	85	8	Trace	12	302	247	0.1	406	500	0.09	0.37	0.2	2
Milk solids added:																
Label claim less than 10 g of protein per cup.	1 cup	245	90	90	9	1	12	316	255	0.1	416	500	0.10	0.43	0.2	2
Label claim 10 or more grams of protein per cup (protein fortified).	1 cup	246	89	100	10	1	14	352	275	0.1	446	500	0.11	0.48	0.2	3
Buttermilk	1 cup	245	90	100	8	2	12	285	219	0.1	371	80[3]	0.08	0.38	0.1	2
Canned:																
Evaporated, unsweetened:																
Whole milk	1 cup	252	74	340	17	19	25	657	510	0.5	764	610[3]	0.12	0.80	0.5	5
Skim milk	1 cup	255	79	200	19	1	29	738	497	0.7	845	1,000[4]	0.11	0.79	0.4	3
Sweetened, condensed	1 cup	306	27	980	24	27	166	868	775	0.6	1,136	1,000[3]	0.28	1.27	0.6	8
Dried:																
Buttermilk	1 cup	120	3	465	41	7	59	1,421	1,119	0.4	1,910	260[3]	0.47	1.90	1.1	7
Nonfat instant:																
Envelope, net wt., 3.2 oz[5]	1 envelope	91	4	325	32	1	47	1,120	896	0.3	1,552	2,160[6]	0.38	1.59	0.8	5
Cup[7]	1 cup	68	4	245	24	Trace	35	837	670	0.2	1,160	1,610[6]	0.28	1.19	0.6	4
Milk beverages:																
Chocolate milk (commercial):																
Regular	1 cup	250	82	210	8	8	26	280	251	0.6	417	300[3]	0.09	0.41	0.3	2
Lowfat (2%)	1 cup	250	84	180	8	5	26	284	254	0.6	422	500	0.10	0.42	0.3	2
Lowfat (1%)	1 cup	250	85	160	8	3	26	287	257	0.6	426	500	0.10	0.40	0.2	2
Egg nog (commercial)	1 cup	254	74	340	10	19	34	330	278	0.5	420	890	0.09	0.48	0.3	4
Malted milk, home-prepared with 1 cup of whole milk and 2 to 3 heaping tsp of malted milk powder (about ¾ oz):																
Chocolate	1 cup of milk plus ¾ oz of powder.	265	81	235	9	9	29	304	265	0.5	500	330	0.14	0.43	0.7	2
Natural	1 cup of milk plus ¾ oz of powder.	265	81	235	11	10	27	347	307	0.3	529	380	0.20	0.54	1.3	2
Shakes, thick:[8]																
Chocolate, container, net wt., 10.6 oz.	1 container	300	72	355	9	8	63	396	378	0.9	672	260	0.14	0.67	0.4	0
Vanilla, container, net wt., 11 oz.	1 container	313	74	350	12	9	56	457	361	0.3	572	360	0.09	0.61	0.5	0

Milk desserts, frozen:															
Ice cream:															
Regular (about 11% fat):															
Hardened	½ gal	1,064	61	2,155	38	115	254	1,406	1,075	1.0	2,052	4,340	0.42	2.63	1.1	6
	1 cup	133	61	270	5	14	32	176	134	0.1	257	540	0.05	0.33	0.1	1
	3-fl oz container	50	61	100	2	5	12	66	51	Trace	96	200	0.02	0.12	0.1	Trace
Soft serve (frozen custard)	1 cup	173	60	375	7	23	38	236	199	0.4	338	790	0.08	0.45	0.2	1
Rich (about 16% fat), hardened.	½ gal	1,188	59	2,805	33	190	256	1,213	927	0.8	1,771	7,200	0.36	2.27	0.9	5
	1 cup	148	59	350	4	24	32	151	115	0.1	221	900	0.04	0.28	0.1	1
Ice milk:															
Hardened (about 4.3% fat)	½ gal	1,048	69	1,470	41	45	232	1,409	1,035	1.5	2,117	1,710	0.61	2.78	0.9	6
	1 cup	131	69	185	5	6	29	176	129	0.1	265	210	0.08	0.35	0.1	1
Soft serve (about 2.6% fat)	1 cup	175	70	225	8	5	38	274	202	0.3	412	180	0.12	0.54	0.2	1
Sherbet (about 2% fat)	½ gal	1,542	66	2,160	17	31	469	827	594	2.5	1,585	1,480	0.26	0.71	1.0	31
	1 cup	193	66	270	2	4	59	103	74	0.3	198	190	0.03	0.09	0.1	4
Milk desserts, other:															
Custard, baked	1 cup	265	77	305	14	15	29	297	310	1.1	387	930	0.11	0.50	0.3	1
Puddings:															
From home recipe:															
Starch base:															
Chocolate	1 cup	260	66	385	8	12	67	250	255	1.3	445	390	0.05	0.36	0.3	1
Vanilla (blancmange)	1 cup	255	76	285	9	10	41	298	232	Trace	352	410	0.08	0.41	0.3	2
Tapioca cream	1 cup	165	72	220	8	8	28	173	180	0.7	223	480	0.07	0.30	0.2	2
From mix (chocolate) and milk:															
Regular (cooked)	1 cup	260	70	320	9	8	59	265	247	0.8	354	340	0.05	0.39	0.3	2
Instant	1 cup	260	69	325	8	7	63	374	237	1.3	335	340	0.08	0	0.3	2
Yogurt															
With added milk solids:															
Made with lowfat milk:															
Fruit-flavored[9]	1 container, net wt, 8 oz	227	75	230	10	3	42	343	269	0.2	439	120[10]	0.08	0.40	0.2	1
Plain	1 container, net wt, 8 oz	227	85	145	12	4	16	415	326	0.2	531	150[10]	0.10	0.49	0.3	2
Made with nonfat milk	1 container, net wt, 8 oz	227	85	125	13	Trace	17	452	355	0.2	579	20[10]	0.11	0.53	0.3	2
Without added milk solids:															
Made with whole milk	1 container, net wt, 8 oz	227	88	140	8	7	11	274	215	0.1	351	280	0.07	0.32	0.2	1
EGGS															
Eggs, large (24 oz per dozen):															
Raw:															
Whole, without shell	1 egg	50	75	80	6	6	1	28	90	1.0	65	260	0.04	0.15	Trace	0
White	1 white	33	88	15	3	Trace	Trace	4	4	Trace	45	0	Trace	0.09	Trace	0
Yolk	1 yolk	17	49	65	3	6	Trace	26	86	0.9	15	310	0.04	0.07	Trace	0

[3] Applies to product without vitamin A added.

[4] Applies to product with added vitamin A. Without added vitamin A, value is 20 International Units (I.U.).

[5] Yields 1 qt fluid milk when reconstituted according to package directions.

[6] Applied to product with added vitamin A.

[7] Weight applied to product with label claim of 1⅓ cups equal 3.2 oz.

[8] Applies to products made from thick shake mixes and that do not contain added ice cream. Products made from milk shake mixes are higher in fat and usually contain added ice cream.

[9] Content of fat, vitamin A, and carbohydrate varies. Consult the label when precise values are needed for special diets.

[10] Applies to product made with milk containing no added vitamin A.

219

Table B-1. (Continued)

Foods, approximate measures, units and weight (edible part unless footnotes indicate otherwise)	Amount	Weight (grams)	Water (percent)	Food Energy (calories)	Protein (grams)	Fat (grams)	Carbohydrate (grams)	Calcium (milligrams)	Phosphorus (milligrams)	Iron (milligrams)	Potassium (milligrams)	Vitamin A Value (I.U.)	Thiamin (milligrams)	Riboflavin (milligrams)	Niacin (milligrams)	Ascorbic Acid (milligrams)
EGGS																
Cooked:																
Fried in butter	1 egg	46	72	85	5	6	1	26	80	0.9	58	290	0.03	0.13	Trace	0
Hard-cooked, shell removed	1 egg	50	75	80	6	6	1	28	90	1.0	65	260	0.04	0.14	Trace	0
Poached	1 egg	50	74	80	6	6	1	28	90	1.0	65	260	0.04	0.13	Trace	0
Scrambled (milk added) in butter. Also omelet.	1 egg	64	76	95	6	7	1	47	97	0.9	85	310	0.04	0.16	Trace	0
FATS, OILS; RELATED PRODUCTS																
Butter																
Regular (1 brick or 4 sticks per lb):																
Stick (½ cup)	1 stick	113	16	815	1	92	Trace	27	26	0.2	29	3,470[11]	0.01	0.04	Trace	0
Tablespoon (about ⅛ stick).	1 tbsp	14	16	100	Trace	12	Trace	3	3	Trace	4	430[11]	Trace	Trace	Trace	0
Pat (1 in square, ⅓ inch high, 90 per lb).	1 pat	5	16	35	Trace	4	Trace	1	1	Trace	1	150[11]	Trace	Trace	Trace	0
Whipped (6 sticks or two 8-oz containers per lb).																
Stick (½ cup)	1 stick	76	16	540	1	61	Trace	18	17	0.1	20	2,310[11]	Trace	0.03	Trace	0
Tablespoon (about ⅛ stick).	1 tbsp	9	16	65	Trace	8	Trace	2	2	Trace	2	290[11]	Trace	Trace	Trace	0
Pat (1¼ inch square, ⅓ inch high; 120 per lb).	1 pat	4	16	25	Trace	3	Trace	1	1	Trace	1	120[11]	0	Trace	0	0
Fats, cooking (vegetable shortenings).	1 cup	200	0	1,770	0	200	0	0	0	0	0	—	0	0	0	0
	1 tbsp	13	0	110	0	13	0	0	0	0	0	—	0	0	0	0
Lard	1 cup	205	0	1,850	0	205	0	0	0	0	0	0	0	0	0	0
	1 tbsp	13	0	115	0	13	0	0	0	0	0	0	0	0	0	0
Margarine:																
Regular (1 brick or 4 sticks per 1 lb):																
Stick (½ cup)	1 stick	113	16	815	1	92	Trace	27	26	0.2	29	3,750[12]	0.01	0.04	Trace	0
Tablespoon (about ⅛ stick)	1 tbsp	14	16	100	Trace	12	Trace	3	3	Trace	4	470[12]	Trace	Trace	Trace	0
Pat (1 inch square, ⅓ inch high; 90 per lb).	1 pat	5	16	35	Trace	4	Trace	1	1	Trace	1	170[12]	Trace	Trace	Trace	0
Soft, two 8-oz containers per lb.	1 container	227	16	1,635	1	184	Trace	53	52	0.4	59	7,500[12]	0.01	0.08	0.1	0
	1 tbsp	14	16	100	Trace	12	Trace	3	3	Trace	4	470[12]	Trace	Trace	Trace	0
Whipped (6 sticks per lb):																
Stick (½ cup)	1 stick	76	16	545	Trace	61	Trace	18	17	0.1	20	2,500[12]	Trace	0.03	Trace	0
Tablespoon (about ⅛ stick)	1 tbsp	9	16	70	Trace	8	Trace	2	2	Trace	2	310[12]	Trace	Trace	Trace	0
Oils, salad or cooking:																
Corn	1 cup	218	0	1,925	0	218	0	0	0	0	0	—	0	0	0	0
	1 tbsp	14	0	120	0	14	0	0	0	0	0	—	0	0	0	0
Olive	1 cup	216	0	1,910	0	216	0	0	0	0	0	—	0	0	0	0
	1 tbsp	14	0	120	0	14	0	0	0	0	0	—	0	0	0	0
Peanut	1 cup	216	0	1,910	0	216	0	0	0	0	0	—	0	0	0	0
	1 tbsp	14	0	120	0	14	0	0	0	0	0	—	0	0	0	0
Safflower	1 cup	218	0	1,925	0	218	0	0	0	0	0	—	0	0	0	0
	1 tbsp	14	0	120	0	14	0	0	0	0	0	—	0	0	0	0

Food	Measure	Grams	Water (%)	Food energy (cal.)	Protein (g)	Fat (g)	Saturated (g)	Oleic (g)	Linoleic (g)	Carbohydrate (g)	Calcium (mg)	Phosphorus (mg)	Iron (mg)	Potassium (mg)	Vitamin A (I.U.)	Thiamin (mg)	Riboflavin (mg)	Niacin (mg)	Ascorbic acid (mg)
Soybean oil, hydrogenated (partially hardened).	1 cup	218	0	1,925	0	218	32	84	75	0	0	0	0	—	—	0	0	0	0
	1 tbsp	14	0	120	0	14	2	5	5	0	0	0	0	—	—	0	0	0	0
Soybean-cottonseed oil blend, hydrogenated.	1 cup	218	0	1,925	0	218	38	63	99	0	0	0	0	—	—	0	0	0	0
	1 tbsp	14	0	120	0	14	2	4	7	0	0	0	0	—	—	0	0	0	0
Salad dressings:																			
Commercial:																			
Blue cheese:																			
Regular	1 tbsp	15	32	75	1	8	2	2	4	1	12	11	Trace	6	30	Trace	0.02	Trace	Trace
Low calorie (5 cal per tsp)	1 tbsp	16	84	10	1	1	Trace	Trace	Trace	1	10	8	Trace	5	30	Trace	0.01	Trace	Trace
French:																			
Regular	1 tbsp	16	39	65	Trace	6	1	1	3	3	2	2	0.1	13	—	—	—	—	—
Low calorie (5 cal per tsp)	1 tbsp	16	77	15	Trace	1	Trace	Trace	Trace	2	2	2	0.1	13	—	—	—	—	—
Italian:																			
Regular	1 tbsp	15	28	85	Trace	9	2	2	4	1	2	1	Trace	2	Trace	Trace	Trace	Trace	—
Low calorie (2 cal per tsp)	1 tbsp	15	90	10	Trace	1	Trace	Trace	Trace	Trace	2	1	Trace	2	Trace	Trace	Trace	Trace	—
Mayonnaise	1 tbsp	14	15	100	Trace	11	2	3	6	Trace	3	4	0.1	5	40	Trace	0.01	Trace	—
Mayonnaise type:																			
Regular	1 tbsp	15	41	65	Trace	6	1	1	3	2	2	4	Trace	1	30	Trace	Trace	Trace	Trace
Low calorie (8 cal per tsp)	1 tbsp	16	81	20	Trace	2	Trace	Trace	1	2	3	4	Trace	1	40	Trace	Trace	Trace	Trace
Tartar sauce, regular	1 tbsp	14	34	75	Trace	8	1	2	4	1	3	4	0.1	11	30	Trace	Trace	Trace	Trace
Thousand Island:																			
Regular	1 tbsp	16	32	80	Trace	8	1	2	4	2	2	3	0.1	18	50	Trace	Trace	Trace	Trace
Low calorie (10 cal per tsp)	1 tbsp	15	68	25	Trace	2	Trace	Trace	1	2	2	3	0.1	17	50	Trace	Trace	Trace	Trace
From home recipe:																			
Cooked type:[13]	1 tbsp	16	68	25	1	2	Trace	Trace	1	2	14	15	0.1	19	80	0.01	0.03	Trace	Trace
FISH, SHELLFISH, MEAT, POULTRY; RELATED PRODUCTS																			
Fish and shellfish:																			
Bluefish, baked with butter or margarine.	3 oz	85	68	135	22	4	—	—	—	0	25	244	0.6	—	40	0.09	0.08	1.6	—
Clams:																			
Raw, meat only	3 oz	85	82	65	11	1	—	—	—	2	59	138	5.2	154	90	0.08	0.15	1.1	8
Canned, solids and liquid	3 oz	85	86	45	7	1	—	—	—	2	47	116	3.5	119	—	0.01	0.09	0.9	—
Crabmeat (white or king), canned, not pressed down.	1 cup	135	77	135	24	3	—	—	—	1	61	246	1.1	149	—	0.11	0.11	2.6	—
Fish sticks, breaded, cooked, frozen (stick, 4 × 1 × ½ inch.	1 fish stick or 1 oz	28	66	50	5	3	—	—	—	2	3	47	0.1	—	0	0.01	0.02	0.5	—
Haddock, breaded, fried[14]	3 oz	85	66	140	17	5	—	—	—	5	34	210	1.0	296	—	0.03	0.06	2.7	2
Ocean perch, breaded, fried[14]	1 fillet	85	59	195	16	11	—	—	—	6	28	192	1.1	242	—	0.10	0.10	1.6	—
Oysters, raw, meat only (13–19 medium Selects).	1 cup	240	85	160	20	4	—	—	—	8	226	343	13.2	290	740	0.34	0.43	6.0	—
Salmon, pink, canned, solids and liquid.	3 oz	85	71	120	17	5	—	—	—	0	167[15]	243	0.7	307	60	0.03	0.16	6.8	—

Note: Dashes (—) denote lack of reliable data for a constituent believed to be present in measurable amount.

[11] Based on year-round average.

[12] Based on average vitamin A content of fortified margarine. Federal specifications for fortified margarine require a minimum of 15,000 International Units (I.U.) of vitamin A per pound.

[13] Fatty acid values apply to product made with regular-type margarine.

[14] Dipped in egg, milk or water, and breadcrumbs; fried in vegetable shortening.

[15] If bones are discarded, value for calcium will be greatly reduced.

Table B-1. (Continued)

Foods, approximate measures, units and weight (edible part unless footnotes indicate otherwise)	Amount	Weight (grams)	Water (per-cent)	Food Energy (cal-ories)	Pro-tein (grams)	Fat (grams)	Carbo-hydrate (grams)	Calcium (milli-grams)	Phos-phorus (milli-grams)	Iron (milli-grams)	Potas-sium (milli-grams)	Vitamin A Value (I.U.)	Thiamin (milli-grams)	Ribo-flavin (milli-grams)	Niacin (milli-grams)	Ascorbic Acid (milli-grams)
FISH, SHELLFISH, MEAT, POULTRY; RELATED PRODUCTS																
Sardines, Atlantic, canned in oil, drained solids.	3 oz	85	62	175	20	9	0	372	424	2.5	502	190	0.02	0.17	4.6	—
Scallops, frozen, breaded, fried, re-heated.	6 scallops	90	60	175	16	8	9	—	—	—	—	—	—	—	—	—
Shad, baked with butter or margarine, bacon.	3 oz	85	64	170	20	10	0	20	266	0.5	320	30	0.11	0.22	7.3	—
Shrimp:																
Canned meat	3 oz	85	70	100	21	1	1	98	224	2.6	104	50	0.01	0.03	1.5	—
French fried[16]	3 oz	85	57	190	17	9	9	61	162	1.7	195	—	0.03	0.07	2.3	—
Tuna, canned in oil, drained solids.	3 oz	85	61	170	24	7	0	7	199	1.6	—	70	0.04	0.10	10.1	—
Tuna salad[17]	1 cup	205	70	350	30	22	7	41	291	2.7	—	590	0.08	0.23	10.3	2
Meat and meat products:																
Bacon, (20 slices per lb, raw), broiled or fried, crisp.	2 slices	15	8	85	4	8	Trace	2	34	0.5	35	0	0.08	0.05	0.8	—
Beef,[18] cooked:																
Cuts braised, simmered or pot roasted (piece, 2½ × 2½ × ¾ inch):																
Lean and fat	3 oz	85	53	245	23	16	0	10	114	2.9	184	30	0.04	0.18	3.6	—
Lean only	2.5 oz	72	62	140	22	5	0	10	108	2.7	176	10	0.04	0.17	3.3	—
Ground beef, broiled:																
Lean with 10% fat	3 oz or patty 3 × ⅝ inch	85	60	185	23	10	0	10	196	3.0	261	20	0.08	0.20	5.1	—
Lean with 21% fat	2.9 oz or patty 3 × ⅝ inch	82	54	235	20	17	0	9	159	2.6	221	30	0.07	0.17	4.4	—
Roast, oven cooked, no liquid added:																
Relatively fat, such as rib (2 pieces, 4⅛ × 2¼ × ¼ inch):																
Lean and fat	3 oz	85	40	375	17	33	0	8	158	2.2	189	70	0.05	0.13	3.1	—
Lean only	1.8 oz	51	57	125	14	7	0	6	131	1.8	161	10	0.04	0.11	2.6	—
Relatively lean, such as heel of round (2 pieces, 4⅛ × 2¼ × ¼ inch):																
Lean and fat	3 oz	85	62	165	25	7	0	11	208	3.2	279	10	0.06	0.19	4.5	—
Lean only	2.8 oz	78	65	125	24	3	0	10	199	3.0	268	Trace	0.06	0.18	4.3	—
Steak:																
Relatively fat sirloin, broiled (piece, 2½ × 2½ × ¾ inch):																
Lean and fat	3 oz	85	44	330	20	27	0	9	162	2.5	220	50	0.05	0.15	4.0	—
Lean only	2 oz	56	59	115	18	4	0	7	146	2.2	202	10	0.05	0.14	3.6	—
Relatively lean round, braised (piece, 4⅛ × 2¼ × ½ inch):																
Lean and fat	3 oz	85	55	220	24	13	0	10	213	3.0	272	20	0.07	0.19	4.8	—
Lean only	2.4 oz	68	61	130	21	4	0	9	182	2.5	238	10	0.05	0.16	4.1	—

	Measure															
Beef, canned:																
Corned beef	3 oz	85	59	185	22	10	0	17	90	3.7	—	—	0.01	0.20	2.9	—
Corned beef hash	1 cup	220	67	400	19	25	24	29	147	4.4	440	—	0.02	0.20	4.6	—
Beef, dried, chipped	2½-oz jar	71	48	145	24	4	0	14	287	3.6	142	—	0.05	0.23	2.7	0
Beef and vegetable stew	1 cup	245	82	220	16	11	15	29	184	2.9	613	2,400	0.15	0.17	4.7	17
Beef potpie (home recipe), baked[19] (piece, ⅓ of 9-inch diam. pie).	1 piece	210	55	515	21	30	39	29	149	3.8	334	1,720	0.30	0.30	5.5	6
Chili con carne with beans, canned.	1 cup	225	72	340	19	16	31	82	321	4.3	594	150	0.08	0.18	3.3	—
Chop suey with beef and pork (home recipe).	1 cup	250	75	300	26	17	13	60	248	4.8	425	600	0.28	0.38	5.0	33
Heart, beef, lean, braised	3 oz	85	61	160	27	5	1	5	154	5.0	197	20	0.21	1.04	6.5	1
Lamb, cooked: Chop, rib (3 per lb with bone), broiled:																
Lean and fat	3.1 oz	89	43	360	18	32	0	8	139	1.0	200	—	0.11	0.19	4.1	—
Lean only	2 oz	57	60	120	16	6	0	6	121	1.1	174	—	0.09	0.15	3.4	—
Leg, roasted (2 pieces, 4⅛ × 2¼ × ¼ inch):																
Lean and fat	3 oz	85	54	235	22	16	0	9	177	1.4	241	—	0.13	0.23	4.7	—
Lean only	2.5 oz	71	62	130	20	5	0	9	169	1.4	227	—	0.12	0.21	4.4	—
Shoulder, roasted (3 pieces, 2½ × 2½ × ¼ inch):																
Lean and fat	3 oz	85	50	285	18	23	0	9	146	1.0	206	—	0.11	0.20	4.0	—
Lean only	2.3 oz	64	61	130	17	6	0	8	140	1.0	193	—	0.10	0.18	3.7	—
Liver, beef fried[20] (slice, 6½ × 2⅜ × ⅜ inch).	3 oz	85	56	195	22	9	5	9	405	7.5	323	45,390[21]	0.22	3.56	14.0	23
Pork, cured, cooked: Ham, light cure, lean and fat, roasted (2 pieces, 4⅛ × 2¼ × ¼ inch)[22]	3 oz	85	54	245	18	19	0	8	146	2.2	199	0	0.40	0.15	3.1	—
Luncheon meat: Boiled ham, slice (8 per 8-oz pkg).	1 oz	28	59	65	5	5	0	3	47	0.8	—	0	0.12	0.04	0.7	—
Canned, spiced or unspiced: Slice, approx. 3 by 2 × ½ inch	1 slice	60	55	175	9	15	1	5	65	1.3	133	0	0.19	0.13	1.8	—
Pork, fresh,[18] cooked: Chop, loin (cut 3 per lb with bone), broiled:																
Lean and fat	2.7 oz	78	42	305	19	25	0	9	209	2.7	216	0	0.75	0.22	4.5	—
Lean only	2 oz	56	53	150	17	9	0	7	181	2.2	192	0	0.63	0.18	3.8	—
Roast, oven cooked, no liquid added (piece, 2½ × 2½ × ¾ inch):																
Lean and fat	3 oz	85	46	310	21	24	0	9	218	2.7	233	0	0.78	0.22	4.8	—
Lean only	2.4 oz	68	55	175	20	10	0	9	211	2.6	224	0	0.73	0.21	4.4	—

Note: Dashes (—) denote lack of reliable data for a constituent believed to be present in measurable amount.

16 Dipped in egg, breadcrumbs, and flour or batter.

17 Prepared with tuna, celery, salad dressing (mayonnaise type), pickle, onion, and egg.

18 Outer layer of fat on the cut was removed to within ½ in of the lean. Deposits of fat within the cut were not removed.

19 Crust made with vegetable shortening and enriched flour.

20 Regular-type margarine used.

21 Value varies widely.

22 About one-fourth of the outer layer of fat on the cut was removed. Deposits of fat within the cut were not removed.

Table B-1. (Continued)

Foods, approximate measures, units and weight (edible part unless footnotes indicate otherwise)	Amount	Weight (grams)	Water (percent)	Food Energy (calories)	Protein (grams)	Fat (grams)	Carbohydrate (grams)	Calcium (milligrams)	Phosphorus (milligrams)	Iron (milligrams)	Potassium (milligrams)	Vitamin A Value (I.U.)	Thiamin (milligrams)	Riboflavin (milligrams)	Niacin (milligrams)	Ascorbic Acid (milligrams)
FISH, SHELLFISH, MEAT, POULTRY; RELATED PRODUCTS																
Shoulder cut, simmered (3 pieces, 2½ × 2½ × ¼ inch):																
Lean and fat	3 oz	85	46	320	20	26	0	9	118	2.6	158	0	0.46	0.21	4.1	—
Lean only	2.2 oz	63	60	135	18	6	0	8	111	2.3	146	0	0.42	0.19	3.7	—
Sausages (see also Luncheon meat):																
Bologna, slice (8 per 8-oz pkg.)	1 slice	28	56	85	3	8	Trace	2	36	0.5	65	—	0.05	0.06	0.7	—
Braunschweiger, slice (6 per 6-oz pkg.)	1 slice	28	53	90	4	8	1	3	69	1.7	—	1,850	0.05	0.41	2.3	—
Brown and serve (10–11 per 8-oz pkg.), browned	1 link	17	40	70	3	6	Trace	—	—	—	—	—	—	—	—	—
Deviled ham, canned	1 tbsp	13	51	45	2	4	0	1	12	0.3	—	0	0.02	0.01	0.2	—
Frankfurter (8 per 1-lb pkg.), cooked (reheated)	1 frankfurter	56	57	170	7	15	1	3	57	0.8	—	—	0.08	0.11	1.4	—
Meat, potted (beef, chicken, turkey), canned	1 tbsp	13	61	30	2	2	0	—	—	—	—	—	Trace	0.03	0.2	—
Pork link (16 per 1-lb pkg.), cooked	1 link	13	35	60	2	6	Trace	1	21	0.3	35	0	0.10	0.04	0.5	—
Salami:																
Dry type, slice (12 per 4-oz pkg.)	1 slice	10	30	45	2	4	Trace	1	28	0.4	—	—	0.04	0.03	0.5	—
Cooked type, slice (8 per 8-oz pkg.)	1 slice	28	51	90	5	7	Trace	3	57	0.7	—	—	0.07	0.07	1.2	—
Vienna sausage (7 per 4-oz can)	1 sausage	16	63	40	2	3	Trace	1	24	0.3	—	—	0.01	0.02	0.4	—
Veal, medium fat, cooked, bone removed:																
Cutlet (4½ × 2¼ × ½ inch, braised or broiled)	3 oz	85	60	185	23	9	0	9	196	2.7	258	—	0.06	0.21	4.6	—
Rib (2 pieces, 4⅛ × 2¼ × ¼ inch), roasted	3 oz	85	55	230	23	14	0	10	211	2.9	259	—	0.11	0.26	6.6	—
Poultry and poultry products:																
Chicken, cooked:																
Breast, fried,[23] bones removed, ½ breast (3.3 oz with bones)	2.8 oz	79	58	160	26	5	1	9	218	1.3	—	70	0.04	0.17	11.6	—
Drumstick, fried,[23] bones removed (2 oz with bones)	1.3 oz	38	55	90	12	4	Trace	6	89	0.9	—	50	0.03	0.15	2.7	—
Half broiler, broiled, bones removed (10.4 oz with bones)	6.2 oz	176	71	240	42	7	0	16	355	3.0	483	160	0.09	0.34	15.5	—
Chicken, canned, boneless	3 oz	85	65	170	18	10	0	18	210	1.3	117	200	0.03	0.11	3.7	3
Chicken a la king, cooked (home recipe)	1 cup	245	68	470	27	34	12	127	358	2.5	404	1,130	0.10	0.42	5.4	12
Chicken and noodles, cooked (home recipe)	1 cup	240	71	365	22	18	26	26	247	2.2	149	430	0.05	0.17	4.3	Trace
Chicken chow mein:																
Canned	1 cup	250	89	95	7	Trace	18	45	85	1.3	418	150	0.05	0.10	1.0	13
From home recipe	1 cup	250	78	255	31	10	10	58	293	2.5	473	280	0.08	0.23	4.3	10
Chicken potpie (home recipe), baked[19] (piece, ⅓ of 9-inch diam. pie)	1 piece	232	57	545	23	31	42	70	232	3.0	343	3,090	0.34	0.31	5.5	5

Food	Measure	Grams	Water (%)	Food energy (cal.)	Protein (g)	Fat (g)	Carbohydrate (g)	Calcium (mg)	Phosphorus (mg)	Iron (mg)	Potassium (mg)	Vitamin A (IU)	Thiamin (mg)	Riboflavin (mg)	Niacin (mg)	Ascorbic acid (mg)
Turkey, roasted, flesh without skin: Dark meat, piece, 2½ × 1⅝ × ¼ inch	4 pieces	85	61	175	26	7	0	—	—	2.0	338	—	0.03	0.20	3.6	—
Light meat, piece, 4 × 2 × ¼ inch	2 pieces	85	62	150	28	3	0	—	—	1.0	349	—	0.04	0.12	9.4	—
Light and dark meat: Chopped or diced	1 cup	140	61	265	44	9	0	11	351	2.5	514	—	0.07	0.25	10.8	—
Pieces (1 slice white meat, 4 × 2 × ¼ inch with 2 slices dark meat, 2½ × 1⅝ × ¼ inch).	3 pieces	85	61	160	27	5	0	7	213	1.5	312	—	0.04	0.15	6.5	—
FRUITS AND FRUIT PRODUCTS																
Apples, raw, unpeeled, without cores: 2¾-inch diam. (about 3 per lb with cores).	1 apple	138	84	80	Trace	1	20	10	14	0.4	152	120	0.04	0.03	0.1	6
3¼ inch diam. (about 2 per lb with cores).	1 apple	212	84	125	Trace	1	31	15	21	0.6	223	190	0.06	0.04	0.2	8
Apple juice, bottled or canned[24]	1 cup	248	88	120	Trace	Trace	30	15	22	1.5	250	—	0.02	0.05	0.2	2[25]
Applesauce, canned: Sweetened	1 cup	255	76	230	1	Trace	61	10	13	1.3	166	100	0.05	0.03	0.1	3[25]
Unsweetened	1 cup	244	89	100	Trace	Trace	26	10	12	1.2	190	100	0.05	0.02	0.1	2[25]
Apricots Raw, without pits (about 12 per lb with pits).	3 apricots	107	85	55	1	Trace	14	18	25	0.5	301	2,890	0.03	0.04	0.6	11
Canned in heavy syrup (halves and syrup).	1 cup	258	77	220	2	Trace	57	28	39	0.8	604	4,490	0.05	0.05	1.0	10
Dried: Uncooked (28 large or 37 medium halves per cup).	1 cup	130	25	340	7	1	86	87	140	7.2	1,273	14,170	0.01	0.21	4.3	16
Cooked, unsweetened, fruit and liquid.	1 cup	250	76	215	4	1	54	55	88	4.5	795	7,500	0.01	0.13	2.5	0
Apricot nectar, canned	1 cup	251	85	145	1	Trace	37	23	30	0.5	379	2,380	0.03	0.03	0.5	36[26]
Avocados, raw, whole, without skins and seeds: California, mid- and late winter (with skin and seed, 3⅛-inch diam.; wt., 10 oz).	1 avocado	216	74	370	5	37	13	22	91	1.3	1,303	630	0.24	0.43	3.5	30
Florida, late summer and fall (with skin and seed, 3⅝-inch diam.; wt., 1 lb).	1 avocado	304	78	390	4	33	27	30	128	1.8	1,836	880	0.33	0.61	4.9	43
Banana without peel (about 2.6 per lb with peel).	1 banana	119	76	100	1	Trace	26	10	31	0.8	440	230	0.06	0.07	0.8	12
Banana flakes	1 tbsp	6	3	20	Trace	Trace	5	2	6	0.2	92	50	0.01	0.01	0.2	Trace
Blackberries, raw	1 cup	144	85	85	2	1	19	46	27	1.3	245	290	0.04	0.06	0.6	30
Blueberries, raw	1 cup	145	83	90	1	1	22	22	19	1.5	117	150	0.04	0.09	0.7	20
Cantaloupe. See Muskmelons																
Cherries: Sour (tart), red, pitted, canned, water packed.	1 cup	244	88	105	2	Trace	26	37	32	0.7	317	1,660	0.07	0.05	0.5	12
Sweet, raw, without pits and stems.	10 cherries	68	80	45	1	Trace	12	15	13	0.3	129	70	0.03	0.04	0.3	7

Note: Dashes (—) denote lack of reliable data for a constituent believed to be present in measurable amount.

19 Crust made with vegetable shortening and enriched flour.
23 Vegetable shortening used.
24 Also applies to pasteurized apple cider.
25 Applies to product without added ascorbic acid. For value of product with added ascorbic acid, refer to label.
26 Based on product with label claim of 45 percent of U.S. RDA in 6 fl oz.

225

Table B–1. (Continued)

Foods, approximate measures, units and weight (edible part unless footnotes indicate otherwise)	Amount	Weight (grams)	Water (percent)	Food Energy (calories)	Protein (grams)	Fat (grams)	Carbohydrate (grams)	Calcium (milligrams)	Phosphorus (milligrams)	Iron (milligrams)	Potassium (milligrams)	Vitamin A Value (I.U.)	Thiamin (milligrams)	Riboflavin (milligrams)	Niacin (milligrams)	Ascorbic Acid (milligrams)
FRUITS AND FRUIT PRODUCTS																
Cranberry juice cocktail, bottled, sweetened.	1 cup	253	83	165	Trace	Trace	42	13	8	0.8	25	Trace	0.03	0.03	0.1	81[27]
Cranberry sauce, sweetened, canned, strained.	1 cup	277	62	405	Trace	1	104	17	11	0.6	83	60	0.03	0.03	0.1	6
Dates:																
Whole, without pits	10 dates	80	23	220	2	Trace	58	47	50	2.4	518	40	0.07	0.08	1.8	0
Chopped	1 cup	178	23	490	4	1	130	105	112	5.3	1,153	90	0.16	0.18	3.9	0
Fruit cocktail, canned, in heavy syrup.	1 cup	255	80	195	1	Trace	50	23	31	1.0	411	360	0.05	0.03	1.0	5
Grapefruit:																
Raw, medium, 3¾-inch diam. (about 1 lb 1 oz):																
Pink or red	½ grapefruit with peel[28]	241	89	50	1	Trace	13	20	20	0.5	166	540	0.05	0.02	0.2	44
White	½ grapefruit with peel[28]	241	89	45	1	Trace	12	19	19	0.5	159	10	0.05	0.02	0.2	44
Canned, sections with syrup	1 cup	254	81	180	2	Trace	45	33	36	0.8	343	30	0.08	0.05	0.5	76
Grapefruit juice:																
Raw, pink, red, or white	1 cup	246	90	95	1	Trace	23	22	37	0.5	399	(29)	0.10	0.05	0.5	93
Canned, white:																
Unsweetened	1 cup	247	89	100	1	Trace	24	20	35	1.0	400	20	0.07	0.05	0.5	84
Sweetened	1 cup	250	86	135	1	Trace	32	20	35	1.0	405	30	0.08	0.05	0.5	78
Frozen, concentrate, unsweetened:																
Undiluted, 6-fl oz can	1 can	207	62	300	4	1	72	70	124	0.8	1,250	60	0.29	0.12	1.4	286
Diluted with 3 parts water by volume.	1 cup	247	89	100	1	Trace	24	25	42	0.2	420	20	0.10	0.04	0.5	96
Dehydrated crystals, prepared with water (1 lb yields about 1 gal).	1 cup	247	90	100	1	Trace	24	22	40	0.2	412	20	0.10	0.05	0.5	91
Grapes, European type (adherent skin), raw:																
Thompson Seedless	10 grapes	50	81	35	Trace	Trace	9	6	10	0.2	87	50	0.03	0.02	0.2	2
Tokay and Emperor, seeded types	10 grapes[30]	60	81	40	Trace	Trace	10	7	11	0.2	99	60	0.03	0.02	0.2	2
Grape juice:																
Canned or bottled	1 cup	253	83	165	1	Trace	42	28	30	0.8	293	—	0.10	0.05	0.5	Trace[25]
Frozen concentrate, sweetened:																
Undiluted, 6-fl oz can	1 can	216	53	395	1	Trace	100	22	32	0.9	255	40	0.13	0.22	1.5	32[31]
Diluted with 3 parts water by volume	1 cup	250	86	135	1	Trace	33	8	10	0.3	85	10	0.05	0.08	0.5	10[31]
Grape drink, canned	1 cup	250	86	135	Trace	Trace	35	8	10	0.3	88	—	0.03[32]	0.03[32]	0.3	(32)
Lemon, raw, size 165, without peel and seeds (about 4 per lb with peels and seeds).	1 lemon	74	90	20	1	Trace	6	19	12	0.4	102	10	0.03	0.01	0.1	39
Lemon juice:																
Raw	1 cup	244	91	60	1	Trace	20	17	24	0.5	344	50	0.07	0.02	0.2	112
Canned, or bottled, unsweetened	1 cup	244	92	55	1	Trace	19	17	24	0.5	344	50	0.07	0.02	0.2	102
Frozen, single strength, unsweetened, 6-fl oz can.	1 can	183	92	40	1	Trace	13	13	16	0.5	258	40	0.05	0.02	0.2	81

Food, approximate measure, and weight	Measure	Weight (g)	Water (%)	Food energy (calories)	Protein (g)	Fat (g)	Carbohydrate (g)	Calcium (mg)	Phosphorus (mg)	Iron (mg)	Potassium (mg)	Vitamin A (I.U.)	Thiamin (mg)	Riboflavin (mg)	Niacin (mg)	Ascorbic acid (mg)
Lemonade concentrate, frozen:																
Undiluted, 6-fl oz can	1 can	219	49	425	Trace	Trace	112	9	13	0.4	153	40	0.05	0.06	0.7	66
Diluted with 4⅓ parts water by volume.	1 cup	248	89	105	Trace	Trace	28	2	3	0.1	40	10	0.01	0.02	0.2	17
Limeade concentrate, frozen:																
Undiluted, 6-fl oz can	1 can	218	50	410	Trace	Trace	108	11	13	0.2	129	Trace	0.02	0.02	0.2	26
Diluted with 4⅓ parts water by volume.	1 cup	247	89	100	Trace	Trace	27	3	3	Trace	32	Trace	Trace	Trace	Trace	6
Lime juice:																
Raw	1 cup	246	90	65	1	Trace	22	22	27	0.5	256	20	0.05	0.02	0.2	79
Canned, unsweetened	1 cup	246	90	65	1	Trace	22	22	27	0.5	256	20	0.05	0.02	0.2	52
Muskmelons, raw, with rind, without seed cavity:																
Cantaloupe, orange-fleshed (with rind and seed cavity, 5-inch diam, 2⅓ lb).	½ melon with rind[33]	477	91	80	2	Trace	20	38	44	1.1	682	9,240	0.11	0.08	1.6	90
Honeydew (with rind and seed cavity, 6½-inch diam, 5¼ lb).	1/10 melon with rind[33]	226	91	50	1	Trace	11	21	24	0.6	374	60	0.06	0.04	0.9	34
Oranges, all commercial varieties, raw:																
Whole, 2⅝-inch diam, without peel and seeds (about 2½ per lb with peel and seeds).	1 orange	131	86	65	1	Trace	16	54	26	0.5	263	260	0.13	0.05	0.5	66
Sections without membranes	1 cup	180	86	90	2	Trace	22	74	36	0.7	360	360	0.18	0.07	0.7	90
Orange juice:																
Raw, all varieties	1 cup	248	88	110	2	Trace	26	27	42	0.5	496	500	0.22	0.07	1.0	124
Canned, unsweetened	1 cup	249	87	120	2	Trace	28	25	45	1.0	496	500	0.17	0.05	0.7	100
Frozen concentrate:																
Undiluted, 6-fl oz can	1 can	213	55	360	5	Trace	87	75	126	0.9	1,500	1,620	0.68	0.11	2.8	360
Diluted with 3 parts water by volume.	1 cup	249	87	120	2	Trace	29	25	42	0.2	503	540	0.23	0.03	0.9	120
Dehydrated crystals, prepared with water (1 lb yields about 1 gal).	1 cup	248	88	115	1	Trace	27	25	40	0.5	518	500	0.20	0.07	1.0	109
Orange and grapefruit juice:																
Frozen concentrate:																
Undiluted, 6-fl oz can	1 can	210	59	330	4	1	78	61	99	0.8	1,308	800	0.48	0.06	2.3	302
Diluted with 3 parts water by volume.	1 cup	248	88	110	1	Trace	26	20	32	0.2	439	270	0.15	0.02	0.7	102
Papayas, raw, ½-inch cubes	1 cup	140	89	55	1	Trace	14	28	22	0.4	328	2,450	0.06	0.06	0.4	78
Peaches:																
Raw:																
Whole, 2½-inch diam, peeled, pitted (about 4 per lb with peels and pits).	1 peach	100	89	40	1	Trace	10	9	19	0.5	202	1,330[34]	0.02	0.05	1.0	7
Sliced	1 cup	170	89	65	1	Trace	16	15	32	0.9	343	2,260[34]	0.03	0.09	1.7	12

Note: Dashes (—) denote lack of reliable data for a constituent believed to be present in measurable amount.

25 Applies to product without added ascorbic acid. For value of product with added ascorbic acid, refer to label.

27 Based on product with label claim of 100 percent of U.S. RDA in 6 fl oz.

28 Weight includes peel and membranes between sections. Without these parts, the weight of the edible portion is 123 g for pink or red and 118 g for white.

29 For white-fleshed varieties, value is about 20 International Units (I.U.) per cup; for red-fleshed varieties, 1,080 I.U.

30 Weight includes seeds. Without seeds, weight of the edible portion is 57 g.

31 Applies to product without added ascorbic acid. With added ascorbic acid, based on claim that 6 fl oz of reconstituted juice contains 45 percent or 50 percent of the U.S. RDA value in milligrams is 108 or 120 for a 6-fl oz can (undiluted), 36 or 40 for 1 cup of juice (diluted).

32 For products with added thiamin and riboflavin but without added ascorbic acid, values in milligrams would be 0.60 for thiamin, 0.80 for riboflavin, and trace for ascorbic acid. For products with only ascorbic acid added, value varies with the brand. Consult the label.

33 Weight includes rind. Without rind, the weight of the edible portion is 272 g for cantaloupe and 149 g for honeydew.

34 Represents yellow-fleshed varieties. For white-fleshed varieties, value is 50 International Units (I.U.) for 1 peach, 90 I.U. for 1 cup of slices.

Table B-1. (Continued)

												Nutrients in Indicated Quantity				
Foods, approximate measures, units and weight (edible part unless footnotes indicate otherwise)	Amount	Weight (grams)	Water (percent)	Food Energy (calories)	Protein (grams)	Fat (grams)	Carbohydrate (grams)	Calcium (milligrams)	Phosphorus (milligrams)	Iron (milligrams)	Potassium (milligrams)	Vitamin A Value (I.U.)	Thiamin (milligrams)	Riboflavin (milligrams)	Niacin (milligrams)	Ascorbic Acid (milligrams)
FRUITS AND FRUIT PRODUCTS																
Canned, yellow-fleshed, solids and liquid (halves or slices):																
Syrup pack	1 cup	256	79	200	1	Trace	51	10	31	0.8	333	1,100	0.03	0.05	1.5	8
Water pack	1 cup	244	91	75	1	Trace	20	10	32	0.7	334	1,100	0.02	0.07	1.5	7
Dried:																
Uncooked	1 cup	160	25	420	5	1	109	77	187	9.6	1,520	6,240	0.02	0.30	8.5	29
Cooked, unsweetened, halves and juice.	1 cup	250	77	205	3	1	54	38	93	4.8	743	3,050	0.01	0.15	3.8	5
Frozen, sliced, sweetened:																
10-oz container	1 container	284	77	250	1	Trace	64	11	37	1.4	352	1,850	0.03	0.11	2.0	116[35]
Cup	1 cup	250	77	220	1	Trace	57	10	33	1.3	310	1,630	0.03	0.10	1.8	103[35]
Pears:																
Raw, with skin, cored:																
Bartlett, 2½-inch diam. (about 2½ per lb with cores and stems).	1 pear	164	83	100	1	1	25	13	18	0.5	213	30	0.03	0.07	0.2	7
Bosc, 2½-inch diam. (about 3 per lb with cores and stems).	1 pear	141	83	85	1	1	22	11	16	0.4	83	30	0.03	0.06	0.1	6
D'Anjou, 3-inch diam. (about 2 per lb with cores and stems).	1 pear	200	83	120	1	1	31	16	22	0.6	260	40	0.04	0.08	0.2	8
Canned, solids and liquid, syrup pack, heavy (halves or slices).	1 cup	255	80	195	1	1	50	13	18	0.5	214	10	0.03	0.05	0.3	3
Pineapple:																
Raw, diced	1 cup	155	85	80	1	Trace	21	26	12	0.8	226	110	0.14	0.05	0.3	26
Canned, heavy syrup pack, solids and liquid:																
Crushed, chunks, tidbits	1 cup	255	80	190	1	Trace	49	28	13	0.8	245	130	0.20	0.05	0.5	18
Slices and liquid:																
Large	1 slice; 2¼ tbsp liquid.	105	80	80	Trace	Trace	20	12	5	0.3	101	50	0.08	0.02	0.2	7
Medium	1 slice; 1¼ tbsp liquid.	58	80	45	Trace	Trace	11	6	3	0.2	56	30	0.05	0.01	0.1	4
Pineapple juice, unsweetened, canned.	1 cup	250	86	140	1	Trace	34	38	23	0.8	373	130	0.13	0.05	0.5	80[27]
Plums:																
Raw, without pits:																
Japanese and hybrid (2⅛-inch diam., about 6½ per lb with pits).	1 plum	66	87	30	Trace	Trace	8	8	12	0.3	112	160	0.02	0.02	0.3	4
Prune-type (1½-inch diam, about 15 per lb with pits).	1 plum	28	79	20	Trace	Trace	6	3	5	0.1	48	80	0.01	0.01	0.1	1
Canned, heavy syrup pack (Italian prunes), with pits and liquid:																
Cup	1 cup[36]	272	77	215	1	Trace	56	23	26	2.3	367	3,130	0.05	0.05	1.0	5
Portion	3 plums; 2¾ tbsp liquid.[36]	140	77	110	1	Trace	29	12	13	1.2	189	1,610	0.03	0.03	0.5	3
Prunes, dried, "softenized," with pits:																

228

Uncooked	Measure	Weight (g)	Water (%)	Food energy (cal)	Protein (g)	Fat (g)	Carbohydrate (g)	Calcium (mg)	Phosphorus (mg)	Iron (mg)	Potassium (mg)	Vitamin A (IU)	Thiamin (mg)	Riboflavin (mg)	Niacin (mg)	Ascorbic acid (mg)
	4 extra large or 5 large prunes,[36]	49	28	110	1	Trace	29	22	34	1.7	298	690	0.04	0.07	0.7	1
Cooked, unsweetened, all sizes, fruit and liquid.	1 cup[36]	250	66	255	2	1	67	51	79	3.8	695	1,590	0.07	0.15	1.5	2
Prune juice, canned or bottled	1 cup	256	80	195	1	Trace	49	36	51	1.8	602	—	0.03	0.03	1.0	5
Raisins, seedless: Cup, not pressed down	1 cup	145	18	420	4	Trace	112	90	146	5.1	1,106	30	0.16	0.12	0.7	1
Packet, ½ oz (1½ tbsp)	1 packet	14	18	40	Trace	Trace	11	9	14	0.5	107	Trace	0.02	0.01	0.1	Trace
Raspberries, red: Raw, capped, whole	1 cup	123	84	70	1	1	17	27	27	1.1	207	160	0.04	0.11	1.1	31
Frozen, sweetened, 10-oz container	1 container	284	74	280	2	1	70	37	48	1.7	284	200	0.06	0.17	1.7	60
Rhubarb, cooked, added sugar: From raw	1 cup	270	63	380	1	Trace	97	211	41	1.6	548	220	0.05	0.14	0.8	16
From frozen, sweetened	1 cup	270	63	385	1	1	98	211	32	1.9	475	190	0.05	0.11	0.5	16
Strawberries: Raw, whole berries, capped	1 cup	149	90	55	1	1	13	31	31	1.5	244	90	0.04	0.10	0.9	88
Frozen, sweetened: Sliced, 10-oz container	1 container	284	71	310	1	1	79	40	48	2.0	318	90	0.06	0.17	1.4	151
Whole, 1-lb container (about 1⅔ cups).	1 container	454	76	415	2	1	107	59	73	2.7	472	140	0.09	0.27	2.3	249
Tangerine, raw, 2⅜-inch diam., size 176, without peel (about 4 per lb with peels and seeds).	1 tangerine	86	87	40	1	Trace	10	34	15	0.3	108	360	0.05	0.02	0.1	27
Tangerine juice, canned, sweetened.	1 cup	249	87	125	1	Trace	30	44	35	0.5	440	1,040	0.15	0.05	0.2	54
Watermelon, raw, 4 × 8 inch wedge with rind and seeds (1/16 of 32⅔-lb melon, 10 × 16 inch).	1 wedge with rind and seeds[37]	926	93	110	2	1	27	30	43	2.1	426	2,510	0.13	0.13	0.9	30

GRAIN PRODUCTS

	Measure	Weight (g)	Water (%)	Food energy (cal)	Protein (g)	Fat (g)	Carbohydrate (g)	Calcium (mg)	Phosphorus (mg)	Iron (mg)	Potassium (mg)	Vitamin A (IU)	Thiamin (mg)	Riboflavin (mg)	Niacin (mg)	Ascorbic acid (mg)
Bagel, 3-inch diam.: Egg	1 bagel	55	32	165	6	2	28	9	43	1.2	41	30	0.14	0.10	1.2	0
Water	1 bagel	55	29	165	6	1	30	8	41	1.2	42	0	0.15	0.11	1.4	0
Barley, pearled, light uncooked	1 cup	200	11	700	16	2	158	32	378	4.0	320	0	0.24	0.10	6.2	0
Biscuits, baking powder, 2-inch diam. (enriched flour, vegetable shortening): From home recipe	1 biscuit	28	27	105	2	5	13	34	49	0.4	33	Trace	0.08	0.08	0.7	Trace
From mix	1 biscuit	28	29	90	2	3	15	19	65	0.6	32	Trace	0.09	0.08	0.8	Trace
Breadcrumbs (enriched):[38] Dry, grated	1 cup	100	7	390	13	5	73	122	141	3.6	152	Trace	0.35	0.35	4.8	Trace
Soft. See White bread.																
Breads: Boston brown bread, canned, slice, 3¼ × ½ inch[38]	1 slice	45	45	95	2	1	21	41	72	0.9	131	0[39]	0.06	0.04	0.7	0

Note: Dashes (—) denote lack of reliable data for a constituent believed to be present in measurable amount.

27 Based on product with label claim of 100 percent of U.S. RDA in 6 fl oz.

35 Value represents products with added ascorbic acid. For products without added ascorbic acid, value in milligrams is 116 for a 10-oz. container, 103 for 1 cup.

36 Weight includes pits. After removal of the pits, the weight of the edible portion is 258 g for 1 cup with liquid, 133 g for 1 portion with liquid, 43 g for 4 or 5 uncooked prunes, and 213 g for 1 cup of cooked unsweetened prunes.

37 Weight includes rind and seeds. Without rind and seeds, weight of the edible portion is 426 g.

38 Made with vegetable shortening.

39 Applied to product made with white cornmeal. With yellow cornmeal, value is 30 International Units (I.U.).

Table B–1. (Continued)

Foods, approximate measures, units and weight (edible part unless footnotes indicate otherwise)	Amount	Weight (grams)	Water (per-cent)	Food Energy (cal-ories)	Pro-tein (grams)	Fat (grams)	Carbo-hydrate (grams)	Calcium (milli-grams)	Phos-phorus (milli-grams)	Iron (milli-grams)	Potas-sium (milli-grams)	Vitamin A Value (I.U.)	Thiamin (milli-grams)	Ribo-flavin (milli-grams)	Niacin (milli-grams)	Ascorbic Acid (milli-grams)
GRAIN PRODUCTS																
Cracked wheat bread (¾ enriched wheat flour, ¼ cracked wheat):[38]																
Loaf, 1 lb	1 loaf	454	35	1,195	39	10	236	399	581	9.5	608	Trace	1.52	1.13	14.8	Trace
Slice (18 per loaf)	1 slice	25	35	65	2	1	13	22	32	0.5	34	Trace	0.08	0.06	0.8	Trace
French or Vienna bread, enriched:[38]																
Loaf, 1 lb	1 loaf	454	31	1,315	41	14	251	195	386	10.0	408	Trace	1.80	1.10	15.0	Trace
Slice:																
French (5 × 2½ × 1 inch)	1 slice	35	31	100	3	1	19	15	30	0.8	32	Trace	0.14	0.08	1.2	Trace
Vienna (4¾ × 4 × ½ inch)	1 slice	25	31	75	2	1	14	11	21	0.6	23	Trace	0.10	0.06	0.8	Trace
Italian bread, enriched:																
Loaf, 1 lb	1 loaf	454	32	1,250	41	4	256	77	349	10.0	336	0	1.80	1.10	15.0	0
Slice, 4½ × 3¼ × ¾ inch	1 slice	30	32	85	3	Trace	17	5	23	0.7	22	0	0.12	0.07	1.0	0
Raisin bread, enriched:[38]																
Loaf, 1 lb	1 loaf	454	35	1,190	30	13	243	322	395	10.0	1,057	Trace	1.70	1.07	10.7	Trace
Slice (18 per loaf)	1 slice	25	35	65	2	1	13	18	22	0.6	58	Trace	0.09	0.06	0.6	Trace
Rye bread:																
American, light (⅔ enriched wheat flour, ⅓ rye flour):																
Loaf, 1 lb	1 loaf	454	36	1,100	41	5	236	340	667	9.1	658	0	1.35	0.98	12.9	0
Slice (4¾ × 3¾ × ⁷⁄₁₆ inch).	1 slice	25	36	60	2	Trace	13	19	37	0.5	36	0	0.07	0.05	0.7	0
Pumpernickel (⅔ rye flour, ⅓ enriched wheat flour):																
Loaf, 1 lb	1 loaf	454	34	1,115	41	5	241	381	1,039	11.8	2,059	0	1.30	0.93	8.5	0
Slice (5 × 4 × ⅜ inch)	1 slice	32	34	80	3	Trace	17	27	73	0.8	145	0	0.09	0.07	0.6	0
White bread, enriched:[38]																
Soft-crumb type:																
Loaf, 1 lb	1 loaf	454	36	1,225	39	15	229	381	440	11.3	476	Trace	1.80	1.10	15.0	Trace
Slice (18 per loaf)	1 slice	25	36	70	2	1	13	21	24	0.6	26	Trace	0.10	0.06	0.8	Trace
Slice, toasted	1 slice	22	25	70	2	1	13	21	24	0.6	26	Trace	0.08	0.06	0.8	Trace
Slice (22 per loaf)	1 slice	20	36	55	2	1	10	17	19	0.5	21	Trace	0.08	0.05	0.7	Trace
Slice, toasted	1 slice	17	25	55	2	1	10	17	19	0.5	21	Trace	0.06	0.05	0.7	Trace
Loaf, 1½ lb	1 loaf	680	36	1,835	59	22	343	571	660	17.0	714	Trace	2.70	1.65	22.5	Trace
Slice (24 per loaf)	1 slice	28	36	75	2	1	14	24	27	0.7	29	Trace	0.11	0.07	0.9	Trace
Slice, toasted	1 slice	24	25	75	2	1	14	24	27	0.7	29	Trace	0.09	0.07	0.9	Trace
Slice (28 per loaf)	1 slice	24	36	65	2	1	12	20	23	0.6	25	Trace	0.10	0.06	0.8	Trace
Slice, toasted	1 slice	21	25	65	2	1	12	20	23	0.6	25	Trace	0.08	0.06	0.8	Trace
Cubes	1 cup	30	36	80	3	1	15	25	29	0.8	32	Trace	0.12	0.07	1.0	Trace
Crumbs	1 cup	45	36	120	4	1	23	38	44	1.1	47	Trace	0.18	0.11	1.5	Trace
Firm-crumb type:																
Loaf, 1 lb	1 loaf	454	35	1,245	41	17	228	435	463	11.3	549	Trace	1.80	1.10	15.0	Trace
Slice (20 per loaf)	1 slice	23	35	65	2	1	12	22	23	0.6	28	Trace	0.09	0.06	0.8	Trace
Slice, toasted	1 slice	20	24	65	2	1	12	22	23	0.6	28	Trace	0.07	0.06	0.8	Trace
Loaf, 2 lb	1 loaf	907	35	2,495	82	34	455	871	925	22.7	1,097	Trace	3.60	2.20	30.0	Trace

Slice (34 per loaf)	1 slice	27	35	75	2	1	14	26	28	0.7	33	Trace	0.11	0.06	0.9	Trace
Slice, toasted	1 slice	23	24	75	2	1	14	26	28	0.7	33	Trace	0.09	0.06	0.9	Trace
Whole-wheat bread:[38]																
Soft-crumb type:[38]																
Loaf, 1 lb	1 loaf	454	36	1,095	41	12	224	381	1,152	13.6	1,161	Trace	1.37	0.45	12.7	Trace
Slice (16 per loaf)	1 slice	28	36	65	3	1	14	24	71	0.8	72	Trace	0.09	0.03	0.8	Trace
Slice, toasted	1 slice	24	24	65	3	1	14	24	71	0.8	72	Trace	0.07	0.03	0.8	Trace
Firm-crumb type:[38]																
Loaf, 1 lb	1 loaf	454	36	1,100	48	14	216	449	1,034	13.6	1,238	Trace	1.17	0.54	12.7	Trace
Slice (18 per loaf)	1 slice	25	36	60	3	1	12	25	57	0.8	68	Trace	0.06	0.03	0.7	Trace
Slice, toasted	1 slice	21	24	60	3	1	12	25	57	0.8	68	Trace	0.05	0.03	0.7	Trace
Breakfast, cereals:																
Hot type, cooked:																
Corn (hominy) grits, degermed:																
Enriched	1 cup	245	87	125	3	Trace	27	2	25	0.7	27	Trace[40]	0.10	0.07	1.0	0
Unenriched	1 cup	245	87	125	3	Trace	27	2	25	0.2	27	Trace[40]	0.05	0.02	0.5	0
Farina, quick-cooking, enriched.	1 cup	245	89	105	3	Trace	22	147	113[41]	(42)	25	0	0.12	0.07	1.0	0
Oatmeal or rolled oats	1 cup	240	87	130	5	2	23	22	137	1.4	146	0	0.19	0.05	0.2	0
Wheat, rolled	1 cup	240	80	180	5	1	41	19	182	1.7	202	0	0.17	0.07	2.2	0
Wheat, whole-meal	1 cup	245	88	110	4	1	23	17	127	1.2	118	0	0.15	0.05	1.5	0
Ready-to-eat:																
Bran flakes (40% bran), added sugar, salt, iron, vitamins.	1 cup	35	3	105	4	1	28	19	125	12.4	137	1,650	0.41	0.49	4.1	12
Bran flakes with raisins, added sugar, salt, iron, vitamins.	1 cup	50	7	145	4	1	40	28	146	17.7	154	2,350	0.58	0.71	5.8	18
Corn flakes:																
Plain, added sugar, salt, iron, vitamins.	1 cup	25	4	95	2	Trace	21	(43)	9	0.6	30	1,180	0.29	0.35	2.9	9
Sugar-coated, added salt, iron, vitamins.	1 cup	40	2	155	2	Trace	37	1	10	1.0	27	1,880	0.46	0.56	4.6	14
Corn, puffed, plain, added sugar, salt, iron, vitamins.	1 cup	20	4	80	2	1	16	4	18	2.3	—	940	0.23	0.28	2.3	7
Corn, shredded, added sugar, salt, iron, thiamin, niacin.	1 cup	25	3	95	2	Trace	22	1	10	0.6	—	0	0.11	0.05	0.5	0
Oats, puffed, added sugar, salt, minerals, vitamins.	1 cup	25	3	100	3	1	19	44	102	2.9	—	1,180	0.29	0.35	2.9	9
Rice, puffed:																
Plain, added iron, thiamin, niacin.	1 cup	15	4	60	1	Trace	13	3	14	0.3	15	0	0.07	0.01	0.7	0
Presweetened, added salt, iron, vitamins.	1 cup	28	3	115	1	0	26	3	14	1.1[44]	43	1,250	0.38	0.43	5.0	15[45]

Note: Dashes (—) denote lack of reliable data for a constituent believed to be present in measurable amount.

[38] Made with vegetable shortening.
[39] Applied to product made with white cornmeal. With yellow cornmeal, value is 30 International Units (I.U.).
[40] Applies to white varieties. For yellow varieties, value is 150 International Units (I.U.).
[41] Applies to products that do not contain di-sodium phosphate. If di-sodium phosphate is an ingredient, value is 162 mg.
[42] Value may range from less than 1 mg to about 8 mg depending on the brand. Consult the label.
[43] Value varies with the brand. Consult the label.
[44] Value varies with the brand. Consult the label.
[45] Applies to product with added ascorbic acid. Without added ascorbic acid, value is trace.

Table B-1. (Continued)

Foods, approximate measures, units and weight (edible part unless footnotes indicate otherwise)	Amount	Weight (grams)	Water (per-cent)	Food Energy (calories)	Protein (grams)	Fat (grams)	Carbohydrate (grams)	Calcium (milligrams)	Phosphorus (milligrams)	Iron (milligrams)	Potassium (milligrams)	Vitamin A Value (I.U.)	Thiamin (milligrams)	Riboflavin (milligrams)	Niacin (milligrams)	Ascorbic Acid (milligrams)
GRAIN PRODUCTS																
Wheat flakes, added sugar, salt, iron, vitamins.	1 cup	30	4	105	3	Trace	24	12	83	(43)	81	1,410	0.35	0.42	3.5	11
Wheat, puffed:																
Plain, added iron, thiamin, niacin.	1 cup	15	3	55	2	Trace	12	4	48	0.6	51	0	0.08	0.03	1.2	0
Presweetened, added salt, iron, vitamins.	1 cup	38	3	140	3	Trace	33	7	52	1.6[44]	63	1,680	0.50	0.57	6.7	20[45]
Wheat, shredded, plain	1 oblong biscuit or 1/2 cup spoon-size biscuits.	25	7	90	2	1	20	11	97	0.9	87	0	0.06	0.03	1.1	0
Wheat germ, without salt and sugar, toasted.	1 tbsp	6	4	25	2	1	3	3	70	0.5	57	10	0.11	0.05	0.3	1
Buckwheat flour, light, sifted	1 cup	98	12	340	6	1	78	11	86	1.0	314	0	0.08	0.04	0.4	0
Bulgur, canned, seasoned	1 cup	135	56	245	8	4	44	27	263	1.9	151	0	0.08	0.05	4.1	0
Cake icings. See Sugars and Sweets.																
Cakes made from cake mixes with enriched flour:[46]																
Angel food:																
Whole cake (9 3/4-inch diam. tube cake).	1 cake	635	34	1,645	36	1	377	603	756	2.5	381	0	0.37	0.95	3.6	0
Piece, 1/12 of cake	1 piece	53	34	135	3	Trace	32	50	63	0.2	32	0	0.03	0.08	0.3	0
Coffeecake:																
Whole cake (7 5/8 × 5 5/8 × 1 1/4 inch).	1 cake	430	30	1,385	27	41	225	262	748	6.9	469	690	0.82	0.91	7.7	1
Piece, 1/6 of cake	1 piece	72	30	230	5	7	38	44	125	1.2	78	120	0.14	0.15	1.3	Trace
Cupcakes, made with egg, milk, 2 1/2-inch diam.:																
Without icing	1 cupcake	25	26	90	1	3	14	40	59	0.3	21	40	0.05	0.05	0.4	Trace
With chocolate icing	1 cupcake	36	22	130	2	5	21	47	71	0.4	42	60	0.05	0.06	0.4	Trace
Devil's food with chocolate icing:																
Whole, 2 layer cake (8- or 9-inch diam.).	1 cake	1,107	24	3,755	49	136	645	653	1,162	16.6	1,439	1,660	1.06	1.65	10.1	1
Piece, 1/16 of cake	1 piece	69	24	235	3	8	40	41	72	1.0	90	100	0.07	0.10	0.6	Trace
Cupcake, 2 1/2-inch diam.	1 cupcake	35	24	120	2	4	20	21	37	0.5	46	50	0.03	0.05	0.3	Trace
Gingerbread:																
Whole cake (8-inch square)	1 cake	570	37	1,575	18	39	291	513	570	8.6	1,562	Trace	0.84	1.00	7.4	Trace
Piece, 1/9 of cake	1 piece	63	37	175	2	4	32	57	63	0.9	173	Trace	0.09	0.11	0.8	Trace
White, 2 layer with chocolate icing:																
Whole cake (8- or 9-inch diam.)	1 cake	1,140	21	4,000	44	122	716	1,129	2,041	11.4	1,322	680	1.50	1.77	12.5	2
Piece, 1/16 of cake	1 piece	71	21	250	3	8	45	70	127	0.7	82	40	0.09	0.11	0.8	Trace
Yellow, 2 layer with chocolate icing:																
Whole cake (8- or 9-inch diam.)	1 cake	1,108	26	3,735	45	125	638	1,008	2,017	12.2	1,208	1,550	1.24	1.67	10.6	2
Piece, 1/16 of cake	1 piece	69	26	235	3	8	40	63	126	0.8	75	100	0.08	0.10	0.7	Trace

Nutrients in Indicated Quantity

Cakes made from home recipes using enriched flour:[47]

Item	Measure	Grams	Water (%)	Food energy	Protein (g)	Fat (g)	Carbohydrate (g)	Calcium (mg)	Phosphorus (mg)	Iron (mg)	Potassium (mg)	Vit. A (IU)	Thiamin (mg)	Riboflavin (mg)	Niacin (mg)	Ascorbic acid (mg)
Boston cream pie with custard filling:[47]																
Whole cake (8-inch diam.)	1 cake	825	35	2,490	41	78	412	553	833	8.2	734[48]	1,730	1.04	1.27	9.6	2
Piece, 1/12 of cake	1 piece	69	35	210	3	6	34	46	70	0.7	61[48]	140	0.09	0.11	0.8	Trace
Fruitcake, dark:																
Loaf, 1 lb (7½ × 2 × 1½ inch).	1 loaf	454	18	1,720	22	69	271	327	513	11.8	2,250	540	0.72	0.73	4.9	2
Slice, 1/30 of loaf	1 slice	15	18	55	1	2	9	11	17	0.4	74	20	0.02	0.02	0.2	Trace
Plain sheet cake:																
Without icing:																
Whole cake (9-inch square)	1 cake	777	25	2,830	35	108	434	497	793	8.5	614[48]	1,320	1.21	1.40	10.2	2
Piece, 1/9 of cake	1 piece	86	25	315	4	12	48	55	88	0.9	68[48]	150	0.13	0.15	1.1	Trace
With uncooked white icing:																
Whole cake (9-inch square)	1 cake	1,096	21	4,020	37	129	694	548	822	8.2	669[48]	2,190	1.22	1.47	10.2	2
Piece, 1/9 of cake	1 piece	121	21	445	4	14	77	61	91	0.8	74[48]	240	0.14	0.16	1.1	Trace
Pound:[49]																
Loaf, 8½ × 3½ × 3¼ inch	1 loaf	565	16	2,725	31	170	273	107	418	7.9	345	1,410	0.90	0.99	7.3	0
Slice, 1/17 of loaf	1 slice	33	16	160	2	10	16	6	24	0.5	20	80	0.05	0.06	0.4	0
Sponge cake:																
Whole cake (9¾-inch diam. tube cake).	1 cake	790	32	2,345	60	45	427	237	885	13.4	687	3,560	1.10	1.64	7.4	Trace
Piece, 1/12 of cake	1 piece	66	32	195	5	4	36	20	74	1.1	57	300	0.09	0.14	0.6	Trace
Cookies made with enriched flour:[50,51]																
Brownies with nuts:																
Home-prepared, 1¾ × 1¾ × ⅞ inch																
From home recipe	1 brownie	20	10	95	1	6	10	8	30	0.4	38	40	0.04	0.03	0.2	Trace
From commercial recipe	1 brownie	20	11	85	1	4	13	9	27	0.4	34	20	0.03	0.02	0.2	Trace
Frozen, with chocolate icing[52] 1½ × 1¾ × ⅞ inch	1 brownie	25	13	105	1	5	15	10	31	0.4	44	50	0.03	0.03	0.2	Trace
Chocolate chip:																
Commercial, 2¼-inch diam., ⅜ inch thick.	4 cookies	42	3	200	2	9	29	16	48	1.0	56	50	0.10	0.17	0.9	Trace
From home recipe, 2⅓-inch diam.	4 cookies	40	3	205	2	12	24	14	40	0.8	47	40	0.06	0.06	0.5	Trace
Fig bars, square (1⅝ × 1⅝ × ⅜ inch or rectangular (1½ × 1¾ × ½ inch).	4 cookies	56	14	200	2	3	42	44	34	1.0	111	60	0.04	0.14	0.9	Trace
Gingersnaps, 2-inch diam., ¼ inch thick.	4 cookies	28	3	90	2	2	22	20	13	0.7	129	20	0.08	0.06	0.7	0
Macaroons, 2¾-inch diam., ¼ inch thick.	2 cookies	38	4	180	2	9	25	10	32	0.3	176	0	0.02	0.06	0.2	0
Oatmeal with raisins, 2⅝-inch diam., ¼ inch thick.	4 cookies	52	3	235	3	8	38	11	53	1.4	192	30	0.15	0.10	1.0	Trace
Plain, prepared from commercial chilled dough, 2½-inch diam., ¼ inch thick.	4 cookies	48	5	240	2	12	31	17	35	0.6	23	30	0.10	0.08	0.9	0
Sandwich type (chocolate or vanilla), 1¾-inch diam., ⅜ inch thick.	4 cookies	40	2	200	2	9	28	10	96	0.7	15	0	0.06	0.10	0.7	0

43 Value varies with the brand. Consult the label.
44 Values varies with the brand. Consult the label.
45 Applies to product with added ascorbic acid. Without added ascorbic acid, value is trace.
46 Excepting angel food cake, cakes were made from mixes containing vegetable shortening; icings, with butter.
47 Excepting sponge cake, vegetable shortening used for cake portion; butter, for icing. If butter or margarine used for cake portion, vitamin A values would be higher.
48 Applies to product made with a sodium aluminum–sulfate–type baking powder. With a low-sodium–type baking powder containing potassium, value would be about twice the amount shown.
49 Equal weights of flour, sugar, eggs, and vegetable shortening.
50 Products are commercial unless otherwise specified.
51 Made with enriched flour and vegetable shortening except for macaroons, which do not contain flour or shortening.
52 Icing made with butter.

Table B-1. (Continued)

Foods, approximate measures, units and weight (edible part unless footnotes indicate otherwise)	Amount	Weight (grams)	Water (percent)	Food Energy (calories)	Protein (grams)	Fat (grams)	Carbohydrate (grams)	Calcium (milligrams)	Phosphorus (milligrams)	Iron (milligrams)	Potassium (milligrams)	Vitamin A Value (I.U.)	Thiamin (milligrams)	Riboflavin (milligrams)	Niacin (milligrams)	Ascorbic Acid (milligrams)
GRAIN PRODUCTS																
Vanilla wafers, 1¾-inch diam., ¼ inch thick.	10 cookies	40	3	185	2	6	30	16	25	0.6	29	50	0.10	0.09	0.8	0
Cornmeal:																
Whole-ground, unbolted, dry form.	1 cup	122	12	435	11	5	90	24	312	2.9	346	620[53]	0.46	0.13	2.4	0
Bolted (nearly whole-grain), dry form.	1 cup	122	12	440	11	4	91	21	272	2.2	303	590[53]	0.37	0.10	2.3	0
Degermed, enriched:																
Dry form	1 cup	138	12	500	11	2	108	8	137	4.0	166	610[53]	0.61	0.36	4.8	0
Cooked	1 cup	240	88	120	3	Trace	26	2	34	1.0	38	140[53]	0.14	0.10	1.2	0
Degermed, unenriched:																
Dry form	1 cup	138	12	500	11	2	108	8	137	1.5	166	610[53]	0.19	0.07	1.4	0
Cooked	1 cup	240	88	120	3	Trace	26	2	34	0.5	38	140[53]	0.05	0.02	0.2	0
Crackers:[38]																
Graham, plain, 2½-inch square	2 wafers	14	6	55	1	1	10	6	21	0.5	55	0	0.02	0.08	0.5	0
Rye wafers, whole-grain, 1⅞ × 3½ inch	2 wafers	13	6	45	2	Trace	10	7	50	0.5	78	0	0.04	0.03	0.2	0
Saltines, made with enriched flour.	4 crackers or 1 packet	11	4	50	1	1	8	2	10	0.5	13	0	0.05	0.05	0.4	0
Danish pastry (enriched flour), plain without fruit or nuts:[54]																
Packaged ring, 12 oz	1 ring	340	22	1,435	25	80	155	170	371	6.1	381	1,050	0.97	1.01	8.6	Trace
Round piece, about 4¼-inch diam., 1 inch thick	1 pastry	65	22	275	5	15	30	33	71	1.2	73	200	0.18	0.19	1.7	Trace
Ounce	1 oz	28	22	120	2	7	13	14	31	0.5	32	90	0.08	0.08	0.7	Trace
Doughnuts, made with enriched flour:[38]																
Cake type, plain, 2½-inch diam., 1 inch high.	1 doughnut	25	24	100	1	5	13	10	48	0.4	23	20	0.05	0.05	0.4	Trace
Yeast-leavened, glazed, 3¾-inch diam., 1¼ inch high.	1 doughnut	50	26	205	3	11	22	16	33	0.6	34	25	0.10	0.10	0.8	0
Macaroni, enriched, cooked (cut lengths, elbows, shells):																
Firm stage (hot)	1 cup	130	64	190	7	1	39	14	85	1.4	103	0	0.23	0.13	1.8	0
Tender stage:																
Cold macaroni	1 cup	105	73	115	4	Trace	24	8	53	0.9	64	0	0.15	0.08	1.2	0
Hot macaroni	1 cup	140	73	155	5	1	32	11	70	1.3	85	0	0.20	0.11	1.5	0
Macaroni (enriched) and cheese:																
Canned[55]	1 cup	240	80	230	9	10	26	199	182	1.0	139	260	0.12	0.24	1.0	Trace
From home recipe (served hot)[56]	1 cup	200	58	430	17	22	40	362	322	1.8	240	860	0.20	0.40	1.8	Trace
Muffins made with enriched flour:[38]																
From home recipe:																
Blueberry, 2⅜-inch diam., 1½ inch high.	1 muffin	40	39	110	3	4	17	34	53	0.6	46	90	0.09	0.10	0.7	Trace
Bran	1 muffin	40	35	105	3	4	17	57	162	1.5	172	90	0.07	0.10	1.7	Trace
Corn (enriched degermed cornmeal and flour), 2⅜-inch diam., 1½ inch high.	1 muffin	40	33	125	3	4	19	42	68	0.7	54	120[57]	0.10	0.10	0.7	Trace

Food	Measure															
Plain, 3-inch diam., 1½ inch high.	1 muffin	40	38	120	3	4	17	42	60	0.6	50	40	0.09	0.12	0.9	Trace
From mix, egg, milk:																
Corn, 2⅜-inch diam., 1½ inch high.[58]	1 muffin	40	30	130	3	4	20	96	152	0.6	44	100[57]	0.08	0.09	0.7	Trace
Noodles (egg noodles), enriched, cooked.	1 cup	160	71	200	7	2	37	16	94	1.4	70	110	0.22	0.13	1.9	0
Noodles, chow mein, canned	1 cup	45	1	220	6	11	26	—	—	—	—	—	—	—	—	—
Pancakes (4-inch diam.):[58]																
Buckwheat, made from mix (with buckwheat and enriched flours), egg and milk added.	1 cake	27	58	55	2	2	6	59	91	0.4	66	60	0.04	0.05	0.2	Trace
Plain:																
Made from home recipe using enriched flour.	1 cake	27	50	60	2	2	9	27	38	0.4	33	30	0.06	0.07	0.5	Trace
Made from mix with enriched flour, egg and milk added.	1 cake	27	51	60	2	2	9	58	70	0.3	42	70	0.04	0.06	0.2	Trace
Pies, pie crust made with enriched flour, vegetable shortening (9-inch diam.):																
Apple:																
Whole	1 pie	945	48	2,420	21	105	360	76	208	6.6	756	280	1.06	0.79	9.3	9
Sector, ⅐ of pie	1 sector	135	48	345	3	15	51	11	30	0.9	108	40	0.15	0.11	1.3	2
Banana cream:																
Whole	1 pie	910	54	2,010	41	85	279	601	746	7.3	1,847	2,280	0.77	1.51	7.0	9
Sector, ⅐ of pie	1 sector	130	54	285	6	12	40	86	107	1.0	264	330	0.11	0.22	1.0	1
Blueberry:																
Whole	1 pie	945	51	2,285	23	102	330	104	217	9.5	614	280	1.03	0.80	10.0	28
Sector, ⅐ of pie	1 sector	135	51	325	3	15	47	15	31	1.4	88	40	0.15	0.11	1.4	4
Cherry:																
Whole	1 pie	945	47	2,465	25	107	363	132	236	6.6	992	4,160	1.09	0.84	9.8	Trace
Sector, ⅐ of pie	1 sector	135	47	350	4	15	52	19	34	0.9	142	590	0.16	0.12	1.4	Trace
Custard:																
Whole	1 pie	910	58	1,985	56	101	213	874	1,028	8.2	1,247	2,090	0.79	1.92	5.6	0
Sector, ⅐ of pie	1 sector	130	58	285	8	14	30	125	147	1.2	178	300	0.11	0.27	0.8	0
Lemon meringue:																
Whole	1 pie	840	47	2,140	31	86	317	118	412	6.7	420	1,430	0.61	0.84	5.2	25
Sector, ⅐ of pie	1 sector	120	47	305	4	12	45	17	59	1.0	60	200	0.09	0.12	0.7	4
Mince:																
Whole	1 pie	945	43	2,560	24	109	389	265	359	13.3	1,682	20	0.96	0.86	9.8	9
Sector, ⅐ of pie	1 sector	135	43	365	3	16	56	38	51	1.9	240	Trace	0.14	0.12	1.4	1
Peach:																
Whole	1 pie	945	48	2,410	24	101	361	95	274	8.5	1,408	6,900	1.04	0.97	14.0	28
Sector, ⅐ of pie	1 sector	135	48	345	3	14	52	14	39	1.2	201	990	0.15	0.14	2.0	4
Pecan:																
Whole	1 pie	825	20	3,450	42	189	423	388	850	25.6	1,015	1,320	1.80	0.95	6.9	Trace
Sector, ⅐ of pie	1 sector	118	20	495	6	27	61	55	122	3.7	145	190	0.26	0.14	1.0	Trace

Note: Dashes (—) denote lack of reliable data for a constituent believed to be present in measurable amount.

[38] Made with vegetable shortening.
[53] Applies to yellow varieties; white varieties contain only a trace.
[54] Contains vegetable shortening and butter.
[55] Made with corn oil.
[56] Made with regular margarine.
[57] Applies to product made with yellow cornmeal.
[58] Made with enriched degermed cornmeal and enriched flour.

235

Table B-1. (Continued)

								Nutrients in Indicated Quantity							
Foods, approximate measures, units and weight (edible part unless footnotes indicate otherwise)	Amount	Weight (grams)	Water (per-cent)	Food Energy (calories)	Protein (grams)	Fat (grams)	Carbohydrate (grams)	Calcium (milligrams)	Phosphorus (milligrams)	Iron (milligrams)	Potassium (milligrams)	Vitamin A Value (I.U.)	Thiamin (milligrams)	Riboflavin (milligrams)	Niacin (milligrams)	Ascorbic Acid (milligrams)
GRAIN PRODUCTS																
Pumpkin:																
Whole	1 pie	910	59	1,920	36	102	223	464	628	7.3	1,456	22,480	0.78	1.27	7.0	Trace
Sector, ⅐ of pie	1 sector	130	59	275	5	15	32	66	90	1.0	208	3,210	0.11	0.18	1.0	Trace
Pie crust (home recipe) made with enriched flour and vegetable shortening, baked.	1 pie shell, 9-inch diam.	180	15	900	11	60	79	25	90	3.1	89	0	0.47	0.40	5.0	0
Pie crust mix with enriched flour and vegetable shortening, 10-oz pkg. prepared and baked.	Piecrust for 2-crust pie, 9-inch diam.	320	19	1,485	20	93	141	131	272	6.1	179	0	1.07	0.79	9.9	0
Pizza (cheese) baked, 4¾-inch sector; ⅛ of 12-inch diam. pie.[19]	1 sector	60	45	145	6	4	22	86	89	1.1	67	230	0.16	0.18	1.6	4
Popcorn, popped:																
Plain, large kernel	1 cup	6	4	25	1	Trace	5	1	17	0.2	—	—	—	0.01	0.1	0
With oil (coconut) and salt added, large kernel.	1 cup	9	3	40	1	2	5	1	19	0.2	—	—	—	0.01	0.2	0
Sugar coated	1 cup	35	4	135	2	1	30	2	47	0.5	—	—	—	0.02	0.4	0
Pretzels, made with enriched flour:																
Dutch, twisted, 2¾ × 2⅝ inch	1 pretzel	16	5	60	2	1	12	4	21	0.2	21	0	0.05	0.04	0.7	0
Thin, twisted, 3¼ × 2¼ × ¼ inch	10 pretzels	60	5	235	6	3	46	13	79	0.9	78	0	0.20	0.15	2.5	0
Stick, 2¼ inch long	10 pretzels	3	5	10	Trace	Trace	2	1	4	Trace	4	0	0.01	0.01	0.1	0
Rice, white, enriched:																
Instant, ready-to-serve, hot	1 cup	165	73	180	4	Trace	40	5	31	1.3	—	0	0.21	(59)	1.7	0
Long grain:																
Raw	1 cup	185	12	670	12	1	149	44	174	5.4	170	0	0.81	0.06	6.5	0
Cooked, served hot	1 cup	205	73	225	4	Trace	50	21	57	1.8	57	0	0.23	0.02	2.1	0
Parboiled:																
Raw	1 cup	185	10	685	14	1	150	111	370	5.4	278	0	0.81	0.07	6.5	0
Cooked, served hot	1 cup	175	73	185	4	Trace	41	33	100	1.4	75	0	0.19	0.02	2.1	0
Rolls, enriched:[38]																
Commerical:																
Brown-and-serve (12 per 12-oz pkg.), browned.	1 roll	26	27	85	2	2	14	20	23	0.5	25	Trace	0.10	0.06	0.9	Trace
Cloverleaf or pan, 2½-inch diam., 2 inch high.	1 roll	28	31	85	2	2	15	21	24	0.5	27	Trace	0.11	0.07	0.9	Trace
Frankfurter and hamburger (8 per 11½-oz pkg.).	1 roll	40	31	120	3	2	21	30	34	0.8	38	Trace	0.16	0.10	1.3	Trace
Hard, 3¾-inch diam., 2 inch high.	1 roll	50	25	155	5	2	30	24	46	1.2	49	Trace	0.20	0.12	1.7	Trace
Hoagie, or submarine, 11½ × 3 × 2½-inch	1 roll	135	31	390	12	4	75	58	115	3.0	122	Trace	0.54	0.32	4.5	Trace
From home recipe:																
Cloverleaf, 2½-inch diam., 2 inch high.	1 roll	35	26	120	3	3	20	16	36	0.7	41	30	0.12	0.12	1.2	Trace
Spaghetti, enriched, cooked:																
Firm stage, "al dente," served hot.	1 cup	130	64	190	7	1	39	14	85	1.4	103	0	0.23	0.13	1.8	0
Tender stage, served hot	1 cup	140	73	155	5	1	32	11	70	1.3	85	0	0.20	0.11	1.5	0

Food	Measure														
Spaghetti (enriched) in tomato sauce with cheese															
From home recipe	1 cup	250	77	260	9	9	37	80	135	2.3	408	1,080	0.25	0.18	2.3	13
Canned	1 cup	250	80	190	6	2	39	40	88	2.8	303	930	0.35	0.28	4.5	10
Spaghetti (enriched) with meat balls and tomato sauce:															
From home recipe	1 cup	248	70	330	19	12	39	124	236	3.7	665	1,590	0.25	0.30	4.0	22
Canned	1 cup	250	78	260	12	10	29	53	113	3.3	245	1,000	0.15	0.18	2.3	5
Toaster pastries	1 pastry	50	12	200	3	6	36	54[60]	67[60]	1.9	74[60]	500	0.16	0.17	2.1	(60)
Waffles, made with enriched flour, 7-inch diam..[38]															
From home recipe	1 waffle	75	41	210	7	7	28	85	130	1.3	109	250	0.17	0.23	1.4	Trace
From mix, egg and milk added	1 waffle	75	42	205	7	8	27	179	257	1.0	146	170	0.14	0.22	0.9	Trace
Wheat flours:															
All-purpose or family flour, enriched:															
Sifted, spooned	1 cup	115	12	420	12	1	88	18	100	3.3	109	0	0.74	0.46	6.1	0
Unsifted, spooned	1 cup	125	12	455	13	1	95	20	109	3.6	119	0	0.80	0.50	6.6	0
Cake or pastry flour, enriched, sifted, spooned.	1 cup	96	12	350	7	1	76	16	70	2.8	91	0	0.61	0.38	5.1	0
Self-rising, enriched, unsifted, spooned.	1 cup	125	12	440	12	1	93	331	583	3.6	—	0	0.80	0.50	6.6	0
Whole-wheat, from hard wheats, stirred.	1 cup	120	12	400	16	2	85	49	446	4.0	444	0	0.66	0.14	5.2	0
LEGUMES (DRY), NUTS, SEEDS; RELATED PRODUCTS															
Almonds, shelled:															
Chopped (about 130 almonds)	1 cup	130	5	775	24	70	25	304	655	6.1	1,005	0	0.31	1.20	4.6	Trace
Slivered, not pressed down (about 115 almonds).	1 cup	115	5	690	21	62	22	269	580	5.4	889	0	0.28	1.06	4.0	Trace
Beans, dry:															
Common varieties as Great Northern, navy, and others:															
Cooked, drained:															
Great Northern	1 cup	180	69	210	14	1	38	90	266	4.9	749	0	0.25	0.13	1.3	0
Pea (navy)	1 cup	190	69	225	15	1	40	95	281	5.1	790	0	0.27	0.13	1.3	0
Canned, solids and liquid:															
White with—															
Frankfurters (sliced)	1 cup	255	71	365	19	18	32	94	303	4.8	668	330	0.18	0.15	3.3	Trace
Pork and tomato sauce	1 cup	255	71	310	16	7	48	138	235	4.6	536	330	0.20	0.08	1.5	5
Pork and sweet sauce	1 cup	255	66	385	16	12	54	161	291	5.9	—	—	0.15	0.10	1.3	—
Red kidney	1 cup	255	76	230	15	1	42	74	278	4.6	673	10	0.13	0.10	1.5	—
Lima, cooked, drained	1 cup	190	64	260	16	1	49	55	293	5.9	1,163	—	0.25	0.11	1.3	—
Blackeye peas, dry, cooked (with residual cooking liquid).	1 cup	250	80	190	13	1	35	43	238	3.3	573	30	0.40	0.10	1.0	—
Brazil nuts, shelled (6-8 large kernels).	1 oz	28	5	185	4	19	3	53	196	1.0	203	Trace	0.27	0.03	0.5	—
Cashew nuts, roasted in oil	1 cup	140	5	785	24	64	41	53	522	5.3	650	140	0.60	0.35	2.5	—

Note: Dashes (—) denote lack of reliable data for a constituent believed to be present in measurable amount.

[19] Crust made with vegetable shortening and enriched flour.
[38] Made with vegetable shortening.
[59] Product may or may not be enriched with riboflavin. Consult the label.
[60] Value varies with the brand. Consult the label.

Table B-1. (Continued)

		Weight (grams)	Water (percent)	Food Energy (calories)	Protein (grams)	Fat (grams)	Carbohydrate (grams)	Calcium (milligrams)	Phosphorus (milligrams)	Iron (milligrams)	Potassium (milligrams)	Vitamin A Value (I.U.)	Thiamin (milligrams)	Riboflavin (milligrams)	Niacin (milligrams)	Ascorbic Acid (milligrams)
Foods, approximate measures, units and weight (edible part unless footnotes indicate otherwise)	Amount															
LEGUMES (DRY), NUTS, SEEDS; RELATED PRODUCTS																
Coconut meat, fresh:																
Piece, about 2 × 2 × ½ inch	1 piece	45	51	155	2	16	4	6	43	0.8	115	0	0.02	0.01	0.2	1
Shredded or grated, not pressed down.	1 cup	80	51	275	3	28	8	10	76	1.4	205	0	0.04	0.02	0.4	2
Filberts (hazelnuts), chopped (about 80 kernels).	1 cup	115	6	730	14	72	19	240	388	3.9	810	—	0.53	—	1.0	Trace
Lentils, whole, cooked	1 cup	200	72	210	16	Trace	39	50	238	4.2	498	40	0.14	0.12	1.2	0
Peanuts, roasted in oil, salted (whole, halves, chopped).	1 cup	144	2	840	37	72	27	107	577	3.0	971	—	0.46	0.19	24.8	0
Peanut butter	1 tbsp	16	2	95	4	8	3	9	61	0.3	100	—	0.02	0.02	2.4	0
Peas, split, dry, cooked	1 cup	200	70	230	16	1	42	22	178	3.4	592	80	0.30	0.18	1.8	—
Pecans, chopped or pieces (about 120 large halves).	1 cup	118	3	810	11	84	17	86	341	2.8	712	150	1.01	0.15	1.1	2
Pumpkin and squash kernels, dry, hulled.	1 cup	140	4	775	41	65	21	71	1,602	15.7	1,386	100	0.34	0.27	3.4	—
Sunflower seeds, dry, hulled	1 cup	145	5	810	35	69	29	174	1,214	10.3	1,334	70	2.84	0.33	7.8	—
Walnuts:																
Black																
Chopped or broken kernels	1 cup	125	3	785	26	74	19	Trace	713	7.5	575	380	0.28	0.14	0.9	—
Ground (finely)	1 cup	80	3	500	16	47	12	Trace	456	4.8	368	240	0.18	0.09	0.6	—
Persian or English, chopped (about 60 halves).	1 cup	120	4	780	18	77	19	119	456	3.7	540	40	0.40	0.16	1.1	2
SUGARS AND SWEETS																
Cake icings:																
Boiled, white:																
Plain	1 cup	94	18	295	1	0	75	2	2	Trace	17	0	Trace	0.03	Trace	0
With coconut	1 cup	166	15	605	3	13	124	10	50	0.8	277	0	0.02	0.07	0.3	0
Uncooked:																
Chocolate made with milk and butter.	1 cup	275	14	1,035	9	38	185	165	305	3.3	536	580	0.06	0.28	0.6	1
Creamy fudge from mix and water.	1 cup	245	15	830	7	16	183	96	218	2.7	238	Trace	0.05	0.20	0.7	Trace
White	1 cup	319	11	1,200	2	21	260	48	38	Trace	57	860	Trace	0.06	Trace	Trace
Candy:																
Caramels, plain or chocolate	1 oz	28	8	115	1	3	22	42	35	0.4	54	Trace	0.01	0.05	0.1	Trace
Chocolate:																
Milk, plain	1 oz	28	1	145	2	9	16	65	65	0.3	109	80	0.02	0.10	0.1	Trace
Semisweet, small pieces (60 per oz).	1 cup or 6-oz pkg	170	1	860	7	61	97	51	255	4.4	553	30	0.02	0.14	0.9	0
Chocolate-covered peanuts	1 oz	28	1	160	5	12	11	33	84	0.4	143	Trace	0.10	0.05	2.1	Trace
Fondant, uncoated (mints, candy corn, other).	1 oz	28	8	105	Trace	1	25	4	2	0.3	1	0	Trace	Trace	Trace	0
Fudge, chocolate, plain	1 oz	28	8	115	1	3	21	22	24	0.3	42	Trace	0.01	0.03	0.1	Trace
Gum drops	1 oz	28	12	100	Trace	Trace	25	2	Trace	0.1	1	0	0	Trace	Trace	0
Hard	1 oz	28	1	110	0	Trace	28	6	2	0.5	1	0	0	0	0	0
Marshmallows	1 oz	28	17	90	1	Trace	23	5	2	0.5	2	0	0	Trace	Trace	0

Food	Measure															
Chocolate-flavored beverage powders (about 4 heaping tsp per oz):																
With nonfat dry milk	1 oz	28	2	100	5	1	20	167	155	0.5	227	10	0.04	0.21	0.2	1
Without milk	1 oz	28	1	100	1	1	25	9	48	0.6	142	—	0.01	0.03	0.1	0
Honey, strained or extracted	1 tbsp	21	17	65	Trace	0	17	1	1	0.1	11	0	Trace	0.01	0.1	Trace
Jams and preserves	1 tbsp	20	29	55	Trace	Trace	14	4	2	0.2	18	Trace	Trace	Trace	Trace	Trace
	1 packet	14	29	40	Trace	Trace	10	3	1	0.1	12	Trace	Trace	0.01	Trace	Trace
Jellies	1 tbsp	18	29	50	Trace	Trace	13	4	1	0.3	14	Trace	Trace	0.01	Trace	1
	1 packet	14	29	40	Trace	Trace	10	3	1	0.2	11	Trace	Trace	Trace	Trace	1
Syrups:																
Chocolate-flavored syrup or topping:																
Thin type	1 fl oz or 2 tbsp	38	32	90	1	1	24	6	35	0.6	106	Trace	0.01	0.03	0.2	0
Fudge type	1 fl oz or 2 tbsp	38	25	125	2	5	20	48	60	0.5	107	60	0.02	0.08	0.2	Trace
Molasses, cane:																
Light (first extraction)	1 tbsp	20	24	50	—	—	13	33	9	0.9	183	—	0.01	0.01	Trace	—
Blackstrap (third extraction)	1 tbsp	20	24	45	—	—	11	137	17	3.2	585	—	0.04	0.04	0.4	—
Sorghum	1 tbsp	21	23	55	—	—	14	35	5	2.6	—	—	0.02	0.02	Trace	—
Table blends, chiefly corn, light and dark.	1 tbsp	21	24	60	0	0	15	9	3	0.8	1	0	—	0	0	0
Sugars:																
Brown, pressed down	1 cup	220	2	820	0	0	212	187	42	7.5	757	0	0	0.07	0.4	0
White:																
Granulated	1 cup	200	1	770	0	0	199	0	0	0.2	6	0	0	0	0	0
	1 tbsp	12	1	45	0	0	12	0	0	Trace	Trace	0	0	0	0	0
	1 packet	6	1	23	0	0	6	0	0	Trace	Trace	0	0	0	0	0
Powdered, sifted, spooned into cup.	1 cup	100	1	385	0	0	100	0	0	0.1	3	0	0	0	0	0
VEGETABLE AND VEGETABLE PRODUCTS																
Asparagus, green:																
Cooked, drained:																
Cuts and tips, 1½- to 2-inch lengths:																
From raw	1 cup	145	94	30	3	Trace	5	30	73	0.9	265	1,310	0.23	0.26	2.0	38
From frozen	1 cup	180	93	40	6	Trace	6	40	115	2.2	396	1,530	0.25	0.23	1.8	41
Spears, ½-inch diam. at base:																
From raw	4 spears	60	94	10	1	Trace	2	13	30	0.4	110	540	0.10	0.11	0.8	16
From frozen	4 spears	60	92	15	2	Trace	2	13	40	0.7	143	470	0.10	0.08	0.7	16
Canned, spears, ½-inch diam. at base.	4 spears	80	93	15	2	Trace	3	15	42	1.5	133	640	0.05	0.08	0.6	12
Beans:																
Lima, immature seeds, frozen, cooked, drained:																
Thick-seeded types (Fordhooks)	1 cup	170	74	170	10	Trace	32	34	153	2.9	724	390	0.12	0.09	1.7	29
Thin-seeded types (baby limas)	1 cup	180	69	210	13	Trace	40	63	227	4.7	709	400	0.16	0.09	2.2	22
Snap:																
Green:																
Cooked, drained:																
From raw (cuts and French style).	1 cup	125	92	30	2	Trace	7	63	46	0.8	189	680	0.09	0.11	0.6	15
From frozen:																
Cuts	1 cup	135	92	35	2	Trace	8	54	43	0.9	205	780	0.09	0.12	0.5	7
French style	1 cup	130	92	35	2	Trace	8	49	39	1.2	177	690	0.08	0.10	0.4	9
Canned, drained solids (cuts)	1 cup	135	92	30	2	Trace	7	61	34	2.0	128	630	0.04	0.07	0.4	5

Note: Dashes (—) denote lack of reliable data for a constituent believed to be present in measurable amount.

Table B-1. (Continued)

		Weight (grams)	Water (percent)	Food Energy (calories)	Protein (grams)	Fat (grams)	Carbohydrate (grams)	Calcium (milligrams)	Phosphorus (milligrams)	Iron (milligrams)	Potassium (milligrams)	Vitamin A Value (I.U.)	Thiamin (milligrams)	Riboflavin (milligrams)	Niacin (milligrams)	Ascorbic Acid (milligrams)
Foods, approximate measures, units and weight (edible part unless footnotes indicate otherwise)	Amount															
VEGETABLE AND VEGETABLE PRODUCTS																
Yellow or wax:																
Cooked, drained:																
From raw (cuts and French style).	1 cup	125	93	30	2	Trace	6	63	46	0.8	189	290	0.09	0.11	0.6	16
From frozen (cuts)	1 cup	135	92	35	2	Trace	8	47	42	0.9	221	140	0.09	0.11	0.5	8
Canned, drained solids (cuts).	1 cup	135	92	30	2	Trace	7	61	34	2.0	128	140	0.04	0.07	0.4	7
Beans, mature. See Beans, dry, and Black-eye peas, dry.																
Bean sprouts (mung):																
Raw	1 cup	105	89	35	4	Trace	7	20	67	1.4	234	20	0.14	0.14	0.8	20
Cooked, drained	1 cup	125	91	35	4	Trace	7	21	60	1.1	195	30	0.11	0.13	0.9	8
Beets:																
Cooked, drained, peeled:																
Whole beets, 2-inch diam.	2 beets	100	91	30	1	Trace	7	14	23	0.5	208	20	0.03	0.04	0.3	6
Diced or sliced	1 cup	170	91	55	2	Trace	12	24	39	0.9	354	30	0.05	0.07	0.5	10
Canned, drained solids:																
Whole beets, small	1 cup	160	89	60	2	Trace	14	30	29	1.1	267	30	0.02	0.05	0.2	5
Diced or sliced	1 cup	170	89	65	2	Trace	15	32	31	1.2	284	30	0.02	0.05	0.2	5
Beet greens, leaves and stems, cooked, drained.	1 cup	145	94	25	2	Trace	5	144	36	2.8	481	7,400	0.10	0.22	0.4	22
Blackeye peas, immature seeds, cooked and drained:																
From raw	1 cup	165	72	180	13	1	30	40	241	3.5	625	580	0.50	0.18	2.3	28
From frozen	1 cup	170	66	220	15	1	40	43	286	4.8	573	290	0.68	0.19	2.4	15
Broccoli, cooked, drained:																
From raw:																
Stalk, medium size	1 stalk	180	91	45	6	1	8	158	112	1.4	481	4,500	0.16	0.36	1.4	162
Stalks, cut into ½-inch pieces	1 cup	155	91	40	5	Trace	7	136	96	1.2	414	3,880	0.14	0.31	1.2	140
From frozen:																
Stalk, 4½ to 5 inch long	1 stalk	30	91	10	1	Trace	1	12	17	0.2	66	570	0.02	0.03	0.2	22
Chopped	1 cup	185	92	50	5	1	9	100	104	1.3	392	4,810	0.11	0.22	0.9	105
Brussels sprouts, cooked, drained:																
From raw, 7–8 sprouts (1¼ to 1½-inch diam.).	1 cup	155	88	55	7	1	10	50	112	1.7	423	810	0.12	0.22	1.2	135
From frozen	1 cup	155	89	50	5	Trace	10	33	95	1.2	457	880	0.12	0.16	0.9	126
Cabbage:																
Common varieties:																
Raw:																
Coarsely shredded or sliced	1 cup	70	92	15	1	Trace	4	34	20	0.3	163	90	0.04	0.04	0.02	33
Finely shredded or chopped	1 cup	90	92	20	1	Trace	5	44	26	0.4	210	120	0.05	0.05	0.3	42
Cooked, drained	1 cup	145	94	30	2	Trace	6	64	29	0.4	236	190	0.06	0.06	0.4	48
Red, raw, coarsely shredded	1 cup	70	90	20	1	Trace	5	29	25	0.6	188	30	0.06	0.04	0.3	43
Savoy, raw, coarsely shredded or sliced.	1 cup	70	92	15	2	Trace	3	47	38	0.6	188	140	0.04	0.06	0.2	39
Cabbage, celery (also called pe-tsi or wong-bok), raw, 1-inch pieces.	1 cup	75	95	10	1	Trace	2	32	30	0.5	190	110	0.04	0.03	0.5	19

Food (description)	Measure															
Cabbage, white mustard (also called bokchoy or pakchoy), cooked, drained.	1 cup	170	95	25	2	Trace	4	252	56	1.0	364	5,270	0.07	0.14	1.2	26
Carrots:																
Raw, without crowns and tips, scraped:																
Whole, 7½ by 1⅛ inch or strips, 2½ to 3 inch long.	1 carrot or 18 strips	72	88	30	1	Trace	7	27	26	0.5	246	7,930	0.04	0.04	0.4	6
Grated	1 cup	110	88	45	1	Trace	11	41	40	0.8	375	12,100	0.07	0.06	0.7	9
Cooked (crosswise cuts), drained	1 cup	155	91	50	1	Trace	11	51	48	0.9	344	16,280	0.08	0.08	0.8	9
Canned:																
Sliced, drained solids	1 cup	155	91	45	1	Trace	10	47	34	1.1	186	23,250	0.03	0.05	0.6	3
Strained or junior (baby food)	1 oz (1¾ to 2 tbsp)	28	92	10	Trace	Trace	2	7	6	0.1	51	3,690	0.01	0.01	0.1	1
Cauliflower:																
Raw, chopped	1 cup	115	91	31	3	Trace	6	29	64	1.3	339	70	0.13	0.12	0.8	90
Cooked, drained:																
From raw (flower buds)	1 cup	125	93	30	3	Trace	5	26	53	0.9	258	80	0.11	0.10	0.8	69
From frozen (flowerets)	1 cup	180	94	30	3	Trace	6	31	68	0.9	373	50	0.07	0.09	0.7	74
Celery, Pascal type, raw:																
Stalk, large outer, 8 × 1½ inch at root end.	1 stalk	40	94	5	Trace	Trace	2	16	11	0.1	136	110	0.01	0.01	0.1	4
Pieces, diced	1 cup	120	94	20	1	Trace	5	47	34	0.4	409	320	0.04	0.04	0.4	11
Collards, cooked, drained:																
From raw (leaves without stems)	1 cup	190	90	65	7	1	10	357	99	1.5	498	14,820	0.21	0.38	2.3	144
From frozen (chopped)	1 cup	170	90	50	5	1	10	299	87	1.7	401	11,560	0.10	0.24	1.0	56
Corn, sweet:																
Cooked, drained:																
From raw, ear 5 × 1¾ inch	1 ear[61]	140	74	70	2	1	16	2	69	0.5	151	310[62]	0.09	0.08	1.1	7
From frozen:																
Ear, 5 inch long	1 ear[61]	229	73	120	4	1	27	4	121	1.0	291	440[62]	0.18	0.10	2.1	9
Kernels	1 cup	165	77	130	5	1	31	5	120	1.3	304	580[62]	0.15	0.10	2.5	8
Canned:																
Cream style	1 cup	256	76	210	5	2	51	8	143	1.5	248	840[62]	0.08	0.13	2.6	13
Whole kernel:																
Vacuum pack	1 cup	210	76	175	5	1	43	6	153	1.1	204	740[62]	0.06	0.13	2.3	11
Wet pack, drained solids	1 cup	165	76	140	4	1	33	8	81	0.8	160	580[62]	0.05	0.08	1.5	7
Cowpeas. See Blackeye peas.																
Cucumber slices, ⅛ inch thick (large, 2⅛-inch diam.; small, 1¾-inch diam.):																
With peel	6 large or 8 small slices	28	95	5	Trace	Trace	1	7	8	0.3	45	70	0.01	0.01	0.1	3
Without peel	6½ large or 9 small pieces	28	96	5	Trace	Trace	1	5	5	0.1	45	Trace	0.01	0.01	0.1	3
Dandelion greens, cooked, drained	1 cup	105	90	35	2	1	7	147	44	1.9	244	12,290	0.14	0.17	1.9	19
Endive, curly (including escarole), raw, small pieces.	1 cup	50	93	10	1	Trace	2	41	27	0.9	147	1,650	0.04	0.07	0.3	5
Kale, cooked, drained:																
From raw (leaves without stems and midribs).	1 cup	110	88	45	5	1	7	206	64	1.8	243	9,130	0.11	0.20	1.8	102
From frozen (leaf style)	1 cup	130	91	40	4	1	7	157	62	1.3	251	10,660	0.08	0.20	0.9	49

Note: Dashes (—) denote lack of reliable data for a constituent believed to be present in measurable amount.

[61] Weight includes cob. Without cob, weight is 77 g for one raw ear (5 inch) and 126 g for one frozen ear (5 inch).

[62] Based on yellow varieties. For white varieties, value is trace.

Table B–1. (Continued)

Foods, approximate measures, units and weight (edible part unless footnotes indicate otherwise)	Amount	Weight (grams)	Water (percent)	Food Energy (calories)	Protein (grams)	Fat (grams)	Carbohydrate (grams)	Calcium (milligrams)	Phosphorus (milligrams)	Iron (milligrams)	Potassium (milligrams)	Vitamin A Value (I.U.)	Thiamin (milligrams)	Riboflavin (milligrams)	Niacin (milligrams)	Ascorbic Acid (milligrams)
VEGETABLE AND VEGETABLE PRODUCTS																
Lettuce, raw:																
Butterhead, as Boston types:																
Head, 5-inch diam.	1 head[63]	220	95	25	2	Trace	4	57	42	3.3	430	1,580	0.10	0.10	0.5	13
Leaves	1 outer or 2 inner or 3 heart leaves	15	95	Trace	Trace	Trace	Trace	5	4	0.3	40	150	0.01	0.01	Trace	1
Crisphead, as iceberg:																
Head, 6-inch diam.	1 head[64]	567	96	70	5	1	16	108	118	2.7	943	1,780	0.32	0.32	1.6	32
Wedge, ¼ of head	1 wedge	135	96	20	1	Trace	4	27	30	0.7	236	450	0.08	0.08	0.4	8
Pieces, chopped or shredded	1 cup	55	96	5	Trace	Trace	2	11	12	0.3	96	180	0.03	0.03	0.2	3
Looseleaf (bunching varieties including romaine or cos), chopped or shredded pieces.	1 cup	55	94	10	1	Trace	2	37	14	0.8	145	1,050	0.03	0.04	0.2	10
Mushrooms, raw, sliced or chopped	1 cup	70	90	20	2	Trace	3	4	81	0.6	290	Trace	0.07	0.32	2.9	2
Mustard greens, without stems and midribs, cooked, drained.	1 cup	140	93	30	3	1	6	193	45	2.5	308	8,120	0.11	0.20	0.8	67
Okra pods, 3 × ⅝ inch, cooked	10 pods	106	91	30	2	Trace	6	98	43	0.5	184	520	0.14	0.19	1.0	21
Onions																
Mature:																
Raw:																
Chopped	1 cup	170	89	65	3	Trace	15	46	61	0.9	267	Trace[65]	0.05	0.07	0.3	17
Sliced	1 cup	115	89	45	2	Trace	10	31	41	0.6	181	Trace[65]	0.03	0.05	0.2	12
Cooked (whole or sliced), drained.	1 cup	210	92	60	3	Trace	14	50	61	0.8	231	Trace[65]	0.06	0.06	0.4	15
Young green, bulb (⅜ inch diam.) and white portion of top.	6 onions	30	88	15	Trace	Trace	3	12	12	0.2	69	Trace	0.02	0.01	0.1	8
Parsley, raw, chopped	1 tbsp	4	85	Trace	Trace	Trace	Trace	7	2	0.2	25	300	Trace	0.01	Trace	6
Parsnips, cooked (diced or 2-inch lengths).	1 cup	155	82	100	2	1	23	70	96	0.9	587	50	0.11	0.12	0.2	16
Peas, green:																
Canned:																
Whole, drained solids	1 cup	170	77	150	8	1	29	44	129	3.2	163	1,170	0.15	0.10	1.4	14
Strained (baby food)	1 oz (1¾ to 2 tbsp)	28	86	15	1	Trace	3	3	18	0.3	28	140	0.02	0.03	0.3	3
Frozen, cooked, drained	1 cup	160	82	110	8	Trace	19	30	138	3.0	216	960	0.43	0.14	2.7	21
Peppers, hot, red, without seeds, dried (ground chili powder, added seasonings).	1 tsp	2	9	5	Trace	Trace	1	5	4	0.3	20	1,300	Trace	0.02	0.2	Trace
Peppers, sweet (about 5 per lb, whole), stems and seeds removed:																
Raw	1 pod	74	93	15	1	Trace	4	7	16	0.5	157	310	0.06	0.06	0.4	94
Cooked, boiled, drained	1 pod	73	95	15	1	Trace	3	7	12	0.4	109	310	0.05	0.05	0.4	70
Potatoes, cooked:																
Baked, peeled after baking (about 2 per lb, raw).	1 potato	156	75	145	4	Trace	33	14	101	1.1	782	Trace	0.15	0.07	2.7	31
Boiled (about 3 per lb, raw):																
Peeled after boiling	1 potato	137	80	105	3	Trace	23	10	72	0.8	556	Trace	0.12	0.05	2.0	22
Peeled before boiling	1 potato	135	83	90	3	Trace	20	8	57	0.7	385	Trace	0.12	0.05	1.6	22

Food	Measure														
French-fried, strip, 2 to 3½ inch long:															
Prepared from raw	10 strips	50	45	135	2	7	18	8	56	0.7	427	Trace	0.07	0.04	1.6	11
Frozen, oven heated	10 strips	50	53	110	2	4	17	5	43	0.9	326	Trace	0.07	0.01	1.3	11
Hashed brown, prepared from frozen.	1 cup	155	56	345	3	18	45	28	78	1.9	439	Trace	0.11	0.03	1.6	12
Mashed, prepared from—															
Raw:															
Milk added	1 cup	210	83	135	4	2	27	50	103	0.8	548	40	0.17	0.11	2.1	21
Milk and butter added	1 cup	210	80	195	4	9	26	50	101	0.8	525	360	0.17	0.11	2.1	19
Dehydrated flakes (without milk), water, milk, butter, and salt added.	1 cup	210	79	195	4	7	30	65	99	0.6	601	270	0.08	0.08	1.9	11
Potato chips, 1¾ by 2½ inch oval cross section.	10 chips	20	2	115	1	8	10	8	28	0.4	226	Trace	0.04	0.01	1.0	3
Potato salad, made with cooked salad dressing.	1 cup	250	76	250	7	7	41	80	160	1.5	798	350	0.20	0.18	2.8	28
Pumpkin, canned	1 cup	245	90	80	2	1	19	61	64	1.0	588	15,680	0.07	0.12	1.5	12
Radishes, raw (prepackaged) stem ends, rootlets cut off.	4 radishes	18	95	5	Trace	Trace	1	5	6	0.2	58	Trace	0.01	0.01	0.1	5
Sauerkraut, canned, solids and liquid.	1 cup	235	93	40	2	Trace	9	85	42	1.2	329	120	0.07	0.09	0.5	33
Southern peas. See Blackeye peas.															
Spinach:															
Raw, chopped	1 cup	55	91	15	2	Trace	2	51	28	1.7	259	4,460	0.06	0.11	0.3	28
Cooked, drained:															
From raw	1 cup	180	92	40	5	1	6	167	68	4.0	583	14,580	0.13	0.25	0.9	50
From frozen:															
Chopped	1 cup	205	92	45	6	1	8	232	90	4.3	683	16,200	0.14	0.31	0.8	39
Leaf	1 cup	190	92	45	6	1	7	200	84	4.8	688	15,390	0.15	0.27	1.0	53
Canned, drained solids	1 cup	205	91	50	6	1	7	242	53	5.3	513	16,400	0.04	0.25	0.6	29
Squash, cooked:															
Summer (all varieties), diced, drained.	1 cup	210	96	30	2	Trace	7	53	53	0.8	296	820	0.11	0.17	1.7	21
Winter (all varieties), baked, mashed.	1 cup	205	81	130	4	1	32	57	98	1.6	945	8,610	0.10	0.27	1.4	27
Sweet potatoes:															
Cooked (raw, 5 × 2 inch; about 2½ per lb):															
Baked in skin, peeled	1 potato	114	64	160	2	1	37	46	66	1.0	342	9,230	0.10	0.08	0.8	25
Boiled in skin, peeled	1 potato	151	71	170	3	1	40	48	71	1.1	367	11,940	0.14	0.09	0.9	26
Candied, 2½ × 2-inch piece	1 piece	105	60	175	1	3	36	39	45	0.9	200	6,620	0.06	0.04	0.4	11
Canned:															
Solid pack (mashed)	1 cup	255	72	275	5	1	63	64	105	2.0	510	19,890	0.13	0.10	1.5	36
Vacuum pack, piece 2¾ × 1 inch	1 piece	40	72	45	1	Trace	10	10	16	0.3	80	3,120	0.02	0.02	0.2	6
Tomatoes:															
Raw, 2⅗-inch diam. (3 per 12 oz pkg.).	1 tomato[66]	135	94	25	1	Trace	6	16	33	0.6	300	1,110	0.07	0.05	0.9	28[67]
Canned, solids and liquid	1 cup	241	94	50	2	Trace	10	14[68]	46	1.2	523	2,170	0.12	0.07	1.7	41
Tomato catsup	1 cup	273	69	290	5	1	69	60	137	2.2	991	3,820	0.25	0.19	4.4	41
	1 tbsp	15	69	15	Trace	Trace	4	3	8	0.1	54	210	0.01	0.01	0.2	2

[63] Weight includes refuse of outer leaves and core. Without these parts, weight is 163 g.

[64] Weight includes core. Without core, weight is 539 g.

[65] Value based on white-fleshed varieties. For yellow-fleshed varieties, value in International Units (I.U.) is 70 for 1 cup chopped raw onions, 50 I.U. for 1 cup sliced raw onions, and 80 I.U. for 1 cup cooked onions.

[66] Weight includes cores and stem ends. Without these parts, weight is 123 g.

[67] Based on year-round average. For tomatoes marketed from November through May, value is about 12 mg; from June through October, 32 mg.

[68] Applies to product without calcium salts added. Value for products with calcium salts added may be as much as 63 mg for whole tomatoes, 241 mg for cut forms.

Table B–1. (Concluded)

Foods, approximate measures, units and weight (edible part unless footnotes indicate otherwise)	Amount	Weight (grams)	Water (percent)	Food Energy (calories)	Protein (grams)	Fat (grams)	Carbohydrate (grams)	Calcium (milligrams)	Phosphorus (milligrams)	Iron (milligrams)	Potassium (milligrams)	Vitamin A Value (I.U.)	Thiamin (milligrams)	Riboflavin (milligrams)	Niacin (milligrams)	Ascorbic Acid (milligrams)
VEGETABLE AND VEGETABLE PRODUCTS																
Tomato juice, canned:																
Cup	1 cup	243	94	45	2	Trace	10	17	44	2.2	552	1,940	0.12	0.07	1.9	39
Glass (6 fl oz)	1 glass	182	94	35	2	Trace	8	13	33	1.6	413	1,460	0.09	0.05	1.5	29
Turnips, cooked, diced	1 cup	155	94	35	1	Trace	8	54	37	0.6	291	Trace	0.06	0.08	0.5	34
Turnip greens, cooked, drained:																
From raw (leaves and stems)	1 cup	145	94	30	3	Trace	5	252	49	1.5	—	8,270	0.15	0.33	0.7	68
From frozen (chopped)	1 cup	165	93	40	4	Trace	6	195	64	2.6	246	11,390	0.08	0.15	0.7	31
Vegetables, mixed, frozen, cooked	1 cup	182	83	115	6	1	24	46	115	2.4	348	9,010	0.22	0.13	2.0	15
MISCELLANEOUS ITEMS																
Baking powders for home use:																
Sodium aluminum sulfate:																
With monocalcium phosphate monohydrate.	1 tsp	3.0	2	5	Trace	Trace	1	58	87	—	5	0	0	0	0	0
With monocalcium phosphate monohydrate, calcium sulfate.	1 tsp	2.9	1	5	Trace	Trace	1	183	45	—	—	0	0	0	0	0
Straight phosphate.	1 tsp	3.8	2	5	Trace	Trace	1	239	359	—	6	0	0	0	0	0
Low sodium	1 tsp	4.3	2	5	Trace	Trace	2	207	314	—	471	0	0	0	0	0
Barbecue sauce	1 cup	250	81	230	4	17	20	53	50	2.0	435	900	0.03	0.03	0.8	13
Beverages, alcoholic:																
Beer	12 fl oz	360	92	150	1	0	14	18	108	Trace	90	—	0.01	0.11	2.2	—
Gin, rum, vodka, whiskey:																
80-proof	1½-fl oz jigger	42	67	95	—	—	Trace	—	—	—	1	—	—	—	—	—
86-proof	1½-fl oz jigger	42	64	105	—	—	Trace	—	—	—	1	—	—	—	—	—
90-proof	1½-fl oz jigger	42	62	110	—	—	Trace	—	—	—	1	—	—	—	—	—
Wines:																
Dessert	3½-fl oz glass	103	77	140	Trace	0	8	8	—	—	77	—	0.01	0.02	0.2	—
Table	3½-fl oz glass	102	86	85	Trace	0	4	9	10	0.4	94	—	Trace	0.01	0.1	—
Beverages, carbonated, sweetened, nonalcoholic:																
Carbonated water	12 fl oz	366	92	115	0	0	29	—	—	—	—	0	0	0	0	0
Cola type	12 fl oz	369	90	145	0	0	37	—	—	—	—	0	0	0	0	0
Fruit-flavored sodas and Tom Collins mixer	12 fl oz	372	88	170	0	0	45	—	—	—	—	0	0	0	0	0
Ginger ale	12 fl oz	366	92	115	0	0	29	—	—	—	0	0	0	0	0	0
Root beer	12 fl oz	370	90	150	0	0	39	—	—	—	0	0	0	0	0	0
Chili powder. See Peppers, hot, red.																
Chocolate:																
Bitter or baking	1 oz	28	2	145	3	15	8	22	109	1.9	235	20	0.01	0.07	0.4	0
Semisweet, see Candy, chocolate.																
Gelatin, dry	one 7-g envelope	7	13	25	6	Trace	0	—	—	—	—	—	—	—	—	—
Gelatin, dessert prepared with gelatin dessert powder and water.	1 cup	240	84	140	4	0	34	—	—	—	—	—	—	—	—	—

Food	Measure	Weight (g)	Water (%)	Food energy (cal)	Protein (g)	Fat (g)	Carbohydrate (g)	Calcium (mg)	Phosphorus (mg)	Iron (mg)	Potassium (mg)	Vitamin A (IU)	Thiamin (mg)	Riboflavin (mg)	Niacin (mg)	Ascorbic acid (mg)
Mustard, prepared, yellow	1 tsp or individual serving pouch or cup.	5	80	5	Trace	Trace	Trace	4	4	0.1	7	—	—	—	—	—
Olives, pickled, canned:																
Green	4 medium or 3 extra large or 2 giant[69]	16	78	15	Trace	2	Trace	8	2	0.2	7	40	—	—	—	—
Ripe, Mission	3 small or 2 large[69]	10	73	15	Trace	2	Trace	9	1	0.1	2	10	Trace	Trace	—	—
Pickles, cucumber:																
Dill, medium, whole, 3¾ inch long, 1¼-inch diam.	1 pickle	65	93	5	Trace	Trace	1	17	14	0.7	130	70	Trace	0.01	Trace	4
Fresh-pack, slices 1½-inch diam., ¼ inch thick.	2 slices	15	79	10	Trace	Trace	3	5	4	0.3	—	20	Trace	Trace	Trace	1
Sweet, gherkin, small, whole, about 2½ inch long, ¾-inch diam.	1 pickle	15	61	20	Trace	Trace	5	2	2	0.2	—	10	Trace	Trace	Trace	1
Relish, finely chopped, sweet	1 tbsp	15	63	20	Trace	Trace	5	3	2	0.1	—	—	—	—	Trace	1
Popcorn. See Popcorn, popped, under Grain products.																
Popsicle, 3-fl oz size	1 popsicle	95	80	70	0	0	18	0	0	Trace	—	—	0	0	0	0
Soups:																
Canned, condensed:																
Prepared with equal volume of milk:																
Cream of chicken	1 cup	245	85	180	7	10	15	172	152	0.5	260	610	0.05	0.27	0.7	2
Cream of mushroom	1 cup	245	83	215	7	14	16	191	169	0.5	279	250	0.05	0.34	0.7	1
Tomato	1 cup	250	84	175	7	7	23	168	155	0.8	418	1,200	0.10	0.25	1.3	15
Prepared with equal volume of water:																
Bean with pork	1 cup	250	84	170	8	6	22	63	128	2.3	395	650	0.13	0.08	1.0	3
Beef broth, bouillon, consomme.	1 cup	240	96	30	5	0	3	Trace	31	0.5	130	Trace	Trace	0.02	1.2	—
Beef noodle	1 cup	240	93	65	4	3	7	7	48	1.0	77	50	0.05	0.07	1.0	Trace
Clam chowder, Manhattan type (with tomatoes, without milk).	1 cup	245	92	80	2	3	12	34	47	1.0	184	880	0.02	0.02	1.0	—
Cream of chicken	1 cup	240	92	95	3	6	8	24	34	0.5	79	410	0.02	0.05	0.5	Trace
Cream of mushroom	1 cup	240	90	135	2	10	10	41	50	0.5	98	70	0.02	0.12	0.7	Trace
Minestrone	1 cup	245	90	105	5	3	14	37	59	1.0	314	2,350	0.07	0.05	1.0	—
Split pea	1 cup	245	85	145	9	3	21	29	149	1.5	270	440	0.25	0.15	1.5	1
Tomato	1 cup	245	91	90	2	3	16	15	34	0.7	230	1,000	0.05	0.05	1.2	12
Vegetable beef	1 cup	245	92	80	5	2	10	12	49	0.7	162	2,700	0.05	0.05	1.0	—
Vegetarian	1 cup	245	92	80	2	2	13	20	39	1.0	172	2,940	0.05	0.05	1.0	—
Dehydrated:																
Bouillon, cube ½ inch	1 cube	4	4	5	1	Trace	Trace	—	—	—	4	—	—	—	—	—
Mixes:																
Unprepared:																
Onion	1½-oz pkg	43	3	150	6	5	23	42	49	0.6	238	30	0.05	0.03	0.3	6
Prepared with water:																
Chicken noodle	1 cup	240	95	55	2	2	8	7	19	0.2	19	50	0.07	0.05	0.5	Trace
Onion	1 cup	240	96	35	1	1	6	10	12	0.2	58	Trace	Trace	Trace	Trace	2
Tomato vegetable with noodles.	1 cup	240	93	65	1	1	12	7	19	0.2	29	480	0.05	0.02	0.5	5
Vinegar, cider	1 tbsp	15	94	Trace	Trace	0	1	1	1	0.1	15	—	—	—	—	—
White sauce, medium, with enriched flour.	1 cup	250	73	405	10	31	22	288	233	0.5	348	1,150	0.12	0.43	0.7	2
Yeast:																
Baker's, dry, active	1 pkg	7	5	20	3	Trace	3	3	90	1.1	140	Trace	0.16	0.38	2.6	Trace
Brewer's, dry	1 tbsp	8	5	25	3	Trace	3	17[70]	140	1.4	152	Trace	1.25	0.34	3.0	Trace

Note: Dashes (—) denote lack of reliable data for a constituent believed to be present in measurable amount.

[69] Weight includes pits. Without pits, weight is 13 g for green, 9 g for ripe.

[70] Value may vary from 6 to 60 mg.

Table B–2. Selected Fast Foods *†

Food	Wt (g)	Energy (kcal)	Food	Wt (g)	Energy (kcal)
ARBY'S			Mr. Misty Kiss	89	70
Roast Beef	140	350	Brazier Chili Dog	128	330
Beef and Cheese	168	450	Brazier Dog	99	273
Super Roast Beef	263	620	Fish Sandwich	170	400
Junior Roast Beef	74	220	Fish Sandwich	177	440
Ham & Cheese	154	380	Super Brazier Dog	182	518
Turkey Deluxe	236	510	Super Brazier Dog with Cheese	203	593
Club Sandwich	252	560	Super Brazier Chili Dog	210	555
			Brazier Fries, small	71	200
BURGER CHEF			Brazier Fries, large	113	320
Hamburger	91	244	Brazier Onion Rings	85	300
Cheeseburger	104	290			
Double Cheeseburger	145	420	JACK IN THE BOX		
Fish Filet	179	547	Hamburger	97	263
Super Shef Sandwich	252	563	Cheeseburger	109	310
Big Shef Sandwich	186	569	Jumbo Jack Hamburger	246	551
TOP Shef Sandwich	138	661	Jumbo Jack Hamburger with Cheese	272	628
Funmeal Feast	—	545	Regular Taco	83	189
Rancher Platter (includes salad)	316	640	Super Taco	146	285
Mariner Platter (includes salad)	373	734	Moby Jack Sandwich	141	455
French Fries, small	68	250	Breakfast Jack Sandwich	121	301
French Fries, large	85	351	French Fries	80	270
Vanilla Shake (12 oz)	336	380	Onion Rings	85	351
Chocolate Shake (12 oz)	336	403	Apple Turnover	119	411
Hot Chocolate	—	198	Vanilla Shake	317	317
			Strawberry Shake	328	323
BURGER KING			Chocolate Shake	322	325
Cheeseburger	—	305	Ham & Cheese Omelette	174	425
Hamburger	—	252	Double Cheese Omelette	166	423
Whopper	—	606	Ranchero Style Omelette	196	414
French Fries	—	214	French Toast	180	537
Vanilla Shake	—	332	Pancakes	232	626
Whaler	—	486	Scrambled Eggs	267	719
Hot Dog	—	291			
			KENTUCKY FRIED CHICKEN		
CHURCH'S FRIED CHICKEN			Original Recipe Dinner		
White Chicken Portion	100	327	Wing & Rib	322	603
Dark Chicken Portion	100	305	Wing & Thigh	341	661
			Drum & Thigh	346	643
DAIRY QUEEN			Extra Crispy Dinner		
Frozen Dessert	113	180	Wing & Rib	349	755
DQ Cone, small	71	110	Wing & Thigh	371	812
DQ Cone, regular	142	230	Drum & Thigh	376	765
DQ Cone, large	213	340	Mashed Potatoes	85	64
DQ Dip Cone, small	78	150	Gravy	14	23
DQ Dip Cone, regular	156	300	Cole Slaw	91	122
DQ Dip Cone, large	234	450	Rolls	21	61
DQ Sundae, small	106	170	Corn (5½-inch ear)	135	169
DQ Sundae, regular	177	290			
DQ Sundae, large	248	400	LONG JOHN SILVER'S		
DQ Malt, small	241	340	Fish with Batter (2 pc)	136	366
DQ Malt, regular	418	600	Fish with Batter (3 pc)	207	549
DQ Malt, large	588	840	Treasure Chest	143	506
DQ Float	397	330	Chicken Planks (4 pc)	166	457
DQ Banana Split	383	540	Peg Legs with Batter (5 pc)	125	350
DQ Parfait	284	460	Ocean Scallops (6 pc)	120	283
DQ Freeze	397	520	Shrimp with Batter (6 pc)	88	268
Mr. Misty Freeze	411	500	Breaded Oysters (6 pc)	156	441
Mr. Misty Float	404	440	Breaded Clams	142	617
"Dilly" Bar	85	240	Fish Sandwich	193	337
DQ Sandwich	60	140	French Fries	85	288

Table B–2. (Concluded)

Food	Wt (g)	Energy (kcal)	Food	Wt (g)	Energy (kcal)
LONG JOHN SILVER'S			TACO BELL		
Cole Slaw	113	138	Bean Burrito	166	343
Corn on the Cob (1 ear)	150	176	Beef Burrito	184	466
Hushpuppies (3)	45	153	Beefy Tostada	184	291
Clam Chowder (8 oz)	170	107	Bellbeefer	123	221
			Bellbeefer with Cheese	137	278
MCDONALD'S			Burrito Supreme	225	457
			Combination Burrito	175	404
Egg McMuffin	138	327	Enchinto	207	454
English Muffin, Buttered	63	186	Pintos 'N Cheese	158	168
Hotcakes with Butter & Syrup	214	500	Taco	83	186
Sausage (Pork)	53	206	Tostada	138	179
Scrambled Eggs	98	180			
Hashbrown Potatoes	55	125			
Big Mac	204	563	WENDY'S		
Cheeseburger	115	307			
Hamburger	102	255	Single Hamburger	200	470
Quarter Pounder	166	424	Double Hamburger	285	670
Quarter Pounder with Cheese	194	524	Triple Hamburger	360	850
Filet-O-Fish	139	432	Single with Cheese	240	580
Regular Fries	68	220	Double with Cheese	325	800
Apple Pie	85	253	Triple with Cheese	400	1040
Cherry Pie	88	260	Chili	250	230
McDonaldland Cookies	67	308	French Fries	120	330
Chocolate Shake	291	383	Frosty	250	390
Strawberry Shake	290	362			
Vanilla Shake	291	352	BEVERAGES		
Hot Fudge Sundae	164	310			
Caramel Sundae	165	328	Coffee	180	2
Strawberry Sundae	164	289	Tea	180	2
			Orange Juice	183	82
			Chocolate Milk	250	213
PIZZA HUT			Skim Milk	245	88
Thin 'N Crispy			Whole Milk	244	159
Beef	—	490	Coca-Cola	246	96
Pork	—	520	Fanta Ginger Ale	244	84
Cheese	—	450	Fanta Grape	247	114
Pepperoni	—	430	Fanta Orange	248	117
Supreme	—	510	Fanta Root Beer	246	103
Thick 'N Chewy			Mr. Pibb	245	95
Beef	—	620	Mr. Pibb without Sugar	236	1
Pork	—	640	Sprite	245	95
Cheese	—	560	Sprite without Sugar	236	3
Pepperoni	—	560	Tab	236	tr
Supreme	—	640	Fresca	236	2

* Adapted from Young, E. A.; Brennan, E. H.; and Irving G. L. (guest eds.): Perspectives on fast foods. *Public Health Currents* 19(1), 1970, published by Ross Laboratories, Columbus, OH 43216.
† *Note:* Fast foods tend to be: (1) high in calories; (2) low in vitamin A; (3) low in fiber; (4) high in sodium; (5) adequate in protein; (6) high in cost compared to a comparable product made at home.

Appendix C

Caloric Costs of Selected Activities (in kcal/min)

Table C–1.

Activity	Body Weight																
	kg 50 lb 110	53 117	56 123	59 130	62 137	65 143	68 150	71 157	74 163	77 170	80 176	83 183	86 190	89 196	92 203	95 209	98 216
Archery	3.3	3.4	3.6	3.8	4.0	4.2	4.4	4.6	4.8	5.0	5.2	5.4	5.6	5.8	6.0	6.2	6.4
Badminton	4.9	5.1	5.4	5.7	6.0	6.3	6.6	6.9	7.2	7.5	7.8	8.1	8.3	8.6	8.9	9.2	9.5
Bakery, general (F)	1.8	1.9	2.0	2.1	2.2	2.3	2.4	2.5	2.6	2.7	2.8	2.9	3.0	3.1	3.2	3.3	3.4
Basketball	6.9	7.3	7.7	8.1	8.6	9.0	9.4	9.8	10.2	10.6	11.0	11.5	11.9	12.3	12.7	13.1	13.5
Billiards	2.1	2.2	2.4	2.5	2.6	2.7	2.9	3.0	3.1	3.2	3.4	3.5	3.6	3.7	3.9	4.0	4.1
Bookbinding	1.9	2.0	2.1	2.2	2.4	2.5	2.6	2.7	2.8	2.9	3.0	3.2	3.3	3.4	3.5	3.6	3.7
Boxing																	
in ring	6.9	7.3	7.7	8.1	8.6	9.0	9.4	9.8	10.2	10.6	11.0	11.5	11.9	12.3	12.7	13.1	13.5
sparring	11.1	11.8	12.4	13.1	13.8	14.4	15.1	15.8	16.4	17.1	17.8	18.4	19.1	19.8	20.4	21.1	21.8
Canoeing																	
leisure	2.2	2.3	2.5	2.6	2.7	2.9	3.0	3.1	3.3	3.4	3.5	3.7	3.8	3.9	4.0	4.2	4.3
racing	5.2	5.5	5.8	6.1	6.4	6.7	7.0	7.3	7.6	7.9	8.2	8.5	8.9	9.2	9.5	9.8	10.1
Card playing	1.3	1.3	1.4	1.5	1.6	1.6	1.7	1.8	1.9	1.9	2.0	2.1	2.2	2.2	2.3	2.4	2.5
Carpentry, general	2.6	2.8	2.9	3.1	3.2	3.4	3.5	3.7	3.8	4.0	4.2	4.3	4.5	4.6	4.8	4.9	5.1
Carpet sweeping (F)	2.3	2.4	2.5	2.7	2.8	2.9	3.1	3.2	3.3	3.5	3.6	3.7	3.9	4.0	4.1	4.3	4.4
Carpet sweeping (M)	2.4	2.5	2.7	2.8	3.0	3.1	3.3	3.4	3.6	3.7	3.8	4.0	4.1	4.3	4.4	4.6	4.7
Circuit-training	9.3	9.8	10.4	10.9	11.5	12.0	12.6	13.1	13.7	14.2	14.8	15.4	15.9	16.5	17.0	17.6	18.1
Cleaning (F)	3.1	3.3	3.5	3.7	3.8	4.0	4.2	4.4	4.6	4.8	5.0	5.1	5.3	5.5	5.7	5.9	6.1
Cleaning (M)	2.9	3.1	3.2	3.4	3.6	3.8	3.9	4.1	4.3	4.5	4.6	4.8	5.0	5.2	5.3	5.5	5.7
Climbing hills																	
with no load	6.1	6.4	6.8	7.1	7.5	7.9	8.2	8.6	9.0	9.3	9.7	10.0	10.4	10.8	11.1	11.5	11.9
with 5-kg load	6.5	6.8	7.2	7.6	8.0	8.4	8.8	9.2	9.5	9.9	10.3	10.7	11.1	11.5	11.9	12.3	12.6
with 10-kg load	7.0	7.4	7.8	8.3	8.7	9.1	9.5	9.9	10.4	10.8	11.2	11.6	12.0	12.5	12.9	13.3	13.7
with 20-kg load	7.4	7.8	8.2	8.7	9.1	9.6	10.0	10.4	10.9	11.3	11.8	12.2	12.6	13.1	13.5	14.0	14.4
Coal mining																	
drilling coal, rock	4.7	5.0	5.3	5.5	5.8	6.1	6.4	6.7	7.0	7.2	7.5	7.8	8.1	8.4	8.6	8.9	9.2
erecting roof supports	4.4	4.7	4.9	5.2	5.5	5.7	6.0	6.2	6.5	6.8	7.0	7.3	7.6	7.8	8.1	8.4	8.6
shoveling coal	5.4	5.7	6.0	6.4	6.7	7.0	7.3	7.7	8.0	8.3	8.6	9.0	9.3	9.6	9.9	10.3	10.6
Cooking (Female)	2.3	2.4	2.5	2.7	2.8	2.9	3.1	3.2	3.3	3.5	3.6	3.7	3.9	4.0	4.1	4.3	4.4
Cooking (Male)	2.4	2.5	2.7	2.8	3.0	3.1	3.3	3.4	3.6	3.7	3.8	4.0	4.1	4.3	4.4	4.6	4.7

250

Activity																	
Cricket																	
batting	4.2	4.4	4.6	4.9	5.1	5.4	5.6	5.9	6.1	6.4	6.6	6.9	7.1	7.4	7.6	7.9	8.1
bowling	4.5	4.8	5.0	5.3	5.6	5.9	6.1	6.4	6.7	6.9	7.2	7.5	7.7	8.0	8.3	8.6	8.8
Croquet	3.0	3.1	3.3	3.5	3.7	3.8	4.0	4.2	4.4	4.5	4.7	4.9	5.1	5.3	5.4	5.6	5.8
Cycling																	
leisure	5.9	6.2	6.6	6.9	7.3	7.6	8.0	8.3	8.7	9.0	9.4	9.7	10.1	10.4	10.8	11.1	11.5
leisure, 5.5 mph	3.2	3.4	3.6	3.8	4.0	4.2	4.4	4.6	4.8	5.0	5.1	5.3	5.5	5.7	5.9	6.1	6.3
leisure, 9.4 mph	5.0	5.3	5.6	5.9	6.2	6.5	6.8	7.1	7.4	7.7	8.0	8.3	8.6	8.9	9.2	9.5	9.8
racing	8.5	9.0	9.5	10.0	10.5	11.0	11.5	12.0	12.5	13.0	13.5	14.0	14.5	15.0	15.5	16.1	16.6
Dancing																	
ballroom	2.6	2.7	2.9	3.0	3.2	3.3	3.5	3.6	3.8	3.9	4.1	4.2	4.4	4.5	4.7	4.8	5.0
choreographed, vigorous	8.4	8.9	9.4	9.9	10.4	10.9	11.4	11.9	12.4	12.9	13.4	13.9	14.4	15.0	15.5	16.0	16.5
"twist," "wiggle"	5.2	5.5	5.8	6.1	6.4	6.7	7.0	7.3	7.6	7.9	8.2	8.5	8.9	9.2	9.5	9.8	10.1
Digging trenches	7.3	7.7	8.1	8.6	9.0	9.4	9.9	10.3	10.7	11.2	11.6	12.0	12.5	12.9	13.3	13.8	14.2
Drawing (standing)	1.8	1.9	2.0	2.1	2.2	2.3	2.4	2.6	2.7	2.8	2.9	3.0	3.1	3.2	3.3	3.4	3.5
Eating (sitting)	1.2	1.2	1.3	1.4	1.4	1.5	1.6	1.6	1.7	1.8	1.8	1.9	2.0	2.0	2.1	2.2	2.3
Electrical work	2.9	3.1	3.2	3.4	3.6	3.8	3.9	4.1	4.3	4.5	4.6	4.8	5.0	5.2	5.3	5.5	5.7
Farming																	
cleaning animal stalls	6.8	7.2	7.6	8.0	8.4	8.8	9.2	9.6	10.0	10.4	10.8	11.2	11.6	12.0	12.4	12.8	13.2
driving harvester	2.0	2.1	2.2	2.4	2.5	2.6	2.7	2.8	3.0	3.1	3.2	3.3	3.4	3.6	3.7	3.8	3.9
driving tractor	1.9	2.0	2.1	2.2	2.3	2.4	2.5	2.6	2.7	2.8	3.0	3.1	3.2	3.3	3.4	3.5	3.6
feeding cattle	4.3	4.5	4.8	5.0	5.3	5.5	5.8	6.0	6.3	6.5	6.8	7.1	7.3	7.6	7.8	8.1	8.3
feeding hens and dogs	3.3	3.4	3.6	3.8	4.0	4.2	4.4	4.6	4.8	5.0	5.2	5.4	5.6	5.8	6.0	6.2	6.4
forking straw bales	6.9	7.3	7.7	8.1	8.6	9.0	9.4	9.8	10.2	10.6	11.0	11.5	11.9	12.3	12.7	13.1	13.5
milking by hand	2.7	2.9	3.0	3.2	3.3	3.5	3.7	3.8	4.0	4.2	4.3	4.5	4.6	4.8	5.0	5.1	5.3
milking by machine	1.2	1.2	1.3	1.4	1.4	1.5	1.6	1.6	1.7	1.8	1.8	1.9	2.0	2.0	2.1	2.2	2.3
shoveling grain	4.3	4.5	4.8	5.0	5.3	5.5	5.8	6.0	6.3	6.5	6.8	7.1	7.3	7.6	7.8	8.1	8.3
Field hockey	6.7	7.1	7.5	7.9	8.3	8.7	9.1	9.5	9.9	10.3	10.7	11.1	11.5	11.9	12.3	12.7	13.1
Fishing	3.1	3.3	3.5	3.7	3.8	4.0	4.2	4.4	4.6	4.8	5.0	5.1	5.3	5.5	5.7	5.9	6.1
Food shopping (F)	3.1	3.3	3.5	3.7	3.8	4.0	4.2	4.4	4.6	4.8	5.0	5.1	5.3	5.5	5.7	5.9	6.1
Food shopping (M)	2.9	3.1	3.2	3.4	3.6	3.8	3.9	4.1	4.3	4.5	4.6	4.8	5.0	5.2	5.3	5.5	5.7
Football	6.6	7.0	7.4	7.8	8.2	8.6	9.0	9.4	9.8	10.2	10.6	11.0	11.4	11.7	12.1	12.5	12.9

251

* From Katch, F. I.; and McArdle, W. D.: *Nutrition, Weight Control, and Exercise.* Boston, Houghton Mifflin, 1977.

Table C-1. (Continued)

Activity	kg / lb																
	50 / 110	53 / 117	56 / 123	59 / 130	62 / 137	65 / 143	68 / 150	71 / 157	74 / 163	77 / 170	80 / 176	83 / 183	86 / 190	89 / 196	92 / 203	95 / 209	98 / 216
Forestry																	
ax chopping, fast	14.9	15.7	16.6	17.5	18.4	19.3	20.2	21.1	22.0	22.9	23.8	24.7	25.5	26.4	27.3	28.2	29.1
ax chopping, slow	4.3	4.5	4.8	5.0	5.3	5.5	5.8	6.0	6.3	6.5	6.8	7.1	7.3	7.6	7.8	8.1	8.3
barking trees	6.2	6.5	6.9	7.3	7.6	8.0	8.4	8.7	9.1	9.5	9.8	10.2	10.6	10.9	11.3	11.7	12.1
carrying logs	9.3	9.9	10.4	11.0	11.5	12.1	12.6	13.2	13.8	14.3	14.9	15.4	16.0	16.6	17.1	17.7	18.2
felling trees	6.6	7.0	7.4	7.8	8.2	8.6	9.0	9.4	9.8	10.2	10.6	11.0	11.4	11.7	12.1	12.5	12.9
hoeing	4.6	4.8	5.1	5.4	5.6	5.9	6.2	6.5	6.7	7.0	7.3	7.6	7.8	8.1	8.4	8.6	8.9
planting by hand	5.5	5.8	6.1	6.4	6.8	7.1	7.4	7.7	8.1	8.4	8.7	9.0	9.4	9.7	10.0	10.4	10.7
sawing by hand	6.1	6.5	6.8	7.2	7.6	7.9	8.3	8.7	9.0	9.4	9.8	10.1	10.5	10.9	11.2	11.6	12.0
sawing, power	3.8	4.0	4.2	4.4	4.7	4.9	5.1	5.3	5.6	5.8	6.0	6.2	6.5	6.7	6.9	7.1	7.4
stacking firewood	4.4	4.7	4.9	5.2	5.5	5.7	6.0	6.2	6.5	6.8	7.0	7.3	7.6	7.8	8.1	8.4	8.6
trimming trees	6.5	6.8	7.2	7.6	8.0	8.4	8.8	9.2	9.5	9.9	10.3	10.7	11.1	11.5	11.9	12.3	12.6
weeding	3.6	3.8	4.0	4.2	4.5	4.7	4.9	5.1	5.3	5.5	5.8	6.0	6.2	6.4	6.6	6.8	7.1
Furriery	4.2	4.4	4.6	4.9	5.1	5.4	5.6	5.9	6.1	6.4	6.6	6.9	7.1	7.4	7.6	7.9	8.1
Gardening																	
digging	6.3	6.7	7.1	7.4	7.8	8.2	8.6	8.9	9.3	9.7	10.1	10.5	10.8	11.2	11.6	12.0	12.3
hedging	3.9	4.1	4.3	4.5	4.8	5.0	5.2	5.5	5.7	5.9	6.2	6.4	6.6	6.9	7.1	7.3	7.5
mowing	5.6	5.9	6.3	6.6	6.9	7.3	7.6	8.0	8.3	8.6	9.0	9.3	9.6	10.0	10.3	10.6	11.0
raking	2.7	2.9	3.0	3.2	3.3	3.5	3.7	3.8	4.0	4.2	4.3	4.5	4.6	4.8	5.0	5.1	5.3
Golf	4.3	4.5	4.8	5.0	5.3	5.5	5.8	6.0	6.3	6.5	6.8	7.1	7.3	7.6	7.8	8.1	8.3
Gymnastics	3.3	3.5	3.7	3.9	4.1	4.3	4.5	4.7	4.9	5.1	5.3	5.5	5.7	5.9	6.1	6.3	6.5
Horse-grooming	6.4	6.8	7.2	7.6	7.9	8.3	8.7	9.1	9.5	9.9	10.2	10.6	11.0	11.4	11.8	12.2	12.5
Horse-racing																	
galloping	6.9	7.3	7.7	8.1	8.5	8.9	9.3	9.7	10.1	10.6	11.0	11.4	11.8	12.2	12.6	13.0	13.4
trotting	5.5	5.8	6.2	6.5	6.8	7.2	7.5	7.8	8.1	8.5	8.8	9.1	9.5	9.8	10.1	10.5	10.8
walking	2.1	2.2	2.3	2.4	2.5	2.7	2.8	2.9	3.0	3.2	3.3	3.4	3.5	3.6	3.8	3.9	4.0
Ironing (F)	1.7	1.7	1.8	1.9	2.0	2.1	2.2	2.3	2.4	2.5	2.6	2.7	2.8	2.9	3.0	3.1	3.2
Ironing (M)	3.2	3.4	3.6	3.8	4.0	4.2	4.4	4.5	4.7	4.9	5.1	5.3	5.5	5.7	5.9	6.1	6.3
Judo	9.8	10.3	10.9	11.5	12.1	12.7	13.3	13.8	14.4	15.0	15.6	16.2	16.8	17.4	17.9	18.5	19.1
Knitting, sewing (F)	1.1	1.2	1.2	1.3	1.4	1.4	1.5	1.6	1.6	1.7	1.8	1.8	1.9	2.0	2.0	2.1	2.2
Knitting, sewing (M)	1.2	1.2	1.3	1.4	1.4	1.5	1.6	1.6	1.7	1.8	1.8	1.9	2.0	2.0	2.1	2.2	2.3

Lock making and lock repairing	2.9	3.0	3.2	3.4	3.5	3.7	3.9	4.0	4.2	4.4	4.6	4.7	4.9	5.1	5.2	5.4	5.6
Lying at ease	1.1	1.2	1.2	1.3	1.4	1.4	1.5	1.6	1.6	1.7	1.8	1.8	1.9	2.0	2.0	2.1	2.2
Machine-tooling																	
machining	2.4	2.5	2.7	2.8	3.0	3.1	3.3	3.4	3.6	3.7	3.8	4.0	4.1	4.3	4.4	4.6	4.7
operating lathe	2.6	2.8	2.9	3.1	3.2	3.4	3.5	3.7	3.8	4.0	4.2	4.3	4.5	4.6	4.8	4.9	5.1
operating punch press	4.4	4.7	4.9	5.2	5.5	5.7	6.0	6.2	6.5	6.8	7.0	7.3	7.6	7.8	8.1	8.4	8.6
tapping and drilling	3.3	3.4	3.6	3.8	4.0	4.2	4.4	4.6	4.8	5.0	5.2	5.4	5.6	5.8	6.0	6.2	6.4
welding	2.6	2.8	2.9	3.1	3.2	3.4	3.5	3.7	3.8	4.0	4.2	4.3	4.5	4.6	4.8	4.9	5.1
working sheet metal	2.4	2.5	2.7	2.8	3.0	3.1	3.3	3.4	3.6	3.7	3.8	4.0	4.1	4.3	4.4	4.6	4.7
Marching, rapid	7.1	7.5	8.0	8.4	8.8	9.2	9.7	10.1	10.5	10.9	11.4	11.8	12.2	12.6	13.1	13.5	13.9
Mopping floor (F)	3.1	3.3	3.5	3.7	3.8	4.0	4.2	4.4	4.6	4.8	5.0	5.1	5.3	5.5	5.7	5.9	6.1
Mopping floor (M)	2.9	3.1	3.2	3.4	3.6	3.8	3.9	4.1	4.3	4.5	4.6	4.8	5.0	5.2	5.3	5.5	5.7
Music playing																	
accordion (sitting)	1.6	1.7	1.8	1.9	2.0	2.1	2.2	2.3	2.4	2.5	2.6	2.7	2.8	2.8	2.9	3.0	3.1
cello (sitting)	2.1	2.2	2.3	2.4	2.5	2.7	2.8	2.9	3.0	3.2	3.3	3.4	3.5	3.6	3.8	3.9	4.0
conducting (standing)	2.0	2.1	2.2	2.3	2.4	2.5	2.7	2.8	2.9	3.0	3.1	3.2	3.4	3.5	3.6	3.7	3.8
drums (sitting)	3.3	3.5	3.7	3.9	4.1	4.3	4.5	4.7	4.9	5.1	5.3	5.5	5.7	5.9	6.1	6.3	6.6
flute (sitting)	1.8	1.9	2.0	2.1	2.2	2.3	2.4	2.5	2.6	2.7	2.8	2.9	3.0	3.1	3.2	3.3	3.4
horn (sitting)	1.5	1.5	1.6	1.7	1.8	1.9	2.0	2.1	2.1	2.2	2.3	2.4	2.5	2.6	2.7	2.8	2.8
organ (sitting)	2.7	2.8	3.0	3.1	3.3	3.4	3.6	3.8	3.9	4.1	4.2	4.4	4.6	4.7	4.9	5.0	5.2
piano (sitting)	2.0	2.1	2.2	2.4	2.5	2.6	2.7	2.8	3.0	3.1	3.2	3.3	3.4	3.6	3.7	3.8	3.9
trumpet (standing)	1.6	1.6	1.7	1.8	1.9	2.0	2.1	2.2	2.3	2.4	2.5	2.6	2.7	2.8	2.9	2.9	3.0
violin (sitting)	2.3	2.4	2.5	2.7	2.8	2.9	3.1	3.2	3.3	3.5	3.6	3.7	3.9	4.0	4.1	4.3	4.4
woodwind (sitting)	1.6	1.7	1.8	1.9	2.0	2.1	2.2	2.3	2.4	2.5	2.6	2.7	2.8	2.8	2.9	3.0	3.1
Painting, inside	1.7	1.8	1.9	2.0	2.1	2.2	2.3	2.4	2.5	2.6	2.7	2.8	2.9	3.0	3.1	3.2	3.3
Painting, outside	3.9	4.1	4.3	4.5	4.8	5.0	5.2	5.5	5.7	5.9	6.2	6.4	6.6	6.9	7.1	7.3	7.5
Planting seedlings	3.5	3.7	3.9	4.1	4.3	4.6	4.8	5.0	5.2	5.4	5.6	5.8	6.0	6.2	6.4	6.7	6.9
Plastering	3.9	4.1	4.4	4.6	4.8	5.1	5.3	5.5	5.8	6.0	6.2	6.5	6.7	6.9	7.2	7.4	7.6
Printing	1.8	1.9	2.0	2.1	2.2	2.3	2.4	2.5	2.6	2.7	2.8	2.9	3.0	3.1	3.2	3.3	3.4
Running, cross-country	8.2	8.6	9.1	9.6	10.1	10.6	11.1	11.6	12.1	12.6	13.0	13.5	14.0	14.5	15.0	15.5	16.0
Running, horizontal																	
11 min, 30 sec per mile	6.8	7.2	7.6	8.0	8.4	8.8	9.2	9.6	10.0	10.5	10.9	11.3	11.7	12.1	12.5	12.9	13.3
9 min per mile	9.7	10.2	10.8	11.4	12.0	12.5	13.1	13.7	14.3	14.9	15.4	16.0	16.6	17.2	17.8	18.3	18.9
8 min per mile	10.8	11.3	11.9	12.5	13.1	13.6	14.2	14.8	15.4	16.0	16.5	17.1	17.7	18.3	18.9	19.4	20.0
7 min per mile	12.2	12.7	13.3	13.9	14.5	15.0	15.6	16.2	16.8	17.4	17.9	18.5	19.1	19.7	20.3	20.8	21.4
6 min per mile	13.9	14.4	15.0	15.6	16.2	16.7	17.3	17.9	18.5	19.1	19.6	20.2	20.8	21.4	22.0	22.5	23.1
5 min, 30 sec per mile	14.5	15.3	16.2	17.1	17.9	18.8	19.7	20.5	21.4	22.3	23.1	24.0	24.9	25.7	26.6	27.5	28.3

Table C-1. (Concluded)

Activity		Body Weight															
kg	50	53	56	59	62	65	68	71	74	77	80	83	86	89	92	95	98
lb	110	117	123	130	137	143	150	157	163	170	176	183	190	196	203	209	216
Scraping paint and sandpapering	3.2	3.3	3.5	3.7	3.9	4.1	4.3	4.5	4.7	4.9	5.0	5.2	5.4	5.6	5.8	6.0	6.2
Scrubbing floors (F)	5.5	5.8	6.1	6.4	6.8	7.1	7.4	7.7	8.1	8.4	8.7	9.0	9.4	9.7	10.0	10.4	10.7
Scrubbing floors (M)	5.4	5.7	6.0	6.4	6.7	7.0	7.3	7.7	8.0	8.3	8.6	9.0	9.3	9.6	9.9	10.3	10.6
Shoe repair, general	2.3	2.4	2.5	2.7	2.8	2.9	3.1	3.2	3.3	3.5	3.6	3.7	3.9	4.0	4.1	4.3	4.4
Sitting quietly	1.1	1.1	1.2	1.2	1.3	1.4	1.4	1.5	1.6	1.6	1.7	1.7	1.8	1.9	1.9	2.0	2.1
Skiing, hard snow																	
level, moderate speed	6.0	6.3	6.7	7.0	7.4	7.7	8.1	8.4	8.8	9.2	9.5	9.9	10.2	10.6	10.9	11.3	11.7
level, walking	7.2	7.6	8.0	8.4	8.9	9.3	9.7	10.2	10.6	11.0	11.4	11.9	12.3	12.7	13.2	13.6	14.0
uphill, maximum speed	13.7	14.5	15.3	16.2	17.0	17.8	18.6	19.5	20.3	21.1	21.9	22.7	23.6	24.4	25.2	26.0	26.9
Skiing, soft snow																	
leisure (F)	4.9	5.2	5.5	5.8	6.1	6.4	6.7	7.0	7.3	7.5	7.8	8.1	8.4	8.7	9.0	9.3	9.6
leisure (M)	5.6	5.9	6.2	6.5	6.9	7.2	7.5	7.9	8.2	8.5	8.9	9.2	9.5	9.9	10.2	10.5	10.9
Skindiving, as frogman																	
considerable motion	13.8	14.6	15.5	16.3	17.1	17.9	18.8	19.6	20.4	21.3	22.1	22.9	23.7	24.6	25.4	26.2	27.0
moderate motion	10.3	10.9	11.5	12.2	12.8	13.4	14.0	14.6	15.2	15.9	16.5	17.1	17.7	18.3	19.0	19.6	20.2
Snowshoeing, soft snow	8.3	8.8	9.3	9.8	10.3	10.8	11.3	11.8	12.3	12.8	13.3	13.8	14.3	14.8	15.3	15.8	16.3
Squash	10.6	11.2	11.9	12.5	13.1	13.8	14.4	15.1	15.7	16.3	17.0	17.6	18.2	18.9	19.5	20.1	20.8
Standing quietly (F)	1.3	1.3	1.4	1.5	1.6	1.6	1.7	1.8	1.9	1.9	2.0	2.1	2.2	2.2	2.3	2.4	2.5
Standing quietly (M)	1.4	1.4	1.5	1.6	1.7	1.8	1.8	1.9	2.0	2.1	2.2	2.2	2.3	2.4	2.5	2.6	2.6
Steel mill, working in																	
fettling	4.5	4.7	5.0	5.3	5.5	5.8	6.1	6.3	6.6	6.9	7.1	7.4	7.7	7.9	8.2	8.5	8.7
forging	5.0	5.3	5.6	5.9	6.2	6.5	6.8	7.1	7.4	7.7	8.0	8.3	8.6	8.9	9.2	9.5	9.8
hand rolling	6.9	7.3	7.7	8.1	8.5	8.9	9.3	9.7	10.1	10.6	11.0	11.4	11.8	12.2	12.6	13.0	13.4
merchant mill rolling	7.3	7.7	8.1	8.6	9.0	9.4	9.9	10.3	10.7	11.2	11.6	12.0	12.5	12.9	13.3	13.8	14.2
removing slag	8.9	9.4	10.0	10.5	11.0	11.6	12.1	12.6	13.2	13.7	14.2	14.8	15.3	15.8	16.4	16.9	17.4
tending furnace	6.3	6.7	7.1	7.4	7.8	8.2	8.6	8.9	9.3	9.7	10.1	10.5	10.8	11.2	11.6	12.0	12.3
tipping molds	4.6	4.9	5.2	5.4	5.7	6.0	6.3	6.5	6.8	7.1	7.4	7.6	7.9	8.2	8.5	8.7	9.0
Stock clerking	2.7	2.9	3.0	3.2	3.3	3.5	3.7	3.8	4.0	4.2	4.3	4.5	4.6	4.8	5.0	5.1	5.3

Swimming																	
backstroke	8.5	9.0	9.5	10.0	10.5	11.0	11.5	12.0	12.5	13.0	13.5	14.0	14.5	15.0	15.5	16.1	16.6
breast stroke	8.1	8.6	9.1	9.6	10.0	10.5	11.0	11.5	12.0	12.5	13.0	13.4	13.9	14.4	14.9	15.4	15.9
crawl, fast	7.8	8.3	8.7	9.2	9.7	10.1	10.6	11.1	11.5	12.0	12.5	12.9	13.4	13.9	14.4	14.8	15.3
crawl, slow	6.4	6.8	7.2	7.6	7.9	8.3	8.7	9.1	9.5	9.9	10.2	10.6	11.0	11.4	11.8	12.2	12.5
side stroke	6.1	6.5	6.8	7.2	7.6	7.9	8.3	8.7	9.0	9.4	9.8	10.1	10.5	10.9	11.2	11.6	12.0
treading, fast	8.5	9.0	9.5	10.0	10.5	11.1	11.6	12.1	12.6	13.1	13.6	14.1	14.6	15.1	15.6	16.2	16.7
treading, normal	3.1	3.3	3.5	3.7	3.8	4.0	4.2	4.4	4.6	4.8	5.0	5.1	5.3	5.5	5.7	5.9	6.1
Table tennis	3.4	3.6	3.8	4.0	4.2	4.4	4.6	4.8	5.0	5.2	5.4	5.6	5.8	6.1	6.3	6.5	6.7
Tailoring																	
cutting	2.1	2.2	2.3	2.4	2.5	2.7	2.8	2.9	3.0	3.2	3.3	3.4	3.5	3.6	3.8	3.9	4.0
hand-sewing	1.6	1.7	1.8	1.9	2.0	2.1	2.2	2.3	2.4	2.5	2.6	2.7	2.8	2.8	2.9	3.0	3.1
machine-sewing	2.3	2.4	2.5	2.7	2.8	2.9	3.1	3.2	3.3	3.5	3.6	3.7	3.9	4.0	4.1	4.3	4.4
pressing	3.1	3.3	3.5	3.7	3.8	4.0	4.2	4.4	4.6	4.8	5.0	5.1	5.3	5.5	5.7	5.9	6.1
Tennis	5.5	5.8	6.1	6.4	6.8	7.1	7.4	7.7	8.1	8.4	8.7	9.0	9.4	9.7	10.0	10.4	10.7
Typing																	
electric	1.4	1.4	1.5	1.6	1.7	1.8	1.8	1.9	2.0	2.1	2.2	2.2	2.3	2.4	2.5	2.6	2.6
manual	1.6	1.6	1.7	1.8	1.9	2.0	2.1	2.2	2.3	2.4	2.5	2.6	2.7	2.8	2.9	2.9	3.0
Volleyball	2.5	2.7	2.8	3.0	3.1	3.3	3.4	3.6	3.7	3.9	4.0	4.2	4.3	4.5	4.6	4.8	4.9
Walking, comfortable pace																	
asphalt road	4.0	4.2	4.5	4.7	5.0	5.2	5.4	5.7	5.9	6.2	6.4	6.6	6.9	7.1	7.4	7.6	7.8
fields and hillsides	4.1	4.3	4.6	4.8	5.1	5.3	5.6	5.8	6.1	6.3	6.6	6.8	7.1	7.3	7.5	7.8	8.0
grass track	4.1	4.3	4.5	4.8	5.0	5.3	5.5	5.8	6.0	6.2	6.5	6.7	7.0	7.2	7.5	7.7	7.9
plowed field	3.9	4.1	4.3	4.5	4.8	5.0	5.2	5.5	5.7	5.9	6.2	6.4	6.6	6.9	7.1	7.3	7.5
Wallpapering	2.4	2.5	2.7	2.8	3.0	3.1	3.3	3.4	3.6	3.7	3.8	4.0	4.1	4.3	4.4	4.6	4.7
Watch repairing	1.3	1.3	1.4	1.5	1.6	1.6	1.7	1.8	1.9	1.9	2.0	2.1	2.2	2.2	2.3	2.4	2.5
Window cleaning (F)	3.0	3.1	3.3	3.5	3.7	3.8	4.0	4.2	4.4	4.5	4.7	4.9	5.1	5.3	5.4	5.6	5.8
Window cleaning (M)	2.9	3.1	3.2	3.4	3.6	3.8	3.9	4.1	4.3	4.5	4.6	4.8	5.0	5.2	5.3	5.5	5.7
Writing (sitting)	1.5	1.5	1.6	1.7	1.8	1.9	2.0	2.1	2.1	2.2	2.3	2.4	2.5	2.6	2.7	2.8	2.8

Appendix D

Fitness Evaluation Worksheets

Evaluation of Cardiorespiratory Fitness (Åstrand-Rhyming Submaximal Bicycle Ergometer Test)

Purpose and Theory

The purpose of this evaluation is to determine your estimated cardiorespiratory fitness based on the Åstrand-Rhyming bicycle ergometer test. This submaximal test is based on the linear relationship that exists between workload (or oxygen consumption) and heart rate. This linear relationship is most reliable between heart rates of approximately 120 and 170 beats per minute. The originators of this evaluation have established an estimated maximal oxygen consumption ($\dot{V}O_2$max) for a heart rate response to a given workload on the bicycle ergometer if correction is made for the subject's age (see Table 9–1).

Procedures

Test administration procedures can be found in Chap. 9.

Work Rate (rpm) _____

Time (min)	*Heart Rate*
1.	_____
2.	_____
3.	_____
4.	_____
5.	_____
6.	_____
7. (if needed)	_____

Average heart rate for last 2 minutes _____ bpm

Estimated $\dot{V}O_2$max (from Figure 9–3) _____ liters/min

Age correction factor (from Table 9–1) _____

Estimated $\dot{V}O_2$max (corrected for age) _____ liters/min

Estimated $\dot{V}O_2$max (ml/kg-min) (from Chap. 9) _____ ml/kg-min

Classification of $\dot{V}O_2$max (ml/kg-min)
   (from Table 9–2) _____

Evaluation of Cardiorespiratory Fitness (The Ohio State University Step Test)

Name _____ Age _____ Date _____

Class _____ Instructor _____

Purpose and Theory

This evaluation is designed to estimate fitness classifications based on heart rate response to bench stepping. The test is designed to be conducted indoors with a minimum of equipment.

Procedure

The procedure for the test is explained in Chapter 9. Equipment needed for the test is identified as well.

Record below the heart rate for each inning completed.

Phase I		*Phase II*		*Phase III*	
Inning	Heart Rate	Inning	Heart Rate	Inning	Heart Rate
1.	_____	1.	_____	1.	_____
2.	_____	2.	_____	2.	_____
3.	_____	3.	_____	3.	_____
4.	_____	4.	_____	4.	_____
5.	_____	5.	_____	5.	_____
6.	_____	6.	_____	6.	_____

Fitness level _____

(see Table 9–3)

Evaluation of Cardiorespiratory Fitness (Cooper's 12-Minute Run)

Name _____ Age _____ Date _____

Class _____ Instructor _____

Purpose and Theory

This field test is designed to estimate your maximal working capacity ($\dot{V}O_2max$) based on the distance run in 12 minutes. Research conducted by Dr. Kenneth Cooper has demonstrated that there is a high correlation between the distance run in 12 minutes and oxygen consumption.

Procedure

On a track measured to indicate distance to the nearest 50 feet cover as much distance as possible in 12 minutes.

Distance covered
    (to nearest hundredth of a mile if possible)   _____

Estimated $\dot{V}O_2max$ (from Figure 9–5)
    (enter graph with distance covered to
    determine $\dot{V}O_2max$ (ml/kg-min).   _____

Classification of $\dot{V}O_2max$ (ml/kg-min)
    (from Table 9–2)   _____

Evaluation of Muscular Strength (Isotonic Testing)

Name _____ Weight _____ Date _____

Class _____ Instructor _____

Purpose and Theory

Strength has been defined as the amount of force produced or resistance overcome during a single maximum effort. Determination of the strength of any given muscle group will be based on the maximal amount of weight that you can move through the range of the exercise one time. This is also known as the single repetition maximum (1 RM). This 1 RM is classified according to the body weight of the individual subject.

Procedure

First be sure you are familiar with the exercise techniques discussed in Chapter 5. To implement the strength evaluation begin with the lowest weight charted in Table 9–4. For example a 120-pound woman being evaluated on the bench press would first attempt 45 percent of her total body weight or 54 pounds. Gradually increase the load after each successful trial, with a 1- to 2-minute rest between trials until the new load can no longer be successfully lifted. Complete the spaces below.

Exercise	1 RM (lbs)	Percentage of Body Weight	Classification*
Bench Press	_____ lbs	_____ %	_____
Standing Press	_____ lbs	_____ %	_____
Arm Curl	_____ lbs	_____ %	_____
Leg Press	_____ lbs	_____ %	_____

* From Table 9–4.

Evaluation of Flexibility
(Sit-and-Reach Test/Shoulder Test)

Name _____   Date _____

Class _____   Instructor _____

Purpose and Theory

The purpose of the sit-and-reach test is to evaluate flexibility (extensibility) of the low back and posterior thighs. The shoulder test is designed to evaluate general flexibility of the shoulder girdle. Evaluation of specific joints is not necessarily indicative of the flexibility of other joints and their associated muscle groups.

Procedure—Sit-and-Reach

The test apparatus is pictured in Chapter 9, Figure 9–7. A description can also be found in Chapter 9.

1. To assume the starting position, remove your shoes and sit down with your knees fully extended and your feet shoulder width apart.
2. Your feet should be flat against the box.
3. Extend your arms forward with your hands placed on top of each other to perform the test.
4. Reach directly forward, palms down, along the measuring scale four times and hold the position of maximum reach on the fourth attempt. The position of maximum reach must be held for 1 second.

Distance reached (cm) _____

Classification
    (from Table 9–5) _____

Procedure—Shoulder Test

Reach behind your back, one arm at a time, and slide each hand up your back as far as possible, keeping the wrist straight.

An evaluator must identify your score based on the information found in Figure 9–8.

Left arm score _____   Right arm score _____

Body Composition Evaluation (Skinfold Method)

Name _____ Age _____ Weight _____

Class _____ Instructor _____ Date _____

Purpose and Theory

The purpose of this evaluation is to determine body composition and an appropriate weight using two different skinfold methods, one from Sloan and Weir and another from Pollock, Schmidt, and Jackson.

Procedure

A complete description of skinfold measurement techniques and use of a caliper can be found in Chapter 9.

Sloan—Weir Data

Men		*Women*	
Anterior Thigh _____ mm		Iliac Crest _____ mm	
Subscapular _____ mm		Tricep _____ mm	

Use the values above in the nomogram in Figure 9–14. For men: anterior thigh (X1), subscapular (X2); for women: iliac crest (X1), triceps (X2).

Density _____

Fat % _____

Classification
  (from Table 9–7) _____

Calculation of "Desired" Weight

1. Fat Weight = Total body weight × Fat %

$$= \underline{\hspace{3cm}} \times \underline{\hspace{1.5cm}}$$

Fat Weight = _____

2. Lean Body Weight (LBW) = Total Weight − Fat Weight

$$= \underline{\hspace{2.5cm}} - \underline{\hspace{2cm}}$$

Lean Body Weight   = _____

3. Desired Weight = $\dfrac{\text{LBW}}{100 - \% \text{ Fat Desired}} \times 100$

Desired Weight = _____ × 100

Desired Weight = _____

263

Pollock, Schmidt, and Jackson Data

Women		*Men*	
Triceps _____ mm		Chest _____ mm	
Suprailiac _____ mm		Abdominal _____ mm	
Anterior Thigh _____ mm		Anterior Thigh _____ mm	

Find the sum of the three measured skinfolds.

Sum of Skinfolds _____ mm   Sum of Skinfolds _____ mm

Enter Table 9–6(A) (Men) or 9–6(B) (Women) using the sum of the three skinfolds and your age.

Fat % _____

Classification
   (from Table 9–7) _____

Calculation of "Desired" Weight

1. Fat Weight = Total body weight × Fat %

   = _____ × _____

   Fat Weight = _____

2. Lean Body Weight (LBW) = Total Weight − Fat Weight

   = _____ − _____

   Lean Body Weight   = _____

3. Desired Weight = $\dfrac{\text{LBW}}{100 - \text{\% Fat Desired}} \times 100$

   Desired Weight = _____ × 100

   Desired Weight = _____

Caloric Intake and Expenditure Evaluation

Purpose and Theory

Ensure that losing weight is appropriate for you by assessing your body fat percentage and following the guidelines in Chapter 8. To lose weight a caloric deficit must be maintained. The form below will allow you to determine the means for weight loss using appropriate procedures.

Procedures

Fill in the blocks below as described.

1. Fill in block A (kilocalories expended per day) using Table 8–2 (men) or Table 8–3 (women).
2. Keep a complete record of everything you eat and drink for two days (don't adjust your habits—keep it honest). Add the total caloric value of the foods eaten over the two days using section B and find the average caloric intake.

A. Kilocalories Expended Per Day

B. Kilocalories Taken in Per Day*

Day 1

	Food	Amount	Caloric Value
Breakfast	_____	_____	_____
	_____	_____	_____
	_____	_____	_____
	_____	_____	_____
	_____	_____	_____
Lunch	_____	_____	_____
	_____	_____	_____
	_____	_____	_____
	_____	_____	_____
	_____	_____	_____

* For caloric value of foods see Appendix B.

Day 1 (Continued)

	Food	Amount	Caloric Value
Dinner	_____	_____	_____
	_____	_____	_____
	_____	_____	_____
	_____	_____	_____
	_____	_____	_____
Snacks	_____	_____	_____
	_____	_____	_____
	_____	_____	_____
	_____	_____	_____
	_____	_____	_____

Total Caloric Intake _____

Day 2

	Food	Amount	Caloric Value
Breakfast	_____	_____	_____
	_____	_____	_____
	_____	_____	_____
	_____	_____	_____
	_____	_____	_____
Lunch	_____	_____	_____
	_____	_____	_____
	_____	_____	_____
	_____	_____	_____
	_____	_____	_____
Dinner	_____	_____	_____
	_____	_____	_____
	_____	_____	_____
	_____	_____	_____
	_____	_____	_____

Day 2 (Continued)

	Food	Amount	Caloric Value
Snacks	_____	_____	_____
	_____	_____	_____
	_____	_____	_____
	_____	_____	_____
	_____	_____	_____

Total Caloric Intake _____

Average Daily Caloric Intake (Day 1 + Day 2 ÷ 2) _____

3. Find the difference by subtracting intake from expenditure.

   A. Expenditure (from A)   _____

   B. Average Caloric Intake (from B) _____

   Difference +/−   _____

   If intake is greater than expenditure circle the (+); this means you have a positive caloric balance. If expenditure is greater, circle the (−); this means you have a negative caloric balance.

4. Remember that to lose 1 pound you must accumulate a total negative caloric balance of 3,500 calories. Plan your weight loss by a combination of reducing caloric intake while maintaining the nutritional guidelines found in Chapters 7 and 8 and increasing your caloric expenditure.

   Choose plan A or plan B and monitor intake and expenditure for 7 days and record each day's caloric intake and expenditure below.

Plan A — One Pound Weight Loss Per Week

*Caloric Intake**			*Caloric Expenditure**		
Day 1. _____	5. _____		Day 1. _____	5. _____	
2. _____	6. _____		2. _____	6. _____	
3. _____	7. _____		3. _____	7. _____	
4. _____			4. _____		

Total For Week _____

Total For Week _____

* *Should be 250 calories less than Average Daily Caloric Intake (see B above).*

* *Should be 250 calories more than A above; see Chapter 4 for suggestions.*

Plan A (Continued)

Total Caloric Intake _____

Total Caloric Expenditure _____

Difference _____

Difference ÷ 3,500 = pounds of weight loss

Weight loss _____ lbs/week.

Plan B — Two Pound Weight Loss Per Week

Caloric Intake*		*Caloric Expenditure**	
Day 1. _____	5. _____	Day 1. _____	5. _____
2. _____	6. _____	2. _____	6. _____
3. _____	7. _____	3. _____	7. _____
4. _____		4. _____	
Total For Week _____		Total For Week _____	

* Should be 500 calories less than Average Daily Caloric Intake (see B above).

* Should be 500 calories more than A above; see Chapter 4 for suggestions.

Total Caloric Intake _____

Total Caloric Expenditure _____

Difference _____

Difference ÷ 3,500 = pounds of weight loss

Weight loss _____ lbs/week.

Stress Management Evaluation

Name _____   Date _____

Class _____   Instructor _____

Purpose and Theory

This evaluation will help you to identify sources of stress and assess your ability to manage stressful situations. The incorporation of regular exercise and a technique to assist in relaxation could be of considerable value in helping you to cope with stress.

Procedures

1. Complete the Self-Scoring Table and have a close friend or relative complete the Evaluator Table. (See Chapter 3 for explanation)

Self-Scoring Test for Stress Determination

Circle the appropriate number for each item.

Conduct	Often	Sometimes	Rarely
1. I experience unexplained headaches and backaches.	2	1	0
2. When I'm nervous I eat/drink/smoke.	2	1	0
3. When problems are not immediately solved I get worried.	2	1	0
4. I feel tired and restless.	2	1	0
5. I work at completion of tasks very close to the deadline.	2	1	0
6. My mood changes.	2	1	0
7. I'm too busy to allow time for physical activity.	2	1	0
8. I'm concerned on more than one problem and can't concentrate well.	2	1	0
9. People at work or home make me feel tense.	2	1	0
10. When people disagree with me I challenge them and feel as though I should not yield.	2	1	0

Maximum Score = 20   My Total Score = _____

Evaluator Table for _____

Circle the appropriate number for each item.

Conduct	Often	Sometimes	Never
1. Seems to be in a hurry, moves and eats fast, hates to wait.	3	2	0
2. Talks very quickly, often interrupts.	3	2	0
3. Seems to worry about things of little consequence.	3	2	0
4. Unable to understand why so many others can't meet their responsibilities.	3	2	0
5. Loses patience quickly.	3	2	0
6. Seems to have a lot to do.	3	2	0

Maximum Score = 18   Score = _____

Total Score (Self-Scoring Table Score plus
Evaluator Table Score) = _____

Circle Below Your Category

Grade	Score	Unmanaged Stress Level
A	0–7	Very Little
B	8–15	Some
C	16–22	Moderate
D	23–29	Too Much
E	30–36	A Great Deal

2. Practice the relaxation technique of Benson (see Chapter 3) twice a day for 3 weeks. Keep a notebook of the time, place, and day for each session and record in the following spaces.

Benson Relaxation Technique performed:

Date	Time	Place	Duration	Date	Time	Place	Duration
_____	_____	_____	_____	_____	_____	_____	_____
_____	_____	_____	_____	_____	_____	_____	_____
_____	_____	_____	_____	_____	_____	_____	_____
_____	_____	_____	_____	_____	_____	_____	_____
_____	_____	_____	_____	_____	_____	_____	_____
_____	_____	_____	_____	_____	_____	_____	_____
_____	_____	_____	_____	_____	_____	_____	_____
_____	_____	_____	_____	_____	_____	_____	_____

Date	Time	Place	Duration	Date	Time	Place	Duration
____	____	____	____	____	____	____	____
____	____	____	____	____	____	____	____
____	____	____	____	____	____	____	____
____	____	____	____	____	____	____	____
____	____	____	____	____	____	____	____
____	____	____	____	____	____	____	____
____	____	____	____	____	____	____	____
____	____	____	____	____	____	____	____
____	____	____	____	____	____	____	____
____	____	____	____	____	____	____	____
____	____	____	____	____	____	____	____
____	____	____	____	____	____	____	____
____	____	____	____	____	____	____	____

3. Reevaluate yourself through the Self-Scoring Table and have the same Evaluator repeat his or her evaluation.

Self-Scoring Test for Stress Determination

Circle the appropriate number for each item.

Conduct	Often	Sometimes	Rarely
1. I experience unexplained headaches and backaches.	2	1	0
2. When I'm nervous I eat/drink/smoke.	2	1	0
3. When problems are not immediately solved I get worried.	2	1	0
4. I feel tired and restless.	2	1	0
5. I work at completion of tasks very close to the deadline.	2	1	0
6. My mood changes.	2	1	0
7. I'm too busy to allow time for physical activity.	2	1	0
8. I'm concerned on more than one problem and can't concentrate well.	2	1	0
9. People at work or home make me feel tense.	2	1	0
10. When people disagree with me I challenge them and feel as though I should not yield.	2	1	0

Maximum Score = 18   My Total Score = _____

Evaluator Table for _____

Circle the appropriate number for each item.

Conduct	Often	Sometimes	Never
1. Seems to be in a hurry, moves and eats fast, hates to wait.	3	2	0
2. Talks very quickly, often interrupts.	3	2	0
3. Seems to worry about things of little consequence.	3	2	0
4. Unable to understand why so many others can't meet their responsibilities.	3	2	0
5. Loses patience quickly.	3	2	0
6. Seems to have a lot to do.	3	2	0

Maximum Score = 18   Score = _____

Total Score (Self-Scoring Table Score plus
Evaluator Table Score) = _____

Circle the Appropriate Category

Grade	Score	Unmanaged Stress Level
A	0–7	Very Little
B	8–15	Some
C	16–22	Moderate
D	23–29	Too Much
E	30–36	A Great Deal

Note any change in your score:

1st Trial Score _____

2nd Trial Score _____

(Remember some change may be influenced by your exercise program.)

Glossary

A band: That area located in the center of the sarcomere containing both actin and myosin.

Acclimatization: Physiological adjustments brought about by continued exposure to a different climate or altitude.

Accommodating resistance: A method of weight training in which the resistance varies throughout the range of motion but is dependent on a fixed accommodation that cannot be tailored to meet individual force production capabilities.

Actin: A protein contained in the myofibril and involved in muscular contraction.

Adaptive response: The process by which a muscle system or other system gradually changes when subjected to an overload.

Adenosine diphosphate (ADP): A complex chemical compound that forms adenosine triphosphate when combined with inorganic phosphate.

Adenosine triphosphate (ATP): A complex chemical compound that is formed with the energy released from food and that is stored in all cells, particularly muscle cells. A cell can perform work only with the energy released from the breakdown of ATP.

Adipocyte: A fat cell.

Aerobic: In the presence of oxygen.

Aerobic base: A person's cardiorespiratory condition.

Aerobic capacity: See Maximal oxygen consumption.

Aerobic power: See Maximal oxygen consumption.

Alveolocapillary membrane: The interface between an alveolus and a pulmonary capillary where gas exchange takes place between the blood and inspired air.

Alveolus (plural: alveoli): A tiny terminal air sac in the lungs through which the transfer of oxygen and carbon dioxide takes place with the blood and inspired air.

Amino acids: Compounds containing nitrogen that are the building blocks of proteins.

Anaerobic: In the absence of oxygen.

Anorexia nervosa: An illness in which there is a nervous loss of appetite. It primarily affects young women and is usually triggered by a stressful situation. Fluid and electrolyte imbalances caused by anorexia nervosa can lead to dehydration and potassium deficiencies, and in some cases, death.

Antagonist muscle groups: Muscle groups in which the various muscles work in opposition to each other. Such groups often have an inherent imbalance.

Aorta: The main artery carrying blood from the left ventricle to the body.

Arrangement of exercises: The principle that weight training exercises should be

273

arranged so that the largest muscle groups are exercised first followed by progressively smaller muscle groups or that exercises should alternate between the upper and lower body.

Åstrand-Rhyming bicycle ergometer test: A submaximal test of cardiorespiratory fitness based on the linear relationship between workload and heart rate.

Atherosclerosis: Narrowing of the lumen of a vessel as a result of the build-up of plaque on the interior surface.

ATP-PC system: An anaerobic energy system in which ATP is manufactured when phosphocreatine (PC) is broken down. This system represents the most rapidly available source of ATP for use by muscle. Activities performed at maximum intensity in a period of 10 seconds or less derive energy (ATP) from this system.

Atrium: One of the two smaller chambers of the heart that pump blood into the ventricles.

Ballistic stretching: Stretching of a muscle through the range of motion of a joint by quick short movements.

Blood clot: Coagulated blood, which can cause a myocardial infarction by lodging in a coronary artery already narrowed by atherosclerotic plaque. A blood clot can also cause a stroke.

Blood fat level: The amount of cholesterol and triglycerides in the blood.

Blood pressure: The force that moves the blood through the circulatory system. Blood pressure has two components: systolic pressure, which is the higher pressure, is created when the heart ejects the blood into the arterial system; diastolic pressure, which is the lower pressure, is the pressure in between heart beats (systoles).

Body composition: The component parts of the body—mainly fat and fat-free weight.

Body fat weight: The total weight of the fat stored in the body.

Borg scale: A formalized system for quantifying feelings of fatigue used to measure perceived exertion.

Bulimia: An illness characterized by binge eating and then purging the gastrointestinal system to alleviate the consequences. Most victims are young women. Bulimics usually maintain near-normal body weights.

Caloric deficit: A situation in which the amount of calories consumed in food is less than the amount of calories expended in activity.

Caloric expenditure: The total number of calories used by the body in maintaining normal function and activity.

Caloric intake: The total number of calories taken into the body in food.

Calorie: A unit of work energy equal to the amount of heat required to raise the temperature of 1 gram of water 1°C.

Carbohydrates: Chemical compounds containing carbon, hydrogen, and oxygen. Some important carbohydrates are the starches, celluloses, and sugars. Carbohydrates are one of the basic foodstuffs.

Carbohydrate loading: See Glycogen loading.

Cardiac hypertrophy: An increase in the size of the heart.

Cardiac output (Q̇): The amount of blood pumped in 1 minute by either the left or right ventricle of the heart; the product of heart rate and stroke volume.

Cardiorespiratory: Pertaining to the circulatory and respiratory systems.

Cardiorespiratory fitness: The physiological and functional capacity of the respiratory and circulatory systems.

Cardiorespiratory system: The respiratory and circulatory systems.

Cardiovascular disease: Disease of the heart muscle and the vessels supplying blood to the heart muscle.

Cardiovascular fitness: The physiological and functional capacity of the vasculature of the heart.

Catecholamines: Substances in the blood that control heart rate and the size of the blood vessels (internal diameter). Catecholamine levels can be increased by inappropriate reactions to stress.

Cerebral hemorrhage: A form of stroke in which an artery in the brain bursts.

Cerebral thrombosis: A form of stroke in which an artery that is already narrowed by atherosclerosis is blocked by a blood clot.

Cholesterol: A fatty compound that is found in animal tissues and in one form is essential to proper functioning of the body. Excess amounts have been linked to atherosclerosis.

Circuit training: A conditioning program consisting of a number of exercises performed at "stations." Usually a given exercise is performed at a station within a specified time; the athlete then moves to the next station, which has its own particular exercise and time frame.

Circulatory efficiency: The relationship between heart rate and stroke volume. When the heart rate is high and the stroke volume low, circulatory efficiency is said to be low. When the heart rate is low and the stroke volume high, circulatory efficiency is said to be high.

Coagulability: The capacity of the blood to clot.

Collateral circulation: Blood vessels that develop as a result of a need for increased blood flow.

Concentric contraction: A muscular contraction in which the muscle shortens while developing tension.

Connective tissue: The tissue that binds together and is the support for the various structures of the body.

Contractility: Having the ability to contract or shorten.

Cool-down: The process of gradually ceasing activity after an exercise session.

Cooper's 12-minute run test: A test of cardiorespiratory fitness based on the distance covered in 12 minutes of running on a track.

Coronary arteries: The blood vessels that supply the heart with blood.

Coronary heart disease: A cardiovascular disease affecting the blood vessels of the heart.

Coronary vasculature: The total network of arteries, veins, and capillaries supplying blood to the heart.

Cross-bridges: Tiny projections extending from myosin filaments toward actin filaments in the sarcomere of a myofibril. The cross-bridges are instrumental in shortening the muscle fiber during contraction.

Daily activity level: The rate at which the body expends calories. It is composed of two parts: the basal rate and the physical activity rate.

Delayed muscle soreness: The pain that peaks about 24 to 48 hours after exercise when a muscle has been overloaded.

Detraining: The cessation of regular exercise after a program of regular appropriate exercise.

Diffusion: The process by which oxygen and carbon dioxide cross the alveolocapillary and the tissue-capillary membranes.

Duration of exercise: One of the four factors in an exercise prescription. It is the amount of time during each exercise session that the appropriate intensity must be continuously maintained.

Dynamic flexibility: The opposition of a joint to motion. See Flexibility.

Eccentric contraction: A muscular contraction in which the muscle lengthens while developing tension.

Ectomorph: A somatotypic classification of the human body denoting linearity, fragility, and delicacy.

Elasticity: The quality of returning to original size and shape after being stretched.

Endomorph: A somatotypic classification of the body denoting roundness and softness; an endomorphic body is predisposed to the development of adipose tissue.

Endomysium: The connective tissue surrounding the muscle fibers in a fasciculus.

Endurance fitness: See Cardiorespiratory fitness.

Energy: The capacity to do work.

Energy continuum: The idea that all three energy-producing systems of the body (ATP-PC, LA, and aerobic) contribute ATP during nearly every activity but that one system usually contributes more to one specific type of activity than the other two.

Energy nutrients: Carbohydrates, fats, and proteins—the only sources of food energy.

Epidemiology: The study of the incidence, distribution, and control of a disease in a human population.

Epimysium: The connective tissue surrounding a muscle.

Ergometer: An apparatus such as a treadmill or stationary bicycle used for measuring the physiological effects of exercise.

Exercise prescription: A determination of the appropriate frequency, intensity, duration, and mode of exercise for a person.

Fad diets: Popular diets that claim to make reducing weight effortless.

Fasciculus: A bundle of muscle fibers.

Fast-twitch fiber: A muscle fiber that has fast contraction time, high anaerobic capacity, and low aerobic capacity, all making the fiber well-suited to activities that require high power output over short time periods.

Fats: The soft tissue of the body other than that making up the skeletal muscle mass and the viscera. Also, those foods, such as oils, butter, margarine, and animal fats that form an important part of the diet.

Fat-free weight: That portion of the total body weight remaining when body fat weight is subtracted; mainly the weight of skeletal muscle. Also known as lean body weight and muscle weight.

Fatty acids: The structural units of fats.

Fiber splitting: The process by which muscle fibers or cells split into two or more fibers or cells as a result of overload, thereby increasing the size of the muscle.

Fibrinolysis: The process by which a blood clot is dissolved by the body. It is believed that the fibrinolytic system is maintained by exercise.

Fitness: A physiological and functional capacity that improves the quality of life.

Flexibility: The range of motion of a joint (static flexibility); opposition or resistance of a joint to motion (dynamic flexibility).

Frequency of exercise: One of the four factors in an exercise prescription. It is the minimum number of times per week that you must exercise in order to obtain a training effect.

Functional capacity: The ability to do work at maximal effort as determined by measures of energy expenditure.

Gas exchange: The transfer of oxygen and carbon dioxide between the blood and inspired air.

Gas transport: The process by which oxygen and carbon dioxide are carried by the blood to and from the lungs and muscle tissues.

Glucose: The only sugar that can be used by the muscles. All other sugars in the body are converted to glucose.

Glycogen loading: An exercise-diet technique that elevates muscle glycogen stores to concentrations two to three times normal. Also known as carbohydrate loading and supercompensation.

Golgi tendon organ: A sensory body located in the tendon of a muscle. Stimulation of the Golgi tendon body results in inhibition of contraction of the muscle group being stretched.

Graded exercise test (GXT): A test that gives a direct measurement of oxygen consumption.

Heart attack: Usually refers to a myocardial infarction but is also used as a general term to refer to damage to the heart muscle.

Heart rate (HR): The number of times the heart beats per minute.

Heart rate method: One of several methods for determining appropriate intensity levels for an exercise prescription.

Heart rate range: A range of heart rates that can be used to assess the intensity of exercise.

Heart rate reserve: The difference between the maximum heart rate and the resting heart rate.

Hemoglobin: The protein in red blood cells that gives them their color and combines with oxygen to transport it to the tissues (1.34 ml of oxygen per gram).

High density lipoprotein (HDL): A fraction of the cholesterol content of the blood thought to contribute to protection against atherosclerosis.

Hypertension: High blood pressure.

Hypertrophy: An increase in the size of a cell or organ.

H zone: The area in the center of the A band where cross-bridges are absent.

I band: That area of the myofibril containing actin and bisected by a Z line.

Intensity of exercise: One of the four factors in an exercise prescription. It is the degree of difficulty imposed on a muscle system.

Isokinetic contraction: A muscular contraction executed at a constant speed and in such a fashion that the tension developed by the muscle while shortening is maximal over the full range of motion of a joint.

Isometric contraction: A muscular contraction in which tension is developed but the muscle does not change in length. Also referred to as a static contraction.

Isotonic contraction: A muscular contraction in which the muscle shortens with varying tension while lifting a constant load.

Joint flexibility: See Flexibility.

Karvonen's formula: A method for determining heart rate reserve.

Kilocalorie: A unit of work energy equal to the amount of heat required to raise the temperature of 1 kilogram of water 1°C.

Kilogram: A metric unit of weight equal to 2.2 pounds.

Lactic acid (LA): A fatiguing metabolite produced by the incomplete breakdown of carbohydrates.

Lactic acid (LA) system: An anaerobic energy system in which ATP is manufactured from the breakdown of carbohydrates to lactic acid. High intensity efforts performed in 1 to 3 minutes require the muscles to draw energy (ATP) primarily from this system.

Lean body weight: See fat-free weight.

Lifetime sports: Sports activities in which a person can participate throughout his or her life.

Liquid pregame meals: An increasingly popular way to eat before a sports event. These commercially packaged meals are nutritious, palatable, easily digested, and readily emptied from the stomach.

Low density lipoprotein (LDL): That fraction of the cholesterol content of the blood thought to promote atherosclerosis.

Maximal aerobic power: See Maximal oxygen consumption.

Maximal heart rate: The upper limit of beats per minute of the heart.

Maximal oxygen consumption ($\dot{V}O_2$max): The maximal rate at which oxygen can be consumed per minute; the power or capacity of the aerobic (oxygen) system.

Mental and emotional fitness: A general rather than specific component of fitness.

Mesomorph: A somatotypic classification of the body denoting a square frame, rugged, hard musculature, large bones, and thick muscles.

Metabolic equivalent (MET): The resting energy requirement, which is estimated to be 3.5 ml of oxygen per kilogram of body weight per minute.

Metabolism: The total of all chemical reactions that occur in the body during the production of energy for work.

Milliliter: One-thousandth of a liter.

Minerals: Inorganic compounds, some of which are important to body functions. Examples of nutrient minerals are calcium, phosphorus, potassium, sodium, iron, and iodine.

Mitochondrion (plural: mitochondria): A subcellular structure that is found in all aerobic cells and in which the reactions of the Kreb's cycle and electron transport system take place.

Mode of exercise: One of the four factors in an exercise prescription. It is the type of exercise that will be performed.

Motor fitness: One or more qualities or abilities associated with physical skills such as endurance, strength, agility, flexibility, balance, and coordination.

Motor unit: An individual motor nerve and all the muscle fibers it innervates.

Muscle bundle: A fasciculus.

Muscle spindle: A sensory organ located in the belly of a muscle. When stimulated it causes the muscle to contract.

Muscle weight: See Fat-free weight.

Muscular endurance: The ability of a muscle or muscle group to perform repeated contractions against a light load for an extended period of time.

Muscular fitness: The ability of the muscle to do work. One aspect of physical fitness.

Muscular strength: The amount of force exerted or resistance overcome by a muscle for a single repetition.

Myocardial infarction: Death of heart muscle tissue caused by the cessation of blood flow to that tissue. A heart attack.

Myofibril: That part of a muscle fiber containing two protein filaments: myosin and actin.

Myosin: A protein contained in the myofibril which with actin causes the fiber to contract.

Negative contraction: See Eccentric contraction.

Negative energy balance: A state in which a person consumes less calories in food than are expended in daily activity.

Nutrients: The substances in food that provide nourishment and are necessary for life.

Nutrition: The process by which the body takes in and uses food for optimal health and performance.

Nutritional fitness: The selection of foods according to their caloric and nutritive values; also, proper eating habits.

Nutritive snacking: Properly selecting foods to be eaten between regular meals to maximize the caloric and nutritional benefits.

Obesity: A condition in which body weight is more than 25 percent above "ideal" body weight for one's height.

Ohio State University Step Test: A submaximal test of cardiorespiratory fitness based on the point at which the subject's heart rate reaches 150 beats per minute while stepping onto and off of a special bench.

Overfat (or overfatness): Having a proportion of body fat that exceeds recommended limits, usually 15 percent for men and 24 percent for women.

Overload: Resistance greater than that which a muscle or muscle group normally encounters. The resistance (load) can be maximal or near-maximal.

Overweight: A condition in which the body weighs more than normal based on height-weight charts.

Oxygen consumption ($\dot{V}O_2$): The volume of oxygen used for energy expenditure. Usually expressed in liters per minute or in a relative term, milliliters per kilogram per minute (ml/kg-min).

Oxygen transport system: The cardiorespiratory system, which is composed of the stroke volume (SV), the heart rate (HR), and the arterial-mixed venous oxygen difference (a − $\bar{v}O_2$diff). Mathematically it is defined as $\dot{V}O_2 = SV \times HR \times a − \bar{v}O_2$diff.

Parcourse: An exercise course for walking or jogging with planned stops that include various calesthenic routines.

Partial pressure: The pressure exerted by one gas in a gas mixture or by a gas in a liquid. Partial pressure permits gases to diffuse across membranes.

Perceived exertion: A rating of the perception of the difficulty of an exercise task. First developed by Borg.

Perimysium: The connective tissue surrounding a fasciculus or muscle bundle.

Phosphagens: Compounds that yield inorganic phosphate and release energy when broken down. ATP and PC are phosphagens.

Phosphocreatine (PC): A chemical compound that is stored in muscle and that when broken down aids in the manufacture of ATP.

Physical activity rate: The rate at which a person uses calories in daily activity. The amount of calories used above the resting or basal rate.

Physical fitness: The overall condition of the body.

Plasma: The liquid portion of blood. It carries the blood cells and plays a small direct role in transport of oxygen.

Positive energy balance: A state in which more calories are consumed as food than are expended in daily activity.

Pregame eating: The techniques involved in wisely selecting and consuming foods to enhance performance in a sports activity.

Progressive resistance: A gradual increase in the overload applied to a muscle.

Proteins: Basic foodstuffs containing amino acids.

Pulmonary artery: The artery that carries blood from the right ventricle to the lungs.

Pulmonary ventilation: See Ventilation.

Pulse: The throbbing that can be felt by applying light pressure with the fingertips to the skin overlying an artery coursing near the surface.

Pulse rate: Heart rate.

PWC$_{170}$ test: A submaximal test of cardiorespiratory fitness based on the amount of work attainable at 85 percent of maximal capacity (170 beats per minute for a 20-year-old).

Range of motion: The degree to which a joint can move.

Relaxation: A conscious release of muscular tension.

Repetition maximum: The maximum load that a muscle or muscle group can lift in a given number of repetitions before fatiguing. For example, an 8-RM load is the maximum load that can be lifted eight times.

Resting or basal rate: The rate at which the body expends calories in a resting state.

Risk factor: A condition, activity, or habit that increases a person's chances of developing coronary heart disease. The most important risk factors are smoking, hypertension, and high blood lipid levels.

Sarcolemma: The cell membrane of a muscle fiber.

Sarcomere: The smallest functional unit of muscle; the distance between two Z lines.

Sarcoplasm: The protoplasm of muscle cells.

Saturated fat: A fat that is usually solid at room temperature, particularly animal fat, eggs, and dairy products. Saturated fat has been linked with cardiovascular diseases and atherosclerosis.

Secondary amenorrhea: Interruption of the normal menstrual cycle resulting from a cause other than one directly associated with the female reproductive tract. For example, low body fat values in female athletes may cause amenorrhea.

Second wind: A sensation characterized by a sudden transition from an ill-defined feeling of distress and fatigue during the early portion of prolonged exercise to a more comfortable, less stressful feeling later in the exercise program.

Sedentary life-style: Exercising rarely and little.

Sets: Groups of repetitions of an exercise.

Sit-and-reach test: A test of flexibility of the low back and hips in which the subject sits on the floor with his or her feet flat against the test box and reaches over a calibrated scale while bending forward at the hips.

Skinfold caliper: An instrument used to measure the thickness of a fold of skin and subcutaneous fat.

Skinfold measurement: Measuring a pinch of skin and subcutaneous fat with a special caliper. The resulting value can be used to estimate total body fat.

Sliding filament theory: The theory that muscle contraction is caused by the actin filament sliding over the myosin filament toward the center of the sarcomere.

Sloan-Weir method: A skinfold measurement technique in which measurements are made at two specified sites for the determination of body density and body fat percentage.

Slow-twitch fiber: A muscle fiber that has slow contraction time, low anaerobic capacity, and high aerobic capacity, all making the fiber suited to activities that require low power output over prolonged periods of time.

Somatotyping: The physical classification of the human body.

Specificity of training: The property of having effects that are directly linked to the particulars of training. For example, a gain in anaerobic power is linked directly to those exercises that involve short intense bouts of work.

Spot reducing: A myth in which it is believed that exercising a certain part of the body will reduce the amount of fat stored in that part.

Static flexibility: The technical term for the range of motion of a joint. See Flexibility.

Static stretching: Stretching of a muscle in a slow progressive fashion and holding at the point of maximum stretch.

Stress management: A learned approach to effectively dealing with stressful situations.

Stress response: Reaction to a stressful situation.

Stroke: Lack of blood flow to a portion of the brain caused by either blockage or rupture of an artery.

Stroke volume (SV): The amount of blood pumped by the left ventricle of the heart in one contraction or beat.

Submaximal exercise: Exercise that demands less than the maximal oxygen consumption of the performer.

Systole: The contraction phase of the left and right ventricles.

Systolic pressure: The pressure of the blood in the arteries during systole.

Target heart rate: A heart rate that is used to assess intensity of exercise.

Testosterone: A hormone that regulates change in muscle size.

Three-site method (of Pollock, Schmidt, and Jackson): A skinfold measurement technique in which measurements are made at three specified sites to determine fat percentage.

Threshold for training: The minimum heart rate at which a training effect will occur. It is normally 60 percent of heart rate reserve.

Tissue-capillary membrane: The interface between the capillary and muscle tissue at which the exchange of oxygen and carbon dioxide takes place.

Triglyceride: The storage form of fats.

Underwater weighing: A technique for determining body composition based on the amount of water displaced by the subject when submerged.

Unsaturated fat: Fat that is generally liquid at room temperature. It is found in vegetable oils and oils of fish origin.

Valsalva maneuver: Forced expiration of air with the glottis closed. It produces reduced venous return and a drop in arterial pressure.

Vegetarian diets: Diets in which no animal products are consumed. Nutrition is derived solely from vegetable products. Two variations of vegetarian diets are the lacto-ovo-vegetarian diet in which milk, milk products, and eggs are also consumed and the lacto-vegetarian diet, in which milk and milk products are also consumed.

Vena cava: The major vessel carrying blood from the body to the right atrium.

Ventilation: The movement of air into and out of the lungs.

Ventricle: One of the two larger chambers of the heart that pump blood to the lungs (right) and the body (left).

Vitamins: Organic nutrients that are important catalysts for metabolic reactions.

Warm-up: The process of preparing to exercise by increasing your activity level with stretching and other exercises designed to warm the muscles.

Water: Probably the most essential of all nutrients for human life.

Z line: A protein band that defines the distance of one sarcomere in the myofibril.

Index